The Baby Sleep Book

Sears Parenting Library

The Baby Book

The Pregnancy Book

The A.D.D. Book

The Attachment Parenting Book

The Baby Sleep Book

The Birth Book

The Breastfeeding Book

The Discipline Book

The Family Nutrition Book

The Fussy Baby Book

The Premature Baby Book

The Successful Child

Parenting.com FAQ Books

Feeding the Picky Eater

The First Three Months

How to Get Your Baby to Sleep

Keeping Your Baby Healthy

Sears Children's Library

Baby on the Way

Eat Healthy, Feel Great

What Baby Needs

You Can Go to the Potty

The
Baby Sleep Book

*The Complete Guide to
a Good Night's Rest for the Whole Family*

WILLIAM SEARS, M.D., ROBERT SEARS, M.D.,
JAMES SEARS, M.D., AND MARTHA SEARS, R.N.

LITTLE, BROWN AND COMPANY
New York   Boston   London

Little, Brown and Company
Hachette Book Group
237 Park Avenue, New York, NY 10017
www.hachettebookgroup.com

FIRST EDITION: OCTOBER 2005

Little, Brown and Company is a division of Hachette Book Group, Inc.
The Little, Brown name and logo are trademarks of Hachette Book
Group, Inc.

Library of Congress Cataloging-in-Publication Data
The baby sleep book : the complete guide to a good night's rest
for the whole family / William Sears . . . et al. — 1st ed.
    p.   cm.
Includes bibliographical references and index.
ISBN 978-0-316-10771-6
1. Infants — Sleep — Popular works. I. Sears, William, M.D.

RJ506.S55S424 2005
649'.122 — dc22   2005002587

10   9   8   7   6

RRD-IN

Designed by Jeanne Abboud
Drawings by Deborah Maze

Printed in the United States of America

To our children — who now all sleep through the night

James
Robert
Peter
Hayden
Erin
Matthew
Stephen
Lauren
— W.S. and M.S.

Andrew
Alex
Joshua
— R.S.

Leanne
Jonathan
— J.S.

Contents

VISIT DR. SEARS ONLINE

www.AskDrSears.com

Now you can access thousands of pages of pediatric medical and parenting information. Our comprehensive online resource, personally written by the Doctors Sears, expands on many of the topics discussed in *The Baby Sleep Book.* We continuously update the health information on our website to provide you with the latest in parenting and health care issues. AskDrSears.com offers valuable insights on such topics as Pregnancy and Childbirth, Infant Feeding, Family Nutrition, Discipline and Behavior, Fussy Babies, and Sleep Problems.

Our website also includes these unique features:

- The Sleep Forum, an interactive forum where parents share their favorite sleep strategies and Dr. Sears adds his comments.
- Dr. Sears's Medicine Cabinet, a comprehensive guide to over-the-counter medications, including specific dose information
- Childhood Illnesses, detailed medical information on many common, and not-so-common, child and family illnesses
- Monthly Pediatric Health News Updates
- Seasonal Pediatric Health Alerts
- Valuable month-by-month parenting and medical advice to complement your child's regular checkups
- Frequently Asked Questions answered
- Personal words of encouragement and humor from the daily lives of the Doctors Sears
- *The Baby Sleep Book* updates. We will post any significant changes to *The Baby Sleep Book* (and all our books) to provide you with the most accurate and up-to-date medical information.

Foreword

I am not aware of any physician authors — or should I say families containing physician authors — who better converse with parents and create respectful partnerships with them than Dr. Bill Sears (now along with his sons). In *The Baby Sleep Book* Dr. Sears, Martha Sears, and their sons Dr. Bob and Dr. Jim make an incredibly useful contribution to our understanding and management of infant and (by association) parent sleep. Years of experience and acquired insight are combined here with a genuinely keen sense of who babies and their families actually are, not who they are supposed to be, a fatal mistake made by authors of most other infant sleep books. Consequently, Dr. Sears reaches just the right balance between what is known to be good for infants and parents from a scientific point of view and what makes sense within individual families. His nonauthoritarian and non-judgmental approach instills trust and just the right mood for parents to fully understand, appreciate, and apply a tremendously impressive range of useful tips, interesting bits of information full of warmth and humor, and strategies that can be put into play if one particular plan doesn't work. Altogether, the information in *The Baby Sleep Book* far exceeds the parental help contained in all the other sleep books that are available. Indeed, the Searses' book sets a new and very high standard against which all other future infant sleep books will be judged. On behalf of parents and babies everywhere, I am delighted to endorse it enthusiastically.

— James J. McKenna, Ph.D., Professor of Anthropology and Director of the Mother-Baby Behavioral Sleep Lab, University of Notre Dame

HOW TO READ THIS BOOK

In response to our "advisers" (sleepless parents), we use chapter 1 to give you the steps and tools to help your baby sleep — you can begin our sleep plan right away. However, nighttime parenting is not just a list of sleep tools, it's a relationship with your baby. So, if you're not too tired, you may want to read chapter 3 first. It will help you understand how babies sleep — or don't! After you've read the first three chapters, then you are ready to put all these sleep tools together into your baby's individual sleep plan (ISP), which we show you how to do in chapter 4. In chapter 5, we share what we Searses do in our families and what many people all over the world do when they learn what their babies need and discover how great it is to be able to meet those needs. The rest of the book gives you a deeper understanding of all the sleep tools discussed in the first four chapters, plus additional sleep tools for handling nighttime challenges such as the all-night nurser. We give you the tools to become *your own* expert in *your* baby and to help you work out *your own* style of nighttime parenting.

A Restful Word from Dr. Bill

Each day in our pediatric practice we hear tired parents say with a sigh, "If only our baby would sleep more." In all our years of writing books and practicing pediatrics, our goal has been to do good things for babies and make life easier for parents. We believe that helping babies sleep better is good not only for them but also for their parents. Parents who get enough sleep at night are happier during the day.

Over the years, we have devoted a lot of time and energy to the sleep problems parents in our practice share with us. We have offered these tired parents many suggestions for helping their babies sleep longer, and we have asked them to report back to us about what worked and what didn't. We have also asked parents who have visited our website (*www.AskDrSears.com*) to share their sleep problems and solutions with us. As a result, much of the advice in this book comes from parents like you. Throughout the book, you will find quotes (in italics) from these parents who have struggled to help their babies sleep, found solutions, and shared them with us.

We've also taken the advice of these parents on how to write a book about sleep. They told us, "Cut right to the plan." This is why the first two chapters of this book contain our step-by-step approach to helping your infant and toddler sleep healthier and happier.

You could lose a lot of sleep reading the many baby sleep books currently on bookstore shelves, most of which are yet another variation on the tired old "let your baby cry it out" theme. This "tough love" method for babies is like training a pet, and this approach to parenting babies at night puts families in a lose-lose situation. Babies may eventually give up crying and go to sleep, but when they do that, they lose trust in their parents to meet their nighttime needs. That can't be good for a baby. Parents lose because this quick ticket to the promised land of sleep keeps them from learning about their baby's individual sleep needs. The other extreme in baby sleep books is the "tough it out" approach, which just pacifies tired parents by reassuring them that baby will eventually sleep through the night. Neither of these approaches is fair to tiny babies or tired parents. Our approach, on the other hand, is a "sleep tools" approach.

If babies could talk, they would say, "Please don't *force* me to sleep; instead, *teach* me to sleep. After all, I'm just a baby!" Sleep is not a state you should try to force a baby into. It's better to set conditions that allow sleep to overtake baby and that make self-settling and lengthy sleeping easier and more attractive to baby. While newborns and young babies need help from parents to relax and fall asleep, older babies can eventually learn to settle themselves. Depending on their temperaments and need levels, different babies will master self-settling skills at different ages, but parents can do a lot to help them along. Teaching your baby how to sleep and how to go back to sleep requires commitment, time, and sensitivity. In this book, we'll show you how.

This is a book of options, not "shoulds." There is no one-bed-fits-all approach to helping babies sleep. We will give you tools and help you select the ones that fit the sleep temperament of your child so that you can create an *individual sleep plan.* Helping your baby learn to sleep better is not like following a diet or exercise regimen. There's a lot of give and take, and the options you choose to try will depend on your baby's personality. Just as there are quiet and more active babies in the daytime, there are sound sleepers and frequent wakers during the night. Some high-strung babies are not fans of sleep in general,

and they need an extra set of tools to help them want to sleep longer.

This is also a book about options for different family lifestyles and different philosophies of nighttime parenting. Realistically, many parents juggle many different sleeping arrangements during the years their children are small. There are co-sleepers, crib sleepers, and families who play musical beds. There is no right arrangement for every family. The one that gets all family members the best night's sleep is the one to follow. The key is to be open to trying various sleeping arrangements at various stages of your child's development until you arrive at one that works for your family. Sleep is important. Higher-quality sleep is associated with happier and healthier babies — and parents. If you keep working at it, you'll find the approach that suits your family best.

Nighttime parenting is a season of child rearing. Yes, your baby will eventually sleep through the night. You may be wondering how to get your infant down to sleep at night, but in a few years, you'll be wondering how to get him up in the morning. Remember, the nights spent with baby in your arms, at your breasts, and in your bed are a very short while in the total life of your child. Yet the memories of your love and availability will last a lifetime.

We wish you and your child years of restful sleep.

The Baby Sleep Book

Five Steps to Get Your Baby to Sleep Better

YOU ARE PROBABLY THINKING, Wow, it's only the first chapter, and the authors are getting right to the point — five ways to get my baby to sleep better! We've arranged the book this way because we assume that you are a tired parent who needs help right away, and you are probably too tired to wade through a lot of facts, theories, and introductory material.

But here's the deal. To get these five steps to work really well for you and your baby, you need to understand more about how babies sleep. They fall asleep and stay asleep differently than adults do. It's important for you to know about this so that your expectations for your family's nightlife are realistic. So, as you put the five steps in this first chapter into action, please read further into this book. The better you understand your baby's nighttime needs, the better everyone in your family will sleep.

This first chapter has many ideas for you to use at bedtime and in the wee hours when baby awakens. These steps will help your baby fall asleep more predictably and go back to sleep faster. Your baby may or may not be ready to sleep through the night, but we promise you that the advice we offer in this chapter will help you develop a plan so that you can all get a better night's sleep.

Here's a preview of the five steps in this chapter:

1. Find out where you and baby sleep best.
2. Learn baby's tired times.
3. Create a safe and comfortable environment conducive to sleep.
4. Create a variety of bedtime rituals.
5. Help baby sleep for longer stretches.

One precaution: If your baby is a newborn (less than two months old), do not jump into this sleep plan or any other sleep plan. Newborn babies are not ready to learn more mature sleep patterns. At this stage, getting to know your baby in a relaxed, intuitive way is more important than establishing a set routine for sleep. Getting attached to your baby in these early weeks will make nighttime parenting easier in the months to come.

Be aware that not everything we suggest will be right for *your* baby. We don't like parenting books that tell parents, "This is how you have to do it. This is the only right way. Tough luck if it doesn't fit with your own ideas or your baby's personality." We believe that parents who know and love their baby are the best judge of how to care for that baby. This is why it's so important to first get attached to your baby. That way, you'll have the wisdom to know what's best for your baby. In this book, we will give you lots of strategies to help your baby develop healthy sleep habits. Which ones you choose depends on your baby's unique sleep temperament.

So let's get started — and here's to a good night's sleep . . . finally!

STEP 1. FIND OUT WHERE YOU AND BABY SLEEP BEST

Where will your baby sleep best? With you in your bed? In a co-sleeper, bassinet, cradle, or crib next to your bed? In a crib in your room? In a crib in his own room? Where do you sleep best? Where do you want your baby to sleep?

Realistically, be prepared to play musical beds with all of these sleeping arrangements as you try to figure out where everyone gets the best night's sleep. And expect these sleeping arrangements to change at various stages of your baby's development. The only persons who can answer the question "Where should baby sleep?" are mom and dad. Listen to what your baby and your inner voice are trying to tell you!

Perhaps you have a new baby (or will have soon) and you are trying to decide where baby will sleep. Or maybe your current sleeping arrangement is one of the reasons you and your baby are not getting a restful night's sleep. Whatever your situation, let's explore your three options:

1. Baby sleeps alone in her own room. This is the traditional picture that many first-time parents envision for their babies. As you flip through baby magazines and furniture catalogs, you see pictures of smiling parents (who look like they've had plenty of sleep) placing their baby in a crib or cradle in the corner of a beautifully decorated nursery with the evening sunset filtering through the drapes. The parents gaze happily at their baby, who smiles up at them. You imagine that this is how your baby will go to sleep, too. You'll pat her little tummy, kiss her on the cheek, and say "night-night." She'll close her eyes, you'll tiptoe out of the room, and you and your husband will enjoy a nice quiet evening together. Your baby will sleep peacefully the whole night through.

Sounds like a fairy tale, doesn't it? Will it all come true? Eventually, but not in the early months. Most, if not all, younger babies need more out of their parents at bedtime than this magazine picture suggests. This is "quality time" for babies. They often do not willingly succumb to quick-to-sleep methods.

Will this sleeping arrangement work? It may work for easygoing babies. Mellow babies tend to fall asleep more easily and awaken less often at night regardless of where they sleep. Some of you parents-to-be are nodding your head. "Yup, that's the kind of baby we are going to have, right, honey?" Yet many of you have already discovered that you have been blessed with a baby who is going to need more nighttime closeness than this distant arrangement offers.

Those of you with crib sleepers are probably in one of two situations right now: (1) your baby had been sleeping well in a crib for months but is now waking up too often, or (2) you have been trying to get your baby to sleep in a crib for months, but she has never slept well in the other room, and you (and she) are tired.

You have two choices. You can either continue to try to teach baby to sleep well in the crib, using the rest of the steps in our plan, or you can explore some other options for where baby will sleep.

Why doesn't your baby sleep well in a crib in her own room? It may be that teething or another temporary physical cause is suddenly rousing her at night. We discuss many such causes of night waking in chapters 3 and 12. But there may be much more to this picture. If your baby has never slept well alone, and nights of stumbling down the hallway to rescue your crying baby every two hours have taken their toll, it may be that your baby is trying to tell you that she needs more nighttime comfort and closeness.

"But our baby sleeps just fine through the night in her own room," your friends may tell you. Every baby has a different personality. Some needier babies simply need more of their parents day and night. On pages 73 to 75 we discuss infant personalities and temperaments and how they relate to baby's nighttime needs. It's time to lose the magazine fantasy and figure out on your own what is best for you and your baby. If we had to pick the single most important message of this book, it would be this: *Trust your own instincts and make your own decisions about what is best for your individual baby and you.*

2. Baby sleeps in your room but not in your bed. This is a common sleep setup for two types of families: those who are living in a one-bedroom apartment (like medical resident Dr. Bob when his second son was born — four people sleeping in one room!), and those who want their baby close by (but not so close that baby's tiny feet are kicking them in the ribs). Maybe you want baby nearby simply for convenient nursing, because baby wakes up several times each night. Or perhaps your baby is a great sleeper, but you prefer having baby sleep near you for your own peace of mind.

Having baby in your room has these advantages:

- When baby wakes, he is within arm's reach or just a step away from you.
- You can get to baby quickly to rock or nurse him back to sleep before he fully wakens.
- If you wake up, you can easily check on baby to reassure yourself all is well.
- You are close to baby, yet you and your spouse have the bed to yourselves.
- Baby enjoys a sense of security.
- You can easily bring baby into your bed to nurse back to sleep, so your comfort is less disturbed.

Of course, there are possible disadvantages as well:

- If you are a light sleeper, you may find yourself disturbed by every sound that baby makes.
- Baby may grow accustomed to your proximity and may wake up more often because there is something to wake up for (nursing) and someone to wake up to.

Here are some common options for finding a safe place for baby to sleep in your room:

The Arm's Reach Co-Sleeper. This is as close as you can get to having baby nearby but not technically in your bed. With the co-sleeper, you can truthfully tell your in-laws, "No, our baby is not sleeping in our bed with us." Since baby is on a separate mattress, he won't feel your every movement, and you won't feel his. You and your spouse can enjoy your intimate space. It also gives you instant access to baby when he wakes (he's within arm's reach), so you can move close to him and nurse or pat him back to sleep before he fully wakes up and cries. (Visit www.armsreach.com and see page 127 for an illustration of the co-sleeper.)

Cradle or bassinet. These baby beds have the advantage of being right next to your bed, but they don't offer the convenience of easy-access nursing, as the co-sleeper does. Cradles and bassinets are portable, however, so you have the flexibility of seeing if baby would sleep well in his own room, too.

Amby Baby Motion Bed. This baby hammock is like a soft-bottom cradle. It hangs from a spring inside a steel frame, so every

---

AAP RECOMMENDS BREASTFED BABIES SLEEP IN PARENTS' ROOM

The 2005 American Academy of Pediatrics policy on breastfeeding states that babies should sleep in the same room as their parents to better facilitate babies' nighttime feeds.

---

time baby moves, the spring gently moves, often lulling baby back to sleep. It, too, has the advantage of being portable, so baby can sleep in any room of the house. It can sit right next to your bed, providing you with easy access to baby at night. (See page 25 for more about this new sleeping tool and how it can help fussy babies sleep more comfortably.)

3. Baby sleeps with you in your bed. Some of you reading this book may be finding that your baby thinks being in the same room with you just isn't close enough. Baby needs to feel you right next to him, and if he doesn't, he wakes up. Or perhaps your baby isn't even born yet, but you've decided that you want to sleep with your baby right from the start. You may feel, "After all, she's a baby. She's been close to me for nine months." Or maybe you are just getting to know your newborn, and you aren't yet sure what you want to do. You may also have encountered this situation: When you put your baby in the crib, he wakes up a lot, but as soon as you bring him into your bed, he sleeps better —

and so do you. Baby is trying to tell you something: "For my well-being I need to sleep closer to you." So, what do you do? You co-sleep!

Sleeping with your baby has some unique advantages:

- You can nurse baby back to sleep while you fall easily back to sleep.
- Baby can fall back to sleep more quickly because you can comfort him before he fully wakes up — and before you fully wake up.
- Baby may sleep longer and better because you are nearby.
- Baby benefits from eight extra hours of closeness each night.
- Working parents get extra "touch time" with baby.
- Studies have shown that even though sleep-sharing babies wake up more to nurse, co-sleeping mothers actually get more restful sleep than moms who don't sleep with their babies.

However, these very advantages can turn out to be disadvantages (depending on how you look at them):

- Baby may actually wake more frequently because he feels you nearby.
- Some parents don't sleep well with a baby in their bed. They want their baby close, but not *that* close.
- Mom may sleep great with baby, but dad may be a light sleeper who can't get used to the extra presence in the bed, so dad may

not sleep well. This may prompt dad to find another room to sleep in (such as the pastel-colored nursery that he painted for the baby).

- Once baby gets used to sleeping with you, he may not want to give it up. For some people, this is an advantage because they welcome this long-term bonding arrangement. For others, co-sleeping may go on longer than they would have liked.

You may have enjoyed sharing sleep with your baby, but now one or all of these disadvantages are interfering with your sleep. If your co-sleeping baby is waking up too often, you can either choose to keep baby in your bed and work through the other steps in our plan or you can consider the other options for where baby may sleep.

Deciding about co-sleeping isn't as simple as weighing a short list of pros and cons. Co-sleeping is part of an attachment-parenting style that can be rewarding for families in many ways. (For a discussion of the Baby B's of attachment parenting, see pages 70 to 73.) Because most parents sleep with their baby at some time in the first couple years, we will later go into detail about sharing sleep with your baby and how to decide if it is the right arrangement for you (see chapter 5).

4. All of the above. Most families play musical beds during their child's early years and juggle bits and pieces of all of these sleeping arrangements. For example, baby may start off in a separate bed or room and then move closer to mom sometime during the night. Remember, it's about what's best for you and your baby, and about adapting to everyone's changing nighttime needs.

Now let's move on to step 2.

STEP 2. LEARN BABY'S TIRED TIMES

When opportunity comes yawning, don't miss it! Watch for signs of drowsiness. Try to catch your baby by the third yawn. Observe her need-to-go-to-sleep signs like you do her hunger cues. When babies begin to show signs of being tired, there is a ten- to fifteen-minute window of opportunity in which they will fall asleep fairly easily. If you miss this window, the tired baby may get progressively more cranky and revved up as she gains the proverbial "second wind." Even though baby is growing more tired by the minute, this cranky mood makes it harder for her to relax and fall asleep.

It's important to figure out when your baby is most likely to be tired so that you can know when to begin your baby's bedtime ritual (see more about bedtime rituals below). If you wait until baby is actually showing signs of being tired and then give him a bath, put on his jammies, feed him, and rock him to sleep, the tired time will be over and baby will be revved up and ready to rock and roll for another hour. A better strategy is to begin the bedtime routine twenty or thirty minutes before the expected tired time. That way, baby will be feeling sleepy just as you get to the part of the bedtime routine when he is supposed to fall asleep. What's more, since

---

SLEEPY SIGNS

Get to know your child's "I need to go to sleep — NOW!" signals. Here are the usual ones:

Baby Signs
- Change in mood. Baby starts to fuss. Some babies become quieter when they are tired or they get less coordinated and their limbs get more "floppy." A great deal of fussing may mean baby is overtired and you missed the earlier signals.
- Drooping eyelids
- Nodding head
- Glazed look, "zoning out"
- Yawning
- Whimpering

Toddler Signs
- Rubbing eyes
- Lying on floor
- Grabbing favorite sleep prop or "lovee"

---

sleepy feelings will begin to creep over baby as you go through the bedtime ritual, he will eventually learn to associate these drowsy feelings with his usual bedtime ritual.

A prompt response at tired times is especially important for energetic, alert babies and toddlers who fight sleep. The baby or child who is tired but who is resisting going to sleep is trying to tell you, "I don't know how to relax. Please help me!" The longer he fights it, the harder it gets. If you can jump in and ease baby off to sleep before he starts to put up a fight, he will go to sleep more easily and stay asleep longer. He will also learn to associate these first signs of being tired with going to sleep immediately — both at nap time and at nighttime.

As soon as he seems tired, I pick up on his cues. I talk very softly, hold him, nurse him, stroke him (but not in a stimulating way), and gradually lower my voice and slow down my lullaby. This is his cue that sleep is expected to follow.

Charting your baby's tired times. On the chart below, write down baby's tired time every evening for one week. Do you see a pattern? Does your baby get sleepy around the same time every night, give or take fifteen

to thirty minutes? Most babies have their natural sleepy time between 6:30 and 7:30 p.m. if they routinely take a nap in the early afternoon, and around 8:30 or 9 p.m. if a late-afternoon nap is the norm.

Or does your baby get sleepy at times that vary by more than an hour? If so, your baby's internal clock may not yet have developed a routine sleepy time, especially if he's still quite young. Or it may be because baby's nap times are not yet consistent. Also, your family's day-to-day schedule may not be predictable.

If your chart is not showing a predictable evening sleepy time after one week of observation, continue charting for another week. Be sure baby's naps are on a fairly routine schedule. If you still don't find a routine

---

TIRED-TIMES CHART

Write down your baby's natural tired times over the course of one week. Tired times are not the times when baby actually falls asleep. They are the times of day and night when you observe tired behavior, regardless of whether or not you get baby to sleep at that time.

Nap Times	Bedtimes
Day 1 _____	_____
Day 2 _____	_____
Day 3 _____	_____
Day 4 _____	_____
Day 5 _____	_____
Day 6 _____	_____
Day 7 _____	_____

If five out of seven of these times are within thirty minutes at nap time and bedtime, then you have likely found your baby's predictable sleepy times.

Baby's predictable tired times at this age are _____ for naps and _____ for bedtime.

TO SCHEDULE OR NOT TO SCHEDULE

A week or two of charting baby's tired times may show you that these times are more predictable than you thought. Or it may show you that your baby's nap times and bedtimes depend a great deal on what else is going on in your household. At this point you may have to make a choice. Either put yourself on a predictable schedule so that baby can take predictable naps and go to bed at the same time every night, or continue to "go with the flow" during the day and give up the idea of baby having a set bedtime. You may not be able to have it both ways.

evening sleepy time, you may need to focus more on nap scheduling. In that case, skip ahead and read chapter 9, Nap-Time Strategies that Work. It takes effort to get a baby on a nap schedule. It may be easier to let baby nap whenever he happens to, but in order to establish a predictable sleepy time in the evening, baby needs to take naps at predictable times as well most of the time.

Changing your baby's tired time. If you have determined your baby's tired time is around 7:30 and you want baby to have an early bedtime, then you're all set. But what if your baby is happily wide awake at 7:30, at 8:30, even at 9 p.m.? What if your baby doesn't act tired until 10 p.m.? You can either accept this and help baby fall asleep at his natural time or you can try to change it. If

you want your baby to be in bed earlier in the evening (for whatever reasons), put baby down for a nap earlier in the afternoon. You may enjoy having baby's company at night, especially if you are away from your baby during the day. In this case, don't worry about working on an earlier bedtime. What if you would rather have your baby stay up late with you but baby is always tired by 7:30? Again, you can adjust baby's afternoon naps. We'll show you how in chapter 9.

To summarize, find your baby's predictable tired time and schedule your baby's naps if needed to get a more predictable bedtime. Start your bedtime ritual about thirty minutes before tired time, and baby will eventually learn to fall asleep easily and predictably.

STEP 3. CREATE A SAFE AND COMFORTABLE ENVIRONMENT CONDUCIVE TO SLEEP

If baby's bedroom (or your bedroom) is too light, too dark, too noisy, too quiet, or too stimulating, your baby may have difficulty going to sleep or staying asleep. Some babies are more sensitive to their sleeping environment than others. The kind of environment that is best for your sleeping baby depends on her sleep temperament. Here are some ideas to help you set the stage for your baby to sleep.

Quiet the bedroom. Most babies can block out some noise, so you don't have to create a noiseless sleeping environment for your baby. Yet, some babies do startle and awaken easily with sudden noises. For noise-sensitive babies, oil the joints and springs of a squeaky crib and the door hinges and shut the windows.

Quiet the house. Quieting the house down at tired time will both give your baby the message that it's time to transition into sleep and also program her to associate this quiet routine with sleepy time. Lower your voice, close the doors, turn off the phone ringer, put the dog outside before he barks, slow down your movements, and minimize distractions. Turn off the TV and put on some calming music. Let your baby sense that the general mood is changing from one of activity to one of quiet. Don't bounce or jiggle baby. Remember, she may already be overstimulated.

I made sure he knew the difference between day and night. During the day I did not try to keep a very quiet house. The phone rang, the dog barked. I kept it dark and quiet at night. I would feed him by night-light, change him by night-light, and everything would be calm. During the day, we would sing at the changing table, at night we wouldn't sing. Now he understands that when the lights go out, it's time for bed and not playtime.

Darken the bedroom. Help your baby learn to associate darkness with sleep. Don't turn on any bright lights during the night, as this can trick baby's internal sleep clock into thinking it's daytime (and wake time!). Use a night-light or install a dimmer switch on the bedroom light so that you can keep the light level low during nighttime diaper changes. If necessary, close the curtains to keep out the morning (or evening) light. Opaque shades, which block out light completely, may get you an extra hour of sleep if you have one of those little roosters who awaken to the first ray of sunlight entering the bedroom.

We used a Redi Shade (available at Home Depot) room-darkening temporary shade, a heavy black pleated paper shade that quickly sticks to the top of the window.

Warm the bed. Always make sure baby's bed (or yours) is warm. Laying baby down on cold sheets is a sure way to shock baby awake. One creative dad told us he used to lie in bed with baby snuggled on his chest for five minutes before scooting over and laying baby down in the warm spot. Before laying baby down in a crib or cradle, warm the sheets with a warm towel from the dryer, a hot-water bottle, a heating pad, or an electric blanket (any of which you should remove before laying baby down, of course, for safety reasons). Use flannel sheets in cold weather.

Lessen physical discomforts. A baby who itches, hurts, or has difficulty breathing is going to wake up. Here are some tonsils-to-toes tips on helping your baby sleep more comfortably:

- *Clear the nose.* Babies need clear nasal passages to breathe. Use nasal saline and gentle suction to clear baby's nose as needed.

- *Remove airborne irritants.* Environmental irritants can cause congested breathing passages and awaken baby. Common household examples are cigarette smoke, baby powder, paint fumes, hair spray, animal dander (keep animals out of an allergic child's bedroom), plants, clothing (especially wool), stuffed animals, dust from a bed canopy, feather pillows, blankets, and fuzzy toys that collect lint and dust. If your baby consistently awakens with a stuffy nose, suspect irritants or allergens in the bedroom. Make your baby's bedroom as dust-free as possible. Besides dusting regularly, remove fuzzy blankets, down comforters, dust-collecting fuzzy toys, and so forth. If your baby is particularly allergy-prone, a HEPA-type air filter will help. As an added nighttime perk, the "white noise" from the hum of the air filter may help baby stay asleep longer.

- *Relieve teething pain.* Teething discomfort may start as early as three months and continue off and on all the way through the two-year molars. A wet bed sheet under baby's head, a drool rash on the cheeks and chin, swollen and tender gums, and a slight fever are telltale clues that baby is teething. If the teething pain seems really bad, with your doctor's advice, give appropriate doses of acetaminophen just before parenting your baby to sleep and again in four hours if baby awakens. (For more on teething pain, see page 228.)

- *Change wet or soiled diapers.* Some babies are bothered by wet diapers at night. Most are not. If your baby sleeps through wet diapers, there is no need to awaken her for a change — unless you're trying to get rid of a persistent diaper rash. Messy nighttime bowel movements do necessitate a diaper change. Here's a nighttime changing tip: If possible, change the diapers just before a feeding, as baby is likely to fall asleep during or after the feeding. Some breastfed babies, however, have a bowel movement during or immediately after a feeding and will need changing again. If you are using cloth diapers, putting two or three diapers on your baby before bedtime will decrease the sensation of wetness. Also, if baby is prone to diaper rash, slather on a hefty layer of barrier cream to protect baby's sensitive skin from the sensation and irritation of wetness. Cold diaper wipes are sure to startle baby awake. Use a wipe warmer or run wipes under warm water (a great job for dad!).

- *Remove irritating sleepwear.* Many infants cannot settle in synthetic sleepwear (some adults, too!). A mother in our practice went through our whole checklist of night-waking causes until she discovered her baby was sensitive to polyester sleepers. Once she changed to 100 percent cotton clothing, her baby slept better. Besides being restless, some babies show skin allergies to new clothing, detergents, and fabric softeners by breaking out in a rash. (For more on dressing your baby safely and comfortably for sleep, see page 76.)

Create a comfortable bedroom temperature. A consistent bedroom temperature of around 70° F is best for sleeping. Also, a relative humidity of around 50 percent is most conducive to sleep. Dry air may leave baby with a stuffy nose that awakens him. Yet humidity that's too high fosters allergy-producing molds. A warm-mist vaporizer can act as a heater in your baby's sleeping area, and it helps maintain an adequate level of humidity in homes with central heating (and the "white noise" of the consistent hum may help baby sleep longer).

Fill tiny tummies. The tinier the tummy, the more frequently a baby needs to be fed — both day and night. Babies have tiny tummies (about the size of their fist), which is why babies under six months of age need one or two night feedings. Some babies (especially breastfed ones) continue to need night feedings even in the second six months of life. You can maximize the amount of time baby will sleep after a feeding by being sure that baby fills his tummy as he feeds off to sleep and again when you feed him in the middle of the night. (See page 139 for how to comfortably fill tiny tummies for longer sleep.)

Swaddle your baby. Swaddling re-creates the womb environment. In the early months, many babies like to "sleep tight," securely swaddled in a cotton baby blanket. Older infants like to sleep "loose," and may sleep for longer stretches with loose coverings that allow them more freedom of movement. Oftentimes, dressing a baby loosely during the day but swaddling him at night can condition the baby to associate sleep with being swaddled. Make sure baby doesn't get too warm.

Once I started swaddling her, she slept through the night. At about three months, she got too strong to swaddle in the traditional way. She would get her arms out and rub her face and startle herself awake. I took a larger thin blanket and wrapped the sides individually over each arm and under her back so she couldn't get loose. It may sound like a cruel thing to do, but she smiled as I did it and slept peacefully all night long.

Babies usually start squirming out of their swaddling wraps by six months. Another possible problem with swaddling is that once babies get used to it, they have a hard time sleeping without being swaddled. The movement of their arms and legs wakes them up.

Dr. Bill cautions: Dr. Robert Salter, professor of orthopedics at the largest children's hospital in the world — the Hospital for Sick Children in Toronto, Canada — literally wrote the book on infant hip development. After the publication of the first edition of *The Baby Book,* in which we extolled the merits of swaddling and showed parents how to swaddle a baby, Dr. Salter wrote me a long letter. He believes leaving babies swaddled for too long, especially in the early months, can interfere with the development of their ball-and-socket hip joint. For this reason, we recommend that parents swaddle their babies only during sleep time. Be sure to give your baby plenty of time to "let loose" when he is awake.

STEP 4. CREATE A VARIETY OF BEDTIME RITUALS

You are learning where baby sleeps, when baby sleeps, and how to create a comfortable sleepy environment, and now we come to the next step in our plan: helping you figure out what bedtime rituals work best for your baby. As you use these same routines night after night (or alternate through several routines consistently), baby will learn to fall asleep easily and stay asleep longer.

Create Healthy and Relaxing Sleep Associations

A sleep association is not a nap-time playgroup or a group of sleepy parents who gather to yawn and complain about their baby's sleep habits. A sleep association refers to a connection made in baby's mind between falling asleep and the various activities, places, experiences, and feelings that precede his nodding off into slumber. The wiring in baby's brain is full of patterns of association. For example, if you usually nurse and sing your baby to sleep in a rocking chair, this setting will become programmed into your baby's mind as a sleep-inducing routine. He will remember the calm and drowsy feelings he gets from rocking and nursing, and this will help him fall asleep.

What kind of sleep associations do you want to teach your baby? Do you want to create attachment-based sleep associations or independence-based sleep associations?

Attachment-based sleep associations. Many parents like to "parent" their babies to sleep — by rocking, feeding, or snuggling while baby drifts off to sleep. Baby learns to associate falling asleep with a parent's presence. The advantage? A closer bond develops between parent and baby. The disadvantage? Mom or dad must be involved with baby

falling asleep for months or even years. Depending on your own instinctive parenting style, you may actually view this as an advantage; certainly your baby would.

Independence-based sleep associations. Some parents strive to help baby learn a more independent way of falling asleep, without the need for parent involvement. The most popular method for getting baby to fall asleep independently is the cry-it-out method. The disadvantage? You don't teach baby to fall asleep, you force him to. Medical research has shown that excessive crying creates stress for a baby. So a baby learns to associate falling asleep with fear, stress, and worry. This is not healthy in the long run. (We will discuss sleep anxiety more on page 104 and the harmful effects of crying it out on pages 210 to 213.) We all want our babies to eventually learn to fall asleep independently using their own self-soothing strategies at an appropriate age. Our sleep plan helps you teach them how to do this rather than forcing them to sleep independently.

In our own families, we chose to create attachment-based sleep associations. We enjoyed the cuddling and closeness of our kids' bedtime routines, and we felt that just being there for our babies was easier than fussing with other stuff. You may feel differently about this, or you may be thinking that it's time for your older baby or toddler to start falling asleep independently. That's okay with us. What is most important is that you help your child develop healthy, happy sleep associations.

Why is it necessary for you to help your baby develop healthy sleep associations? Why not just put baby down in her crib, walk out of the room, and let her fall asleep on her own? Won't she learn that being in the crib means there's nothing to do now but sleep? Well, yes, she will begin to associate being left alone in the crib with sleep. Her developing brain is busy building patterns of association all the time. That's what brains do. But in the early months, babies do not have the developmental capacity to transition without help from a state of being awake to one of being asleep. A tiny baby left alone in her crib to fall asleep on her own is likely to cry fearfully and then sleep anxiously. Going to sleep anxiously defeats one of the goals of your sleep plan: *to teach baby a healthy attitude about sleep — that sleep is a pleasant state to enter and a happy state to remain in.*

Babies need to be parented to sleep so that they can form pleasant sleep associations. What kind of activities, experiences, and feelings do you want your baby to associate with going to sleep? Babies who fall asleep while breast- or bottlefeeding will learn to associate warm milk, rhythmic sucking, and being cuddled close to mom with sleep. Babies who are carried around or rocked to sleep will learn that motion and comfort, as well as contact with mom or dad, are what send them into dreamland. Babies who are put in a crib to cry themselves to sleep learn that sleep is a lonely time when they need to comfort themselves.

Remember, you want your baby to sleep not only longer but also happier. So, in considering any advice about sleep, including the advice in this book, ask yourself this:

> "If I were my baby, how would I want to go to sleep?"

Getting behind the eyes of your baby and imagining how you would want your parents to act in a certain situation is one of the most important parenting tools that we have learned during our years as parents and pediatricians. You will nearly always make wise decisions about how to parent your children if you begin your decision process by trying to understand the situation from your child's point of view. If you were a baby, would you rather be parented to sleep at the breast of your mother or in the arms of your father or just put down all alone in a crib and left to cry yourself to sleep?

We are now going to show you ways to create sleep associations that have one goal in mind — to help baby learn that sleep is a pleasant state to enter and a happy state to remain in.

Sleep associations and sleep tools. It's helpful to develop a repertoire of sleep associations and sleep-inducing tools that work for you. Think of your baby's primary sleep association as your main method of putting baby to sleep. Sleep tools are additional things such as soft music, dim lights, or stories that may help to calm a child and prepare her for sleep. Some parents will choose one primary sleep association as the foundation, and use several sleep tools to help. Others like to get baby used to several different primary associations for sleep so that they have more options at bedtime.

AND THE SLEEP ASSOCIATION WINNERS ARE:

Primary Sleep Associations

- feeding to sleep (breast or bottle)
- feeding almost to sleep
- parenting down to sleep without feeding
- rocking or walking down
- wearing down in a sling
- putting down to fall asleep independently

Additional Sleep Tools

- soft music
- singing lullabies
- dimmed light
- white noise
- pacifier or "lovee"
- patting
- sucking
- stroking (massage)
- swinging
- driving
- dancing in arms
- scent of mother
- verbal sleep cues (e.g., "nighty-night")
- stories
- a combination of several

Which primary sleep association is going to work best for your baby? You won't know until you've tried them all. We suggest you go through a trial period of a few weeks to see what primary method of putting baby to sleep works the best. Try feeding baby to sleep a few nights, then try rocking or walking. Try snuggling with baby but not feeding him to sleep. Involve dad in the routine as well. Try a variety of methods until you learn what works best.

Primary Sleep Associations

Here are the primary associations to consider as you decide what will work best in your family: feeding baby to sleep, including feeding baby almost to sleep; lulling baby to sleep by rocking or walking; wearing baby down to sleep in a sling; and putting baby down to fall asleep independently.

Breastfeeding or bottlefeeding your baby to sleep. If babies could vote, going off to sleep the *warm way* would win the Best Transition Award. A high-touch continuum from warm bath, to warm arms, to warm breast, to warm bed is a winning recipe for sleep. Snuggle next to your baby in your bed and nurse her off to sleep. If you nurse baby to sleep in your arms, be sure to wait until she is fully asleep before you try to transfer her into her own bed. Once baby is asleep, just ease away. Check out Martha's de-latch technique (page 140) to learn more.

Breastfeeding seems to be nature's plan for comforting babies and helping them fall asleep. In fact, breast milk contains a sleep-inducing protein that helps lull baby into dreamland. (As an added advantage, as baby relaxes, so does mother, thanks to the hormones released when baby sucks at the breast.) Young babies also fall asleep very easily while bottlefeeding. (For related strategies, see also page 179, where dad adds the finishing touch to mother's nursing.)

We recommend that you not place any limitations on your baby's nursing to sleep during the early weeks of breastfeeding. In the first four to six weeks after baby's birth, you are learning to read your baby's hunger cues, your baby is learning to tell you when he is hungry, and your milk supply is adjusting to baby's needs. Relax and enjoy the breastfeeding experience.

A smart baby will come to love this feeding-to-sleep association and enjoy and expect it for as long as you breastfeed or use bottles. On the one hand, this means that you will be able to count on feeding as an easy way to get baby off to sleep. Even a baby who is fighting sleep will eventually succumb to the relaxing feelings that come from sucking. On the other hand, mom's breasts (or the bottle) have to be there at bedtime, and again later, when baby awakens in the middle of the night. Even if feeding is your baby's number-one primary sleep association, you may want to help him learn other associations so you have other ways to put him to bed.

In developing our sleep plan, we asked mothers of frequent night wakers, "For your next baby, what will you do differently?" The following answer, from our daughter Hayden (formerly the star of our *Fussy Baby* book and now a new mother), is representative of what many moms told us:

I cherish those precious times of nursing Ashton to sleep, as I realize they will pass all too soon. Yet, for our next baby, I will not use just one way of putting her to sleep. I'll do a variety of things so she's not so set on only one way of falling asleep. This will include my husband, Jason, putting her to sleep now and then, so that when she's older, he can put her to sleep in his own way.

Many parents tell us that nursing baby at bedtime and a couple more times during the night works very well for them if they are co-sleeping. Baby is content, and mother manages to get enough sleep because baby is sleeping close by and she can nurse baby back to sleep without waking up completely herself. Mom may wake a little more often, but she feels that the benefits outweigh any inconvenience for her.

Some moms, however, have told us that at age six months, twelve months, even eighteen months, their babies continue to wake up (sometimes several times!) each night to nurse and that they can no longer cope with this much night nursing. They wish that their babies would learn that there is more than one way to fall asleep. Well, babies *can* learn other ways to sleep, and later in this book we will share ways to teach a baby new sleep associations. For now, we want you to know that many mothers nurse their babies to sleep for many months, including during the night, and still manage to get enough rest. If you currently enjoy nursing your baby to sleep, we don't want to get in the way of a good thing. One of the lessons we want you to learn about parenting is to *enjoy the moment.* We want you to get attached to your baby without worrying about a lot of what-ifs. (If frequent night nursing is a top concern, you will welcome the tips offered in chapter 6.)

Feeding baby *almost* to sleep. Many breastfeeding moms who want dad to also be able to put baby to sleep teach their baby sleep associations beyond breastfeeding. Baby breastfeeds at bedtime, settles down, and starts to feel drowsy. Then, using walking or rocking while patting baby's back and other methods for easing the transition into sleep, dad takes over while baby drifts off to sleep (see our nighttime fathering tips in chapter 8). Bottlefeeding parents can use this approach, too, if they don't want their baby falling asleep with a bottle in her mouth. This approach helps baby learn that there are other ways to fall asleep besides relying on the comfort of sucking. When you use this approach with an older infant who no longer needs two or three nighttime feedings, baby may be less likely to wake up at night and may be more willing to go back to sleep with just some gentle patting or snuggling from either mom or dad.

The main reason for getting baby used to other sleep associations is to avoid mother burnout from frequent night nursing of an older infant (the most common sleep concern we encounter in our pediatric practice). In the wonderful world of night nursing, babies absolutely love going fully to sleep at mother's breast and having instant access to this warm and cozy prop when they wake up. If it's working for you, please don't change. Yet, it often helps to add the finishing touch of another prop after nursing to help baby go from being awake but drowsy through light sleep into a state of deep sleep. Try these finishing touches:

- *Nurse, then pat, sing, or rock baby to sleep.* Instead of nursing baby completely to sleep, nurse until she starts to slow down her sucking and closes her eyes but is not yet asleep. Ease your nipple out of her mouth (see Martha's unlatching trick, page 140) and then rock, pat, or sing her down until she is completely asleep.

- *Mother-nurse, plus father-nurse.* Near the end of the nursing, ease baby gently into father's arms to add the finishing touch (for a complete discussion of how fathers can do this, see page 179). Then, hopefully, when baby wakes up, she will be more likely to accept dad or another caregiver putting her back to sleep by using the same finishing touch.

- *Add a variety of sleep tools.* You can use any of the tools listed on page 16 and discussed in this section to lull your baby to sleep after feeding. If these techniques are not working and baby insists on feeding to sleep, consider that a baby who is not willing is not yet ready. Give your baby a few weeks for her sleep patterns to mature and then try again.

Parenting baby down to sleep without feeding. This is more easily said than done. Because of the sleep-association principle discussed above, if baby always falls fully asleep the same way, especially at the breast, he will expect, demand, or even scream for the same prop — usually the breast — to get back to sleep. Occasionally try putting your baby down in his bed when he is sleepy but not totally asleep. Use the various sleep-inducing tools from pages 20 to 26 to lull baby to sleep. Showing him how to fall asleep without feeding teaches him that it's okay to go to sleep in other ways. Your baby may fuss when you first try some of the sleep-inducing tools. If he fusses more than just a little, remember this important parenting principle: *Don't persist with a bad experiment.* Yet, even if just once or twice a week you try to put your baby down when he is only partially asleep, at least you've planted a bit of the "I can do it" association.

Rocking or walking down. Try rocking baby to sleep in a bedside rocking chair, or walk with baby, patting her back and singing. To keep the motion going (and keep baby asleep), ease her into a cradle and continue the rocking motion at a rate of about sixty rocks per minute. This is the heartbeat rhythm your baby was used to in the womb.

Wearing down in a sling. Place your baby in a baby sling and wear her around the house for a half hour or so before the designated bedtime. When she is fully asleep in the sling, ease her out of the sling onto your bed. Or, if she's not fully asleep, lie down with her in the neck nestle or warm fuzzy position on your chest (see page 177). When baby is fully asleep, roll over on your side, slip yourself out of the sling, and let baby lie on the bed on her back using the sling as a cover. Wearing down (or what we also dub "slinging down") is particularly useful for the reluctant napper. When baby falls asleep in the sling, you can both lie down and enjoy a much-needed mutual nap.

Putting baby down to sleep independently. Some parents like to set up a more independent sleep arrangement early on, in which, hopefully, baby learns to settle himself down to sleep without much parental interaction. They reason that a baby who learns to fall asleep on his own will also be able to settle himself back to sleep on his own when he wakes during the night. This type of sleep training has become popular with some parents because it results in a "low maintenance" baby at night. It has also received a great deal of criticism because of the amount of crying that babies experience during the training phase. It ignores the fact that babies are born with an innate need for comfort and security while falling asleep, upon waking, while going back to sleep, and in some cases even while sleeping.

Ideally, the comfort they seek is supplied by a human caregiver. Babies who sleep independently usually need to have various sleep-inducing tools handy to calm them when they are falling asleep and again when they awaken. They may need motion, such as the rocking, swinging, or bouncing movements of a cradle, swing, or baby hammock. They

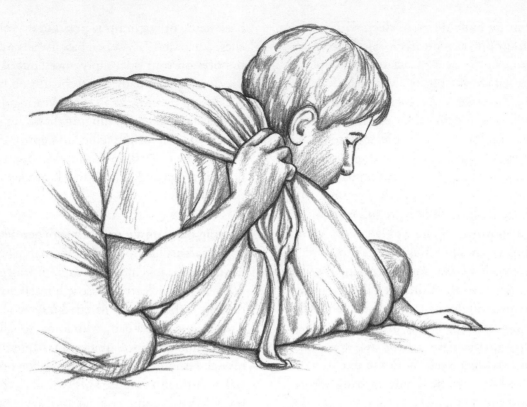

may depend on a pacifier. Perhaps they learn to associate soft music or other sounds with sleep. Parents develop a routine that lulls baby into dreamland. Use the variety of sleep-association tools we discuss on the following pages to help your baby learn to fall asleep independently.

To train babies to fall asleep lying in a crib by themselves without any comforting sleep associations would be very tough on them. In chapter 10 you will learn why we discourage this "tough love" approach to sleep training when it involves crying it out. Research shows that a sleep-training method that involves extended crying alone (without parent comforting) is not emotionally or physically

healthy for babies — or for parents. Very easygoing babies may be able to learn to fall asleep independently with only minimal fuss, and in chapter 4 we will offer suggestions for how this can be done in an appropriately sensitive way. Remember, our goal is for you to create stress-free sleep associations for your baby that result in a happy, healthy sleeper.

Sleep Tools — Transitioning Tips

Babies don't come equipped with the type of sleep switch that you can suddenly turn off at nap time and bedtime. Yet, a transitioning-to-sleep ritual can be like a dimmer switch that gradually tunes out and turns down stimula-

VARYING BABY'S SLEEP ASSOCIATIONS

Get baby used to a variety of sleep associations at bedtime. The way your baby goes to sleep is the way she expects to go back to sleep when she awakens. When baby is older, you and your spouse may want to take turns putting baby to sleep. Baby will learn mom's way of getting him to sleep (probably nursing) and dad's way of getting him to sleep (walking, "wearing down" in the baby sling, rocking and humming, and so on). You may decide that you want to have your baby sleep in your bed with you but you want to vary what you do to help her fall asleep. Some nights mom will nurse baby to sleep. Other nights dad will soothe baby to sleep. You can both vary your soothing techniques. Some nights wear baby down to sleep by walking her around in a baby sling carrier. Other nights lull her to sleep in a baby swing. Mom has the option of not nursing baby to sleep, instead using dad's "wearing down" technique. You can even vary where baby sleeps. Some nights, put baby in her cradle. On other nights, put her in a crib and bring her into bed with you when she wakes. Or share the whole night in your big bed together.

tion in baby's environment. In sleep psychology, this is known as "fading" (like what happens when you are listening to a dull lecture). You can't expect a baby to go from his excit-ing waking life right into sleep. (You don't fall asleep this way, do you?) There has to be a transition time. Here are some favorites that have worked in our families:

Fathering down. "Nursing" implies comforting, not only breastfeeding. Fathers can and should "nurse" their babies down to sleep. Place baby in the neck nestle position (see page 177) and "dance" or rock your baby to sleep.

One day after we explained the concept of sleep associations to a tired mother, she replied, "My baby has only one sleep

SEARS SLEEP TIP FOR DADS

Avoid the quick release (sounds like a quarterback throwing a pass!) in getting your baby to sleep. Have patience. Sometimes a too-quick release from being securely attached to a parent can bother babies and cause them to jerk back awake. If baby continues to wake up when you try to transition him from your arms into his bed or is not falling completely asleep in your arms while being rocked or walked, try putting him down on your chest in the neck nestle position or next to you. Once he is fully asleep (you can tell by observing the limp-limb sign — hands unclenched, arms dangling loosely at his side, facial muscles still), then ease yourself away. If baby's hands are clenched and limbs are flexed, chances are he is still in the state of light sleep and will awaken if you try to put him down too quickly.

association — ME!" If this sounds like you, read — with your husband — chapter 8, Twenty-three Nighttime Fathering Tips.

Nestling down. Transferring the sleeping baby from your arms to his bed can prove to be tricky. An abrupt change from being nestled next to a parent's body to lying alone on a mattress will awaken some babies. To ease your baby through this transition, try the intermediate step of lying down on your bed with your sleeping baby still in your arms. We call this the "teddy bear snuggle." Once he's sound asleep (see limp-limb sign, page 21), you can ease yourself away or move him to wherever he sleeps.

Feet down. When transitioning your sleeping baby from your arms to his bed or crib, set him down so his feet touch the bed first, then his body, then his head. If baby is tipped head down first, he may startle and wake up.

Sucking down. Sucking is soothing, yet the human pacifier can wear out. Besides the breast or bottle, try your finger or teach baby to find his own hand to suck on.

Patting down. After you ease baby onto her bed, pat her chest or tummy gently and rhythmically, around sixty pats per minute (like your heartbeat). Gradually lighten and slow the patting as she succumbs to sleep. Add some verbal sleep cues (see page 27).

As she was just about to sleep, I'd run my fingers across her face, over her eyes, and down her nose so that her eyes would close.

Touching down. Oh, how babies love to be touched as they fall asleep. Here are some ideas for soothing, loving touches:

- *Patting.* Pat baby's back or bottom gently and rhythmically while she is being held in your arms. Gentle patting on her tummy can also be used to soothe a baby who is lying in bed, especially when picking her up might be too stimulating.

- *Massage.* Light stroking of baby's head and back is a favorite. A gentle full-body massage before bed may also help baby relax into bedtime mode.

- *Skin-to-skin.* Young babies especially love the familiar feel of your skin on theirs.

- *Transitional touch.* If baby starts to stir as you try to slip her out of your arms or ease away from her in bed, offer the laying on of hands. Place your hand on baby's chest or tummy and leave it there until she drifts back to sleep. This extra touch is especially important in babies who have a hard time transitioning from your arms into the bassinet or crib. They need this transitional touch to stay fully asleep. It can save you a trip back to the rocking chair to soothe an awakened baby back to sleep.

Swinging down. Try a baby hammock, as shown on page 25. For most babies, motion, not stillness, signals sleep. Remember how your baby used to sleep during the day when you were pregnant but kept you awake at night when you lay down to sleep. When you were up and around, the motion of your body soothed her into sleep. When you were still, she woke up.

Wind-up swings for winding down babies are a boon to parents when their arms are wearing out. Some infants find the mechanical swing less interesting, if not downright boring, compared with being in the arms of a human being, and off to sleep they go. Yet some babies are notoriously resistant to mechanical mother substitutes and will protest anything less than the real mom. Before you actually spend money on a swing, you might want to borrow one for a week or two to see if the spell of the swing will work for your baby. You may discover that you are uncomfortable with mechanical mothering and decide that your baby is better off in your arms.

Driving down. If you've tried all of the above transitioning techniques and baby still resists falling asleep, place baby in a car seat and drive around until he falls asleep. When you return home and baby is in a deep sleep, carry the sleeping baby (car seat and all) into your bedroom and let baby remain in the car seat until the first night waking. If he is in a deep sleep, you may be able to ease him out of the car seat into his own bed.

Using props. Called transitional objects or "lovees," these are favorite toys that help children more easily transition from the familiar and interesting waking world to the world of sleep. Transitional objects should be cuddly but safe. Rolling over on plastic toys may awaken baby.

The scent of mother. Leaving in the crib a breast pad or T-shirt that mother wore all day may help baby transition from the whole mother at night.

Sounds to sleep by. A parent softly singing a lullaby is the classic sound cue for babies to go to sleep. Quiet instrumental music is another traditional favorite. Here are some creative ways you can use sound to soothe your baby to sleep:

- *Mom's musical voice.* The soft sounds of mom's voice, either in song or in quiet words will mesmerize baby. That's why they're called lullabies.

- *Dad's deep tones.* Some babies really take to dad's full, rumbly tones. Besides hearing his voice, they can feel the vibrations from the voice box when held on dad's chest. (See the neck nestle, page 177.)

- *Rhythmic music.* Music with simple repeating words and rhythms is soothing to babies. Nursery rhymes and lullabies are the classic examples. Even quiet pop music with a steady beat can get baby into the rhythm of sleep. Peaceful classical music is another favorite. Complex classical music or turbulent-sounding rap or rock, on the other hand, can be overstimulating.

- *A medley of tunes.* Put together a medley of easy-listening lullabies on a CD or tape and set the player for continuous play. You won't have to worry about running out of music and breaking the sleepy mood. Then tape a medley of you singing baby's favorite lullabies. Your familiar voice may help baby settle when she is being put down to sleep by someone else.

- *A musical mobile.* For babies in a cradle or crib, turn on a musical mobile to help baby associate the gentle movement and the sound with going to sleep. If the mobile helps to get him to sleep, restart it when he wakes to get him back to sleep.

I saved one song, our sleep song, for when it was time to go to sleep. She learned to associate that song with falling asleep.

For some suggestions from the Sears family library of music, see Appendix A.

White noise. These are monotonous sounds that block out other noises and bore a baby to sleep. Besides the continuous monotone humming or "shhhh" of a parent, here are some white-noise sounds that work:

- the hum of a fan or air conditioner
- tape recording of the vacuum cleaner or running water from a faucet or shower
- a bubbling fish tank
- a loudly ticking clock or a metronome set at sixty beats a minute (which can also be tape-recorded)
- recordings of waterfalls or ocean sounds

I wore my baby in a sling while vacuuming. The sounds lulled him to sleep and I got some cleaning done.

◆

Our son loves to nurse to sleep and sometimes will prolong the nursing as much as thirty to forty minutes. My husband realized one evening

that our son had fallen asleep after only ten minutes while nursing and listening to a quiet mommy and daddy conversation. I decided to tape our conversation one evening. Now, when I want our son to go to sleep a little faster and my husband isn't around to talk to, I just play our mommy-and-daddy tape.

◆

If baby is restless and won't nurse off to sleep, my husband turns on the dishwasher for white noise and then walks baby for a time.

Motion for sleep. What baby doesn't like motion? This is why babies fall asleep in swings, rockers, cars, and while being held and walked. Here are suggestions for slings, swings, and other things you can use to lull baby to sleep:

- *Rocking.* Mom's or dad's arms and the steady motion of a rocking chair have been putting babies to sleep for ages.

- *Cradle.* Gently rock baby's cradle to lull baby to sleep or back to sleep.

- *Baby swing.* Many babies will drift off to sleep in a baby swing at nap time or bedtime.

- *Baby slings.* Wearing baby in a sling or other infant carrier while you move about simulates the womb environment and will soothe baby to sleep (see pages 19 and 20).

- *Dancing.* You can combine all kinds of sensory input in a dance that will envelop baby in a soothing environment. This works great for fussy babies and those who fight sleep. Snuggle baby in your arms,

A MOVING BABY BED

Motion is a time-tested sleep inducer for babies. That's why babies fall asleep so easily while being carried or rocked. Cradles and baby swings have been the traditional way to soothe babies to sleep without being in a parent's arms, but there is a new way parents can soothe baby off into dreamland. If you've already tried the usual props to help your baby sleep, try the Amby Baby Motion Bed. Here are some of the unique features of the Amby that make it such a helpful sleep tool:

- *It uses three-dimensional motion.* This cradle-size hammock hangs from a sturdy spring, allowing parents to gently rock baby in all three directions — up and down, back and forth, and from side to side. This is the same motion baby experienced while in the womb and now feels when being carried.

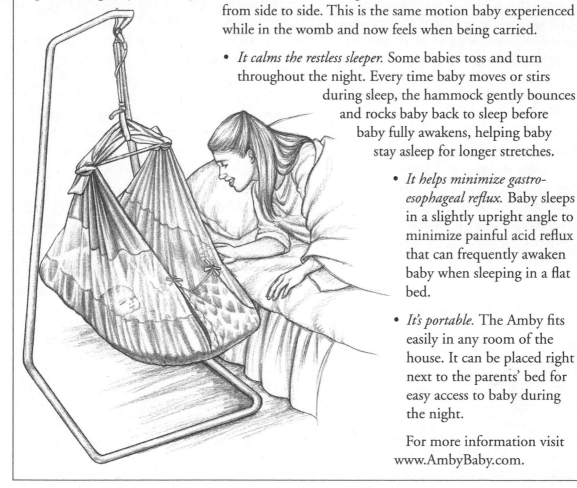

- *It calms the restless sleeper.* Some babies toss and turn throughout the night. Every time baby moves or stirs during sleep, the hammock gently bounces and rocks baby back to sleep before baby fully awakens, helping baby stay asleep for longer stretches.

- *It helps minimize gastro-esophageal reflux.* Baby sleeps in a slightly upright angle to minimize painful acid reflux that can frequently awaken baby when sleeping in a flat bed.

- *It's portable.* The Amby fits easily in any room of the house. It can be placed right next to the parents' bed for easy access to baby during the night.

  For more information visit www.AmbyBaby.com.

either in the cradle hold, up on your shoulder, or draped tummy down over your forearm. Move around gently in all directions — up, down, and back and forth — and pat baby's bottom as you hum, sing, or make other gentle sounds. All this gentle stimulation blocks out the anxious, fretful feelings coming from inside of baby and really takes baby back to the womb.

A box full of tricks. While most babies need a predictable routine to get to sleep, some enjoy novelty. And even your best transitioning tricks may not work when baby enters a new stage of development. You'll need a box full of sleep strategies to see you through the first year or two of your baby's life. Keep trying new things.

Consider winding-down routines as an opportunity to spend quality time with your child. Enjoy this peaceful time together. Don't look at your watch. Don't think about everything else you have to do. If you relax, your baby will pick up on your attitude and probably go to sleep more easily.

Figuring Out What Works for Your Baby

During the first week or two of your sleep plan, you will be trying to determine which sleep associations and tools work for your baby.

For newborns and younger babies, you will be learning one or two routines that you can depend on to get your baby off to sleep. This will likely involve some combination of feeding, rocking, or walking.

For older infants who already have a strong primary sleep association, you may be ready to make a change because it is no longer working for you. You will be trying to establish one or two new sleep associations so your baby can learn to fall asleep in other ways. Your baby will probably protest or fight this change and want you to go back to his preferred routine. Use various sleep tool ideas from the list on page 16 along with whatever new primary sleep associations you are trying to establish. Be sure to try new ideas you have never considered before — you may be pleasantly surprised at what works for your baby. Write down your observations to help you remember what has worked:

Primary Sleep Association	Additional Sleep Tools	Time It Took to Fall Asleep
Day 1 _____	_____	_____
Day 2 _____	_____	_____
Day 3 _____	_____	_____
Day 4 _____	_____	_____
Day 5 _____	_____	_____
Day 6 _____	_____	_____
Day 7 _____	_____	_____

Baby's favorite sleep-association combo is _____.

Now that you have figured out a variety of ways to happily parent your baby to sleep, let's learn ways of helping baby enjoy sleeping longer.

STEP 5. HELP BABY SLEEP FOR LONGER STRETCHES

Babies — and parents — enjoy a more restful night if their sleep is not cut short. As you will learn in chapter 3, babies are wired to wake up during the night, and they usually need a parent's help to settle back into sleep. As babies mature, so do their sleep patterns, so that they are able to sleep for longer stretches and resettle themselves. When this blissful time happens varies greatly from baby to baby. While you can't force your baby to sleep through the night, you can provide conditions that will help your child attain sleep maturity to sleep for longer stretches.

Why do babies wake up so much? Answer: They're babies! In chapter 3 and chapter 12, we'll discuss the many developmental, medical, and physical reasons babies wake up. Keeping in mind that breastfeeding babies under one year typically need to nurse twice a night, and those over a year at least once, here are some ideas for lengthening the stretch of time between feeds.

Change where baby sleeps. In step 1 you chose where you wanted baby to sleep. Hopefully it is working for both of you. However, the bed that baby starts the night in may not necessarily be the same bed she wakes up in each morning. Consider this: Is your baby waking during the night because she is alone

in another room and wants to be closer to you? If you think this may be the case, try moving baby closer to you at the first night waking. (See Baby Sleeps in Your Room but Not in Your Bed, page 5, and Baby Sleeps with You in Your Bed, page 6.) Or is baby already in your bed and waking up because you are right there? If so, try moving baby farther away from you when you come to bed or at the first night waking.

"Coach" baby to sleep. Repeating cue words, sounds that baby associates with going to sleep, will often help baby get back to sleep. Offer these cues as the last sound baby hears before drifting off to sleep and use these same words again when she awakens in the middle of the night (e.g., "night-night," "sleepy-sleepy," "happy nappy," or "shhhh"). Using the sleep-associations principle, baby learns to associate these sounds with both going to sleep and going back to sleep. The time-tested sound *shhhh,* which mothers naturally do, has a biological basis. It is similar to the sound of uterine blood flow that baby was used to while in the womb.

When he made his first peep, we quickly issued reminders, such as "Shhhh . . . sleepy-sleepy." We let him know that it wasn't time to get up yet.

Lay on hands. When baby stirs, gently lay your hands on her without picking her up. Stay with her and continue laying on a comforting hand as you say or sing your favorite sleep cues, such as "night-night" or "sleepy-sleepy." Stay with it until she settles. If she starts to wake up again right away, you can give it another try. Again lay your hands on her and give her your "sleepy-sleepy" sleep cue. If she just can't fall asleep, pick her up and walk around the bedroom for a while, holding her in a sleep-inducing position such as the neck nestle (see page 177). By this time you will know whether you can get her to stretch out her sleep more or whether it's simply time to feed her.

Leave a little bit of mother behind. To help baby stay asleep when you are not there, have something nearby that smells like you. This might be a breast pad that has the odor of your milk or an item of your clothing. Your bed will naturally have your scent. You can also sleep with baby's crib or cradle sheets for a night (use them for a pillowcase) and then place them on baby's mattress. Your scent should last for a few days.

I nurse and wear my baby a lot during the day. He actually sleeps better if I take off the shirt that I have worn all day and cover him with it before I put the blanket on him at night.

Offer a thumb or a pacifier. "Pacifier" literally means peacemaker. Giving baby something to suck on will often bring peace to both baby and parents. You can actually help your baby learn to suck his hand or thumb. These are "handier" than pacifiers. They are warm, soft, and easily available. They don't fall on the floor, they are just the right size for baby's mouth, and they don't obstruct the nose or need to be clipped on with a cord. Babies feel more in control of their hands.

As you're putting baby down to sleep, ease her thumb or hand into her mouth, and do this again each time she wakes up. This way she learns to associate sucking with going to sleep — and back to sleep. If baby continues to suck but wakes up anyway, she's probably hungry and needs you, not just a milkless thumb. During checkups, when I need tiny babies to be quiet so that I can listen to their hearts, I sometimes coax their thumbs into their mouths. Sometimes I notice mothers raise their eyebrows as if they didn't realize they could do this. Babies in the womb suck their thumbs. In the early months, babies who can't quite find their thumbs will suck on their wrists or even forearms. They are born with their own natural pacifier. Take advantage of it. And don't overuse artificial pacifiers. If, when baby cries, you find yourself by reflex reaching for the binky instead of the baby, remember our advice: "Use it, don't abuse it, and quickly try to lose it."

Some parents worry that teaching baby to suck his thumb will lead to a long-term habit that will be hard to break (you can't just throw the thumb away like you can the pacifier). While this can happen, if it gets you a better night's sleep for now, it's probably worth it.

Try both the quick and the delayed response. Should you come running as soon as you hear your baby awaken in the night? Or should you hold off to see if baby goes back to sleep? Some parents find it easier if they get to baby quickly and help baby back to sleep before the cries escalate and baby gets revved up. If you wait too long, it can be much harder for both mother and baby to get back to sleep. With co-sleeping babies, a half-awake mother can simply roll over and nurse her half-awake baby, and the nursing pair can drift back to sleep without either one getting worked up.

Sometimes in the middle of the night I quickly offer her a breast or a "soothie" pacifier and she doesn't fully wake up.

◆

The trick is to never let him fully wake up and to never let him cry. If he cries, he's wide awake.

Other parents find that if they let their baby squirm and fuss a bit, baby is able to re-settle without intervention. This is a waking-by-waking call. It helps to remember that not all noises that sleeping babies make are cries for help. (See Normal Night Noises Sleeping Babies Make, page 65.) If you think your baby can settle himself back to sleep, delay rushing in and picking him up. Give him a chance to work things out on his own. He will let you know if he needs help.

Keep it simple and quick. No middle-of-the-night entertainment, please. You're there as a comforter, not a playmate. Nighttime is for sleeping, not for playing. If baby needs your help to resettle, try to do it quickly, calmly, and comfortably. Even though you're tired — and perhaps frustrated — try using what we dub the "Caribbean approach" — "no problem, baby." If baby senses your anxiety and irritation, she is less likely to resettle. Try to resettle baby with a simple song or

LEARN WHEN TO LET SLEEPING BABIES LIE

One of the most difficult lessons for new co-sleeping breastfeeding mothers is to develop a balance between "I nurse my baby at the first whimper" and "Oh, that's just a normal sleep noise — she'll go back to sleep by herself." If you nurse your baby right away, you will probably both get back to sleep sooner. Yet, if you nurse every time she awakens, you may end up with a baby who wants to nurse all night long and doesn't know any other way of falling back to sleep. You have to try to find the balance that works best for you and your baby. We discuss this dilemma in detail in chapter 5.

patting with your hands. If you need to pick up baby for a bit of swaying or rocking, don't make the routine too interesting. Your goal is to lull her back to sleep.

Someday your child will find the promised land of sleeping through the night. Babies do eventually wean! This high-maintenance stage of nighttime parenting will pass. Again, the time in your arms, at your breast, and in your bed is a relatively short while in the life of a child, yet the memories of love and availability will last forever.

YOUR CHECKLIST OF SLEEP TOOLS

Here's a checklist of topics we covered in this chapter, plus some that we'll cover in subsequent chapters, to help your baby sleep happier, healthier, and longer.

☐ sleep safety (page 76)
☐ different sleeping arrangements (page 4)
☐ charting baby's tired times (page 9)
☐ sleep associations (page 14)
☐ sounds to sleep by (page 23)
☐ a loving touch (page 22)
☐ a familiar scent (page 23)
☐ a pacifier (page 28)
☐ motion for sleep (page 24)
☐ feeding baby partially to sleep (page 18)
☐ back-to-sleep cues (pages 27 and 40)
☐ bedtime rituals (pages 13 and 37)
☐ nursing down (page 16)
☐ wearing down (pages 19 and 20)
☐ fathering down (pages 21 and 177)
☐ nestling down (page 22)
☐ patting down (page 22)
☐ walking/rocking down (page 19)
☐ swinging down (page 22)
☐ offering a "lovee" (pages 23 and 40)
☐ quieting the bedroom (page 10)
☐ quieting the house (page 11)
☐ darkening the bedroom (page 11)
☐ warming the bed (page 11)
☐ lessening physical discomforts (page 11)
☐ filling tiny tummies (page 13)
☐ swaddling (page 13)
☐ creating a comfortable bedroom temperature (page 12)
☐ dressing baby comfortably for sleep (page 12)

KEEP A SLEEP LOG

While most mothers would rather spend their free time resting than filling in charts, sleep logs can help in many ways. Charts give you a visual picture of your child's individual twenty-four-hour sleep patterns. You may be surprised to discover that he sleeps more than you thought. A sleep log can help you spot problem times and track progress to see if your sleep strategies are working. When discussing your sleep concerns with your pediatrician, show your doctor the sleep log and point out the problem areas that you've identified. In this way, you and your doctor can see at a glance your baby's sleep patterns and where certain sleep strategies may be applied. Photocopy the sample sleep log on the next page. As you try all the sleep-inducing strategies described in chapters 1 and 2, fill in the sleep log and chart your baby's progress.

10-DAY SLEEP LOG

DAY	8 a.m.	9 a.m.	10 a.m.	11 a.m.	12 p.m.	1 p.m.	2 p.m.	3 p.m.	4 p.m.	5 p.m.	6 p.m.	7 p.m.	8 p.m.	9 p.m.	10 p.m.	11 p.m.	12 a.m.	1 a.m.	2 a.m.	3 a.m.	4 a.m.	5 a.m.	6 a.m.	7 a.m.	Total Hours of Sleep	Number of Night Wakings	Sleep Stretch at Night*	What You Tried
1																												
2																												
3																												
4																												
5																												
6																												
7																												
8																												
9																												
10																												

Directions: Color black each hour of sleep, including daytime naps. Mark ↑ each time your baby wakes up. Mark F each time you feed your baby.

Comments:

*"Sleep stretch" refers to the number of hours of uninterrupted sleep.

Fifteen Tips to Help Toddlers and Preschoolers Sleep

THE FIVE STEPS to happy sleeping that we described in the previous chapter apply to toddlers as well as to babies. Yet, as babies turn into toddlers, their nighttime needs change, and parents need to learn more sleep strategies. Toddlers still need your presence at bedtime, and their bedtime rituals will reflect their need for closeness. Sometime between two and three years of age, children begin to form conscious memories that will stay with them for the rest of their lives. What bedtime memories do you want your child to file away?

WHAT TODDLERS LEARN AT BEDTIME

It's good to have goals as a parent. When you know what you want for your children in the long term, it's easier to do the things you have to do right now to reach that goal. What are your sleep goals for your child? Three important sleep goals are:

- Children should learn that sleep is a pleasant state to enter and a peaceful state to stay in.
- Children should eventually learn to go to sleep happily on their own.
- Children should have pleasant memories of how they were parented to sleep.

Children need to develop a pleasant attitude toward falling asleep and staying asleep. We believe that your child's ability to sleep well in the future depends on his having happy, stress-free, positive experiences at bedtime when he is young. Eventually, these positive experiences will translate into sleep independence — the ability to fall asleep and to go back to sleep on his own. And all these good sleep experiences will help your child grow up to be a happier, less stressed, and healthier person.

Many well-meaning parents push their kids into sleep independence too soon. After a long day at work and caring for the kids, parents need a break and want the evening for themselves. Their whole goal at bedtime is for their child between the ages of one and four to fall asleep on his own, and to do so quickly and quietly. When this is achieved, parents feel they have finally succeeded in creating a "good sleeper."

But what if a child isn't quite ready for this? Or, what happens when a child has been shown that bedtime is a time when she is forced to stay in a dark room alone and told to be quiet and go to sleep? This is a child who will procrastinate because she fears or resents the isolation at bedtime. She will make up all kinds of reasons why she wants mom or dad's attention at bedtime. She will get up to find you because she's thirsty or because there's a monster under her bed. She will ask you to leave the light on or the door open. She will use every stalling tactic she can think of when what she really means is she just wants *you*. This is a child who is more likely to grow up with a fear of bedtime, of the dark, and of being alone. She may feel anxious and insecure because her parents have pushed her into nighttime independence before she was truly ready. Imagine how you as an adult would feel if you went to bed every night feeling stressed, scared, and unfulfilled. There is one more ingredient that parents often add to this bedtime picture without realizing it — anger or hostility. Even if there is no anger in your voice, phrases like "Get back to bed," "If you get out of bed one more time . . . ," and "Stop your whining and go to sleep" used night after night over the years add up to a child who resents and fears bedtime.

Ask yourself this: Are you willing to put in some time now to help your kids achieve the long-term goal of a healthy attitude about sleep and a trusting, secure attitude toward life? While most of what is in this chapter assumes that you are going to be nearby while your toddler drifts off to sleep, one of your long-term goals is that your child will eventually go to sleep happily on his own. So keep in mind that while you are *parenting* (not just putting) your toddler to sleep, you are also teaching him the skills and attitudes that he will someday use to help himself fall asleep without you there. No, you are not a victim of childish manipulation. When you rub your child's back at bedtime to help her relax or when you soothe your tearful toddler with quiet talking in the middle of the night, you are modeling self-help skills. When your child is ready to cope with these challenges on his own, he will call up images of the good feelings he had while falling asleep in your presence. And *bingo*, he'll fall asleep on his own.

FIFTEEN TIPS FOR EASING YOUR TODDLER OFF TO DREAMLAND

We'll begin with fifteen tips that apply to nearly all toddlers. These are practical strategies aimed at (1) getting little ones off to dreamland, and (2) teaching them a healthy attitude toward sleep. The second half of this chapter turns the spotlight (or a very dim night-light — we don't want to wake the kids) on common toddler sleep concerns that tired parents have shared with us — and our solutions.

SEASONS OF NIGHTTIME PARENTING

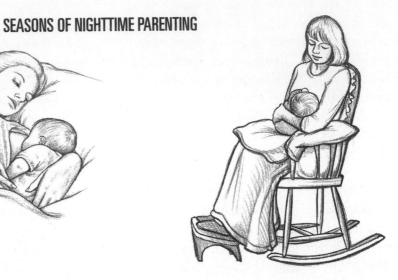

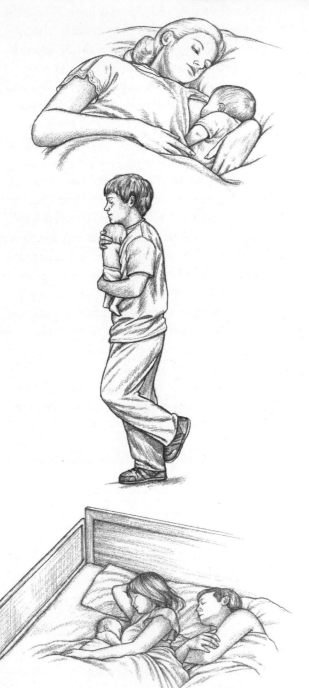

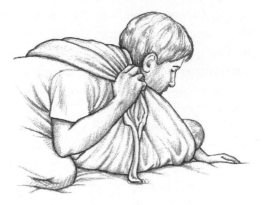

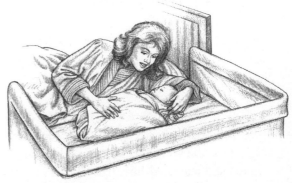

MOVING FROM ONENESS TO SEPARATENESS

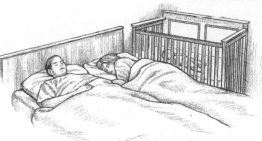

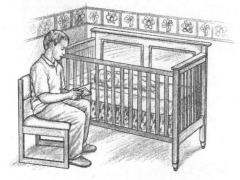

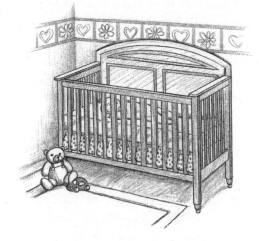

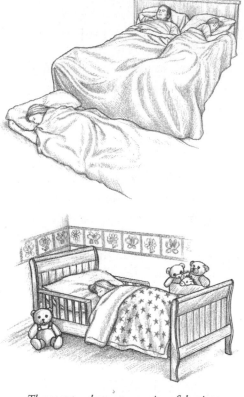

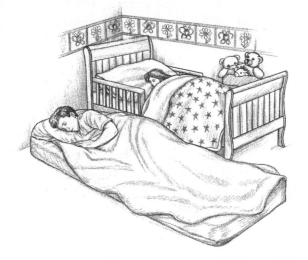

These seasons show a progression of sleeping arrangements from oneness to separateness. The age at which children develop various stages of sleep maturity varies greatly. The important point is that children can go through this progression and develop a healthy attitude toward sleep — that it is a pleasant state to enter and a fearless state to remain in.

*One night my daughter called out, "Mama,
I need you!" I went right away to her room,
nursed her, and she sleepily said, "Thank you,
Mama," and drifted off to sleep. I praise God
that she knows we are here for her and that she
uses us when she needs us. I pray that this will
be a lifelong pattern, not just in sleep but in her
everyday life.*

1. Tire Out Your Toddler

Encourage your child to be active during the
day. The more physical activity that
children — and adults — get during the day,
the better they sleep at night. Babies who are
not yet walking can be encouraged to play on
the floor, cruise, and crawl. Take your toddler
to the park to run, jump, and bounce on the
playground equipment. Toddlers get their
exercise in bursts of activity. They don't take
long walks or set out to jog three miles, as
adults do. Toddlers are active and busy all day
long, but they take frequent rests. The American Academy of Pediatrics, for a variety of
reasons, including the epidemic of childhood
obesity, has wisely issued the advisory "no TV
for tots under two." Toddlers should not be
plugged in for more than a half hour a day to
video games or television.

SEARS SLEEP TIP

Kids who are couch potatoes by day tend
to sleep less at night.

2. Set Consistent Bedtimes

Toddlers generally go to bed too late. Or
they go to bed at different times every
night. Modern families' busy daytime
lifestyles encourage this "whenever"
approach to bedtime. Unless your family's
lifestyle allows for your toddler to sleep
later in the morning, try to set an early and
consistent bedtime for your little one.
Even if a later bedtime is what works best
in your family, try to be consistent about
when your child goes to bed. By putting
kids to bed at the same time night after
night you are programming their internal
sleep clock so that they can fall asleep easily
at a set time.

3. Set the Stage

Toddlers and preschoolers are not going to
go to bed willingly if there is a lot of activity
in your household. They don't like to miss
anything. When it's time for your toddler to
go to bed, turn down the lights all over the
house, turn off the television (you can record
what you're missing), and channel older children's energy into quiet activities. As you
turn down the household activity level, let
your child know that bedtime is coming.
Set the kitchen timer for ten or fifteen minutes and tell your child that when the timer
goes off, it's bedtime. Or use an egg timer and
say "When all the sand hits the bottom, it's
time to start getting ready for bed." Kids are
less likely to argue with a timer than with a
parent.

NIGHTTIME PROPS FOR TOTS

While a mother's breast, a father's arms, and a familiar voice singing a lullaby will always be your child's favorite sleep inducers, there are times when parents need some reinforcements. Try these:

- *An aquarium.* The bubbles, the gracefully swimming fish, the hum of the pump, and the slowly changing lights and shadows are mesmerizing. They will calm toddlers and eventually lull them to sleep.

- *White noise machines.* A favorite of adults, these bedside sound machines allow you to choose various monotonous sounds that soothe young and old into sleep, such as a babbling brook, ocean waves, rainfall, and melodious chants. (See Sounds to Sleep By, page 23.)

- *An air filter.* A HEPA air filter not only rids the bedroom air of dust, allergens, and other nose-stuffing and night-waking irritants but also produces white noise that blocks out other sounds that can awaken a light sleeper.

- *A dimmer switch.* Gradually dimming the lights as you lie together will help ease your toddler into sleep. See if you can find a dimmer that can be operated with a remote control so that you don't have to get up to dim the lights. Or put the dimmer on the reading lamp next to the bed.

4. Enjoy a Variety of Bedtime Rituals

Bedtime rituals are all the things you do consistently, every night, starting a half hour to an hour before tired time. Bedtime rituals help the busy toddler wind down and make the transition from an exciting and active evening to the quietness and relative boredom of going to sleep.

You can't force your child to sleep, but you can create a quiet, soothing environment that allows sleep to overtake your child. For a while before bedtime, avoid stimulating activities, such as wrestling or running around the house. Save exciting activities that rev up a child's mind and body for late afternoon. Children need a buffer zone between a busy day and bedtime. Quiet activities and a regular bedtime routine can help kids make the transition from awake time to sleepy time.

Bedtime routines don't have to be exactly the same from one night to the next. Toddlers enjoy novelty. Bedtime with mom may be different from bedtime with dad, but that's a good thing. Bedtime rituals need to be creative and include quality time with parents because even children who are very tired may not be willing to give up and go to bed. They don't want to be separated from you or miss anything. Bedtime routines should be interesting and special, even as they wind children down from an active day.

Ritual tips. Different babies enjoy different rituals at different ages. Be flexible. What works one month may not necessarily work the next. Here are some tried-and-true favorites:

- The Bedtime B's: bath, breast or bottle, back rub, book, and clean bottom. (If bathtime revs up your child, bathe her during the day.)
- Strolling through the house with baby in a sling (see wearing down, pages 19 and 20).
- Reading a poem or singing "Twinkle, Twinkle Little Star."
- Saying good night to everyone. Toddlers love long good-night lists: ("Good night toys, good night pets, good night Mama, good night Grandpa," and so on).
- A bath followed by a favorite calming book.
- A back rub. Give your child a massage and gradually lighten your touch as he drifts off to sleep. Or "plant a garden" on your child's back, using different touches for the different kinds of seeds your child asks to plant. Gradually lighten your strokes as you smooth out the soil.
- Playing music and humming or singing along. Choose quiet, gentle songs, not get-up-and-dance music. You may find that playing or singing one special song becomes part of your settling-down-to-sleep routine.
- Your child may fall asleep more easily if there is quiet background activity in the

household instead of complete quiet. A little bit of noise reassures her that you are close by if you exit before she's asleep.
- Nursing to sleep — a perennial favorite.

I'd save all my phone calls and return them when I knew my toddler was ready for sleep. Toddlers always want to nurse when you're on the phone, so take advantage of that and let the quiet ebb and flow of your voice lull baby right to sleep.

Signing off. The bedtime ritual that worked best for us with our toddler Matthew, who had a hard time winding down and leaving the excitement of daytime activities, was one we called "signing off." When it was near his bedtime, we made the rounds: "Say night-night to the toys, night-night to Mommy, night-night to Princess (the cat), night-night to Honey Bee (the dog)." As we walked upstairs, we said night-night to the relatives in the photos on the wall and to whatever else we encountered between the family room and the bedroom. When we finally arrived in the bedroom, we completed the wind-down ritual by saying night-night to the toys and pictures on the wall. This slow signing off seems to help children who are so engrossed in their play that they have a hard time transitioning to bedtime.

The fish story. When Matthew was three, an evening of exciting activity often meant that he would have a hard time falling asleep. So after he climbed into bed, I would tell him a "fish story." It was not an exciting tale about the one that got away. Instead, it went like this: "When I was a young boy, I used to go fishing . . . and I would catch one fish (and tell about it), two fish, three fish . . ." With each fish my voice got lower and slower. Some nights it was ten fish, other nights twenty fish before Matthew was peacefully asleep. Basically, I was boring him to sleep.

Before-bed prayers. Nighttime prayers are a way to share your faith with your child. We have always felt that the words children hear as they drift off to sleep are imprinted more deeply in their minds than words spoken during the day. You can say the same prayer every night, either a traditional child's prayer or one you make up in your family, or use a basic prayer with variations based on the child's day ("Thank you, God, for . . ."). This prayer is likely to stay in your child's memory for the rest of his life.

5. Respond to Sleepy Signs

Throughout this book, we urge you to respond to signs that your baby is tired. Toddlers, like babies, go to sleep more easily when they are feeling sleepy. Watch for these signs that your child is tired and ready to wind down and go to sleep:

- activity slows and he lies on floor, rubs eyes, yawns (younger toddler)
- activity picks up in an attempt to fend off the sendoff (older, wiser toddler)
- picks up lovee and ambles toward bedroom (fairy-tale toddler)

If you wait to start your ritual until after the tired signs appear, you'll miss your win-dow of opportunity. For some toddlers, preparations for going to sleep can wind them up. If you wait until he's tired to start getting ready for bed, he may be all charged up again by the time he's clean, dry, and in pajamas. Bathe him, brush his teeth, put his jammies on, and get him all ready for bed before the usual time the drowsy signs occur. Let your child become drowsy while you do the quiet part of your ritual, such as stories, a massage, and snuggling.

Rather than do the whole ritual thing, we simply did quiet things until our toddler gave tired signals. If she wasn't in her pajamas, it was no big deal. I'd nurse her to sleep, and that was it. As long as her clothes were clean and comfortable, anything could be pajamas. And if we got caught by tired time and her clothes were dirty, we'd just change them once she was asleep. Teeth brushing could be anytime, too. My advice is to nurse your child off to sleep when the window of opportunity opens, or it will close while you're fiddling around with toothbrushes and outfits.

6. Enjoy Bedtime Stories

A story tops off the day, like dessert at the end of a meal. Reading to your child is an important part of nighttime parenting, one that most parents enjoy most of the time. (There may be one or two stories that your child absolutely loves that you might get a *little* tired of.) If you treasure the time you spend reading bedtime stories, you will radiate patience and relaxation as you read them. If your child senses you are tense and just trying to get to the last page (or if you actually skip pages), she won't fall asleep as quickly. Here's how to get the most out of reading books to toddlers:

Love your books. Since you're going to spend a lot of time reading, pick stories that you enjoy, too, so that when your little one pleads "Read it again," you won't mind. Martha and I have been reading bedtime stories for over thirty years. Our last child, Lauren, was no longer breastfeeding as a toddler (she's ours by adoption), so it took a large stack of books, and she loved every one. It was a great way to get our biggest night owl to lie still long enough to get relaxed and drift off. Some of our favorites that are appropriate for children ranging from toddlers to preschoolers are listed in Appendix B.

Use your sleepy-soothing voice. Speak gently, quietly, and in a monotonous voice. Avoid exaggerated facial expressions or a sudden change in volume, which can startle a child awake. Gradually pause longer between sentences and read more slowly and softly toward the end of the story.

Keep it simple. Read age-appropriate stories with simple pictures. Try to keep to one book. Otherwise, your child may awaken during the pause while you search for another book.

Position for sleep. Have your child lie in her most common sleeping position while you read to her.

Don't stop too soon. Even though a child's eyes may be closing, his ears are very keen to follow a story. We once heard a child instruct his mother, "Keep reading — I can still hear you even when I'm sleeping."

I read to my three-year-old daughter at bedtime, and then she tells me "good night, love you, sweet dreams" and rolls over and goes to sleep on her own.

7. Put a "Lovee" to Bed, Too

As you tuck in your toddler, put a favorite stuffed toy, doll, or other "lovee" to bed next to her. Help her tuck her little friend under the covers and give her lovee a hug or a kiss good night. Parenting her doll or toy off to sleep the same way you help her go to sleep will aid her in winding down. On nights when your child is reluctant to go to bed, tell her, "Let's go put dolly to bed." As she shares in dolly's bedtime ritual, she will get ready for sleep herself.

Once when she was resisting, I stumbled upon a way to get Ashton to fall asleep. I went cheek to cheek with her as if I were giving her a hug and I nibbled her earlobe with my lips. I immediately felt her body relax and saw her eyelids start to droop. The rhythmic nibbling combined with the warmth of my breath and our closeness to each other sent her quickly into dreamland. It was also very soothing for me and a good tool for my husband to try.

8. Offer Verbal Sleep Cues

Find a few favorite phrases that relax your child. Say them over and over in a singsong voice as your child is falling asleep or when he needs assistance in getting back to sleep. Your child will hear your soothing voice but not have to think about what you are saying. Dr. Bob used to repeat "Rest your eyes" to his son over and over again. Try these phrases:

"Nighty-night"
"Go night-night"
"Sleepy-sleepy"
"Time for sleep"
"Sleep now"

Find a phrase that is reassuring to your child during the day and use it consistently to help him recover from a meltdown, something like, "It's okay." Soon your child will learn to associate "It's okay" with settling. When he awakens from a scary dream or for some other reason, hearing the familiar "It's okay" may quickly resettle him back to sleep.

Our two-year-old loves trains. Sometimes he wakes up during the night fussy and upset and we say, "Can you hear the train?" and we make train noises. He listens, nods, and stops crying. He knows there isn't a real train, but at least he stops crying to listen carefully.

9. Enlist Help from a Sibling

At age six, our daughter Hayden could easily "mother" her two-year-old sister, Erin, to sleep (because she had had plenty of mothering when she was little). We would occasionally encourage Hayden to lie down with Erin and sing to her or look at a picture book and get her to sleep "just like Mommy and Daddy

did with you." Erin would fall asleep, and sometimes Hayden would, too. We got a lot of mileage from sibling co-sleeping. When we had two close-in-age children that we wanted to go to bed at the same time, we would announce, "Whoever is in bed first picks the story."

10. Make Peace Before Bedtime

Children, like adults, have difficulty sleeping when they are angry or upset. If children have been arguing during the day, help them make up before bedtime and go to bed friends. If you and your child have been at odds all day, or if it has been an upsetting day for other reasons, take time to talk it out briefly and then do something pleasant with your child before bedtime. Maybe this is a night for an extra bedtime story or for a tale from your adventures as a child. Cuddle your child off to sleep and help him clear his mind of upsetting thoughts. This can even be a part of your sign-off prayer.

11. Try a Reward Chart

If bedtime is not going well at your house, try a reward chart. Set the timer to announce bedtime, and tell your child that if he goes to bed without complaining, he will get a gold star on his chart. After three good nights in a row, take him out for a fun reward (fun as in play, not as in a junky treat). When you've had a success or two, change the reward schedule to once every seven days. Soon he'll forget all about the chart.

12. Water Your Child

"I need a drink of water" is a classic stall tactic. Head it off by giving your child a drink of water in the bathroom before bed. Call it the "last drink" so she knows she can't keep asking for water. Or put a sippy cup or water bottle next to your child's bed to quench the thirst that invariably hits as soon as she is under the covers. She'll enjoy the independent feeling of having it at hand, especially if she feels she's gotten a good dose of hands-on nighttime parenting.

13. Use a Night-Light

Sleep researchers have shown that the brain is able to sleep better at night with no light on, but some children are afraid of complete darkness. Try using a dim night-light in your child's room. An older child may feel more secure with his own flashlight or a reading light next to his bed that he can turn on if he wakes up. When our daughter Lauren was older and in her own room, we found that she was happier going to sleep with the light on. We then turned it off when we went to bed.

14. Try "Fade-Away" Strategies

Getting your baby to sleep independently implies helping your baby get used to needing less of you and comfortably relying on his own self-settling abilities. "Fading away" means gradually weaning your child from breast, bottle, arms, voice, and eventually your presence at his bedside as he falls asleep. (See pages 161 to 163 for examples of this getting-baby-to-sleep-alone strategy.)

15. Just Go to Bed!

You know your child is tired, you've been through the whole wind-down ritual, but he will not go to sleep. In this case, tell your child he must lie in his bed and either look at books or play quietly. If he still needs you close by, read your own book or magazine in his room. If he has to entertain himself, he will probably soon be ready to sleep. It may help to put on some soothing music.

The rule is he doesn't have to go to sleep. He just needs to stay in bed. He is allowed to read for as long as he wants. He seems to get to sleep earlier and more easily when he feels he has some control over his sleep time.

TEACHING YOUR YOUNG CHILD TO FALL ASLEEP ALONE AND HAPPY

Putting your child to bed while you are there snuggling with her is easy. The challenge that most parents face is getting their child to learn to fall asleep without mom or dad there.

All the steps so far in this chapter are designed to help your child feel comfortable and happy at bedtime, but how do you move toward sleep independence in a way your child will accept?

A better question is this: Is it realistic for parents to expect most young kids to fall asleep alone? In our experience the answer is no. When children are around age three, their imagination kicks in and they develop a fear of being alone in the dark at night. They can imagine monsters in the closet or under the bed. Or they may simply want their parent there for no particular reason. This is normal behavior for a child. But because these fears are irrational, most parents don't take them seriously and simply expect their child to get over them. Even kids who slept alone as babies or toddlers can begin to fear sleeping alone later on.

How can parents get their kids to be happy falling asleep alone? Slowly, gradually, and as peacefully as possible. Getting your child to sleep independently involves helping her get used to needing less of you and to comfortably rely on her own self-settling abilities. It means gradually weaning your child from your arms, voice, and eventually your presence at her bedside as she falls asleep.

If until now you have been staying with your child while she falls asleep, you'll probably find that there is very little stress to overcome. If your child used to fall asleep alone but has since stopped, she may have experienced some months of stress while you were trying to accomplish sleep independence again. In this case, you will probably need

to take a step backward in the weaning process, reconnect with your child, spend a few weeks or months letting your child fall asleep worry-free with you right there next to her, and then begin what we call the "fading-away" process.

On pages 161 through 163 we go into detail on how to slowly fade out of your child's bedroom. Skip ahead and read those pages now if you are currently trying to achieve this goal.

For the purposes of this chapter, here is a summary of the fading-away method:

- Snuggle your child to sleep. Lie in bed with your child while he falls asleep.
- Camp out next to the bed. Sit on the floor next to your child while she goes to sleep.
- Move in and out. Leave the room for brief intervals but come back frequently.
- Check on your child. Hang out in the hallway or next room but peek your head in to let your child know you're there. Come back to your child's room every five or ten minutes until he's asleep.

If you re-create a stress-free bedtime, your child will be less likely to have nighttime fears, anxiety, and stress in the years to come. Put in a little time now. View this as a short season in your parenting career. In the long run, your child will be better for it.

In chapter 7 we will go into more detail about how to transition a toddler from needing your presence to falling asleep on his own. We will also discuss how to move a child out of your room and into his own.

FOOD FOR SLEEP

Toddlers have small tummies. They usually need a snack before going to bed. Just remember that what children eat affects how they sleep. Some foods contribute to restful sleep — we call them "sleepers." Other foods — "wakers" — get in the way of a good night's sleep. Wakers are caffeine- and sugar-containing foods that stimulate neurochemicals that perk up the brain. Sleepers are foods that contain tryptophan, an amino acid that the body uses to make serotonin and melatonin, neurochemicals that slow down nerve traffic and relax the busy brain.

It's a good idea to eat tryptophan-containing foods with complex carbo-hydrates (those that are high in fiber). The carbs help usher more tryptophan into the brain so it can manufacture more sleep-inducing neurotransmitters. Without carbs to help, other amino acids that ride along with tryptophan, such as tyrosine, can perk up the brain and keep the child awake. High-protein, low-carb menus are best

saved for breakfast, when it's time for the sleeping brain to wake up and be busy.

Carbs all by themselves are not good sleeper foods. There's no tryptophan in these foods, and sugary, junk-food carbs (fiberless carbs) eaten all by themselves can set you up for a blood-sugar roller-coaster ride. First, you get a jolt of energy from the sugar. A couple hours later, when your blood sugar falls, causing your body to release stress hormones, you feel restless. If you're sleeping, you may wake up.

Calcium is another sleeper nutrient. It helps the brain use tryptophan to manufacture melatonin. Magnesium, another sleep-inducing mineral, is found especially in whole-grain cereal, sunflower seeds, spinach, tofu, and nuts.

So what makes a good bedtime snack? The best sleeper snacks contain protein, healthy carbs, and some calcium and magnesium. So how about grandma's classic bedtime snack of homemade oatmeal cookies and milk? The glass of

QUESTIONS AND ANSWERS ABOUT TODDLER SLEEP

You'll run into many detours on the road to getting your toddler to sleep. Some of them can exhaust your patience. If you can manage to hang on to your sense of humor, some of them are actually pretty funny. Here are the

most common questions we get asked in our medical practice and on our website:

BEDTIME PROCRASTINATOR

We begin putting our two-and-a-half-year-old to bed at eight o'clock, but he always has a bunch of excuses that prolong milk contains tryptophan, healthy carbs (lactose), and calcium. Homemade oatmeal cookies contain healthy carbs to partner with the proteins in the milk.

Don't worry, be sleepy! Stress stimulates the body to release cortisol, which can rev up the sleepy brain and deplete it of tryptophan. This is one of many bio-chemical ways in which stress keeps you awake. So give your child bedtime snacks in a peaceful environment in order to get the maximum benefit from tryptophan.

Best sleeper snacks. For good snacks to sleep by, try these protein-carb-calcium combos:

- milk and whole-grain cookie (e.g., raisin oatmeal)
- milk and whole-grain cereal
- a hard-boiled egg and a slice of whole-grain toast
- a half peanut butter sandwich on whole-grain bread
- apple slices and cheddar cheese (our favorite)
- tofu and fruit

These snacks contain just enough carbs, calcium, and protein to relax rather than perk up the brain. It takes about an hour for all these sleep inducers to reach the brain.

Best dinners for sleep. The foods you serve your child at dinner can help him get to sleep, too. Here are some dinners to help wind down your family. (These foods, in small portions, make great bedtime snacks, too, even if they're a bit unconventional.)

- chili with beans, not spicy
- sesame seeds (rich in tryptophan) ground and sprinkled on salad with tuna chunks, and whole-wheat crackers
- tuna salad on whole wheat bread
- tofu stir-fry with hazelnuts
- scrambled eggs and cheese
- meats or poultry with veggies
- hummus with whole wheat pita bread
- whole-grain pasta with salmon
- whole-grain pasta with parmesan cheese

the routine: he needs a drink of water, he has to go to the bathroom, he asks us to read again (and again). Sometimes it takes me an hour to an hour and a half to get him to sleep. We're tired after a day's work, and we could often fall asleep before he does. Where should we draw the line?

The main reason kids procrastinate at bedtime is stress. They aren't worried about the actual getting-ready-for-bed routine. They are anxious about the very end of the routine — when you leave them alone to fall asleep. Fear of going to bed alone makes the whole routine stressful, and your child is much more likely to act out in any way he can to delay the impending alone-in-bed time. This makes the whole bedtime hour less enjoyable for you, too.

Get behind the eyes of your child and understand bedtime procrastination from his viewpoint. Ask yourself, "If I were my child, what would I need from my parents at bedtime?" Answer: My parents! Instead of regarding bedtime as a chore, think of this prolonged going-to-bed ritual as *quality time* you spend with your child. This may be the only time during the whole day when he has your focused attention, so, of course, he wants to make the most of it and reconnect with you. If you can relax and enjoy this time, you will both be happier.

Parents in this situation usually need to take a step backward and spend a few weeks or months sitting by their child's bedside using the fade-away technique introduced on page 43.

This can be difficult, since you are tired, and your tired child is being very demanding. You may be wanting some time with your spouse or time just for yourself. Take it as a compliment that your child enjoys this special time with you. We worry more about babies who are not so demanding of their parents at night. And keep it in perspective — those early years fly by all too quickly.

Develop a consistent bedtime ritual using the tips discussed earlier in this chapter. On nights when you know you don't have enough patience for the whole routine, call in a crutch. Listen to an audiotape of your child's favorite story, or watch a calm video together. You can snuggle up on the couch

> ## SEARS SLEEP TIP
>
> It's all about attitude. Instead of dreading prolonged bedtime rituals, view them as treasured times that you are storing up so that you can all sleep better later on.

with your child, enjoying bedtime closeness without expending a lot of energy. Many nights when Matthew was three or four years old, he and I snuggled together in a beanbag chair and he dozed off while watching *Lady and the Tramp*. Meanwhile, Martha was free to be with baby Stephen.

After one or two stories, if she wanted more, I said something like, "Mommy needs to go put on her pajamas now, and I'll be back to check on you in a few minutes." I encouraged her to look at the books we had just read together. She was okay with that and would often be asleep by the time I got back.

WANTS TO STAY UP LATE

Our two-year-old fights going to bed until ten or eleven o'clock. I know he's tired; certainly we are. How can I get him to sleep earlier?

The most important aspects of helping a toddler go to bed early, especially when you know he is tired and is just fighting it, are to learn when his tired time is (see page 8), anticipate it, get into the bedtime routine early, and set the stage for sleep (see

TUCK ME IN WITH A TALE

Little minds are in a receptive state at bedtime. Bedtime stories can help a child reflect on her life, and you can tuck a little teaching into the stories you tell. Events from your growing-up years are a great source of bedtime tales.

You can also use bedtimes as teachable moments to implant pleasant thoughts and admirable values into your child as she drifts off to sleep. Do this night after night and these bits of wisdom will be filed away in her library of experiences. Years later these bedtime lessons will be an important influence in her life.

Bedtime prayers are a time-honored tradition for smoothing out the wrinkles of life and for passing on parental values and beliefs. Teach your child a familiar prayer, or make up your own prayers of gratitude and concern for others.

Toddler Andrew used to ask Dr. Bob while snuggling to sleep, "Tell me good things, Daddy." Bob would create peaceful scenes for Andrew to imagine, such as, "We are sitting next to a quiet river in the warm sunshine with little fish swimming by." Four or five little images would help Andrew settle into sleep peacefully.

Also, take inventory of what else is going on in your family. Does your child miss you during the day and want to make up for it at night? Are changes in your routine, such as a move, a change in childcare providers, or the arrival of a new baby, upsetting your child? Some children don't want to go to bed because they are afraid of going to sleep. Others resist bedtime because they don't want to be separated from their parents or because they want more quality time with their parents. In our family we noticed that the busier and more preoccupied we were during the day, the more our children lobbied for quality time at night.

You know that your son needs to get to bed earlier so that he can get enough sleep. And you and your spouse may need some couple time in the evening. So how do you take what you have figured out about why your child is resisting bedtime and use this insight to get him to sleep earlier?

If there are stressful situations that make it hard for your child to sleep, try to remedy them. Make an effort to spend quality time with your child at hours other than bedtime. Encourage lots of active play so that your child will be tired at night. Turn off the television.

Plan ahead for an earlier bedtime. Start your winding-down-for-bed routine earlier. Have your child take a bath and get his pajamas on earlier in the evening. Then at least he is ready for bed, and you don't have to hurry through the whole routine when you are both tired and cranky. Use the time between bath and bed for quiet games and other activities that you do together.

page 13)— and to do this consistently night after night. You may also need to eliminate or reschedule afternoon naps (see page 191).

It may be that your child is just not ready to go to sleep before ten o'clock. Throughout this book we stress the importance of earlier bedtimes, especially for toddlers and children. Yet an early bedtime may not work well in your family. With today's busy schedules, parents may not have much time with their children during the day. As a result, children demand more attention from their parents in the evening and balk at bedtime. If your child is, on the whole, well rested (maybe he's taking a long afternoon nap that helps him stay awake at night), a later bedtime may be more realistic. The hour when your child goes to bed is not as important as going to bed at the same hour every night.

Instead of wasting your whole evening struggling to put your toddler to bed, let him stay up and play quietly while you and your spouse have your own time together. Make it a late-night rule that you don't play games or have fun. It's up to your child to entertain himself. These "boring" evenings can eventually lead to an earlier bedtime.

WAKES UP TOO EARLY

Our almost-three-year-old wakes up at 5 a.m. to play. He's bright-eyed and bushy-tailed and ready to go, but I'm not.

Some children are like roosters. They wake up and are ready to go with the first ray of sunlight on their little faces. This doesn't necessarily mean you have to get up at the crack of dawn. Here are some suggestions for staying in bed longer in the morning:

- Put blackout curtains on the windows in your child's room. This should keep the little rooster asleep for an extra hour or two. But you will probably have to let him stay up an hour later at night. To do that, he may need a slightly later afternoon nap. In other words, everything gets pushed forward clockwise — later rising, later nap, later bedtime. You have to decide if you want more time for yourself in the morning or in the evening. You won't get both.

- If dad gets up early, your toddler can tag along with him while he does all the guy things — shower, shave, dress, fix breakfast — so that you'll get to sleep longer. It's good father-son "alone together" time.

- Get up and lie with your toddler on the floor on a futon. While he plays quietly, you can snooze or at least be horizontal long enough to feel more rested once the clock says it's a more reasonable hour. By modeling that it's still sleepy time for you, you'll give your toddler the message that it's a good idea to play quietly. Of course, this strategy assumes that your house is thoroughly child-proofed, the doors to the outside are locked, and any off-limit areas are gated off. Even though most youngsters won't wander all over the house when they could be by you, you'll rest easier knowing he won't get into trouble if you really do doze off. Dr. Bob's wife positioned herself on the floor in a way that the toddler would have to crawl over her to get away, so she'd know if he was on the move.

- Try a safety gate in the bedroom doorway. Set up a water bottle and small snack (something nonchokable) next to your child's bed before you go to bed. Teach your child to play and eat quietly and safely in the room when he wakes. You can even set a quiet alarm clock and tell him he can call for you when the alarm goes *ding*. Even better is a music player with a timer that you can set to come on with your child's favorite music (a regular alarm buzzer may be too scary).

WAKES UP TO PLAY

Our eighteen-month-old baby sleeps in a crib next to us, and sometimes she wakes up in the middle of the night, eager to play. It's cute, but we're not in the mood to play at 3 a.m. How can we stop this habit?

First, you can be encouraged to hear that this is usually just a phase as baby discovers new milestones. It often passes within a few weeks. Despite this, your toddler needs to learn that nighttime is for sleeping, not for playing. Here's how we discouraged our middle-of-the-night playmates. Whenever our toddler who was sleeping close to us woke us up in the night, we acknowledged her presence but then told her, "Time to sleep." Then we pretended to go back to sleep. If we "played dead" long enough, she would decide that it wasn't very interesting to be awake in the dark, and she would go back to sleep. If your baby protests this silent treatment, you can cuddle her close to you (use a firm hand) and

repeat the sleep cue ("Time to sleep" or "Sleepy-sleepy"). Or roll over and lie with your back to baby. Most babies eventually give up and after a few nights go back to sleep easily.

If this phase lasts too long and is obviously not going away, in the interests of letting one of you actually get to stay asleep, the person who is feeling generous can get up and walk or rock baby back to sleep. Don't turn on any lights (there will be enough night light coming in to find your way around). After she gets good and bored she'll be ready to go back to sleep. Then you can both make your way back to her crib or your bed.

DISCOURAGING THE MIDNIGHT VISITOR

Our two-year-old comes into our room, where he used to sleep, at all hours of the night. Short of locking him in, which I obviously don't want to do, how can I get him to stay in his room?

Like salmon returning to their birthplace to spawn, children often naturally gravitate back to their preferred sleeping place. Those middle-of-the-night visits, though disrupting, are a typical developmental stage, especially if your child is making the transition from sleeping in your room to sleeping solo in his own. Here's how to give your child extra nighttime security without disrupting your sleep:

Have an open-door policy, but set some rules. Put a futon, mattress, or a cute sleeping bag at the foot of your bed and market this as his "special bed." Then show and tell him this rule: "You can come into Mommy and Daddy's room at night if you need to and sleep in your special bed, but you must tip-toe in as quietly as a mouse and not wake up Mommy and Daddy. Mommy and Daddy need our sleep, otherwise we will be cranky the next day. And a cranky Mommy and Daddy are no fun to be with."

To reinforce both your availability and the message that nighttime is when everyone sleeps, go on to tell him, "If you wake Mommy and Daddy up, you'll have to go back into your room." Try another show-and-tell game. During the day, walk with him from his room into yours and show him how to slip quietly into his special bed without waking you up.

Here's how some parents in our practice negotiated with their midnight visitor:

After we moved, our four-year-old, Josh, wanted to sleep with us all the time. Even after he fell asleep in his own bed, he'd creep in with us at about three o'clock in the morning. Even though we enjoy cuddling with him, especially as we all fall asleep, he's an after-midnight kicker, and we'd spend most of the night crossing our arms over our sensitive body parts. So we made a deal. We told Josh that we loved sleeping with him, but now that he was bigger, we didn't sleep well when he was in our bed all the time, and this made us tired and grumpy parents. We further explained that we could probably handle feeling that way once a week. So we made up a chart and told Josh that if he stayed in his own bed all night Monday through Saturday, he

could sleep with us all night on Sunday. Now Josh is eager to sleep "well" on his own so that we can all enjoy our Sunday-night snuggles.

Try not to view this nighttime visit as bad behavior. It is natural and normal. It will diminish in time without your even needing to discourage it.

WEANING OFF NIGHTTIME BOTTLES

Our two-year-old still insists on a bottle at bedtime and if he wakes during the night. I know this isn't good for his teeth, but he really seems to need the comfort. I also wish he'd stop needing the bottle during the night. What can I do?

This is a common dilemma. A toddler who is used to the comfort of sucking on a bottle to sleep won't give this up easily, but it's true that milk or juice sugar that stays on the teeth at night can cause cavities. In chapter 6 we'll discuss this situation in detail, but here's the basic approach we recommend:

- Go sugar-free. Slowly dilute the milk or juice with water over a couple weeks until it is all water. If your child clues in to this trick, back off for a few days, then continue again. This at least eliminates the risk of cavities.

- Have a bye-bye-bottle party. Have a ceremony where you toss the bottles into the outside recycling bin, watch the truck take them away, and then celebrate with songs, dancing, cake, and presents. Encourage your child by reminding him that he is all grown up now and that tonight he will "go night-night as a big boy." (Have a hidden spare bottle handy in case your child decides he doesn't like this idea come bedtime and his protests go beyond what you feel is okay.) Some of his presents can be other bedtime props, like a musical stuffed toy, new pillow, or a blanket.

- Substitute yourself. You may find that once you've taken the bottle away, you need to find something to take its place. Your child may declare that that something is you. You may need to spend a few weeks helping your child go to sleep.

- If you're using other substitute props, make sure your child knows how to find them during the night when he wakes up and asks for the bottle.

If you feel your child really needs the comfort of a bottle with water, that's okay. You'll know best when to be rid of the bottle once and for all.

BECOMING A BED HOG

Our thirteen-month-old has been sharing our bed, and up until now it has been great. But lately he has started moving around while he sleeps. It's like he thinks he owns the bed. My husband and I are starting to feel the effects of a third person in our bed. Help!

Funny — and not so funny — things happen when baby shares your bed. Three familiar,

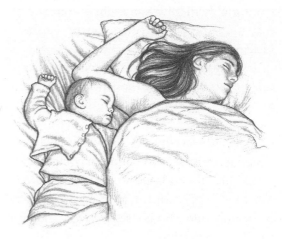

though sometimes annoying, sleep positions that family-bed babies seem to enjoy are the heat-seeking missile, the starfish, and the H-sleeper.

The *heat-seeking missile* snuggles comfortably into a parental armpit or a breast and refuses to back off. Like a mother hen, you instinctively put your wing (your arm) over the top of your baby's head. He may want to stay in touch with, or actually attached to, your warm body all night long. Baby sleeps great, but you may not. No worries, though, about this baby falling out of bed.

The *starfish baby* stretches his arms and legs out as far as they can go, sometimes so much that they almost force you right off the bed. Starfish sometimes become thrashers.

The *H-sleeper* enjoys physical contact with both parents. He falls asleep between the parents, parallel with their bodies, and then strategically rotates himself until he is perpendicular to his parents, resting his head on one parent and his feet on the other. (Isn't that nice? He loves you both!) Again, baby sleeps comfortably that way all night — but you may not, especially if you're the one getting kicked in the ribs.

Usually when an infant or toddler starts taking over the bed in these positions, dad announces, "It's time for a big-boy bed!" Is dad right?

Here are your options. If everybody is sleeping reasonably well, you may be able to laugh this off and hope it's a passing phase. Yet if baby's nighttime frolicking means baby is the only one who is sleeping well, you need to take some action.

- "Draw the line." Put a line of pillows between you and your toddler. He gets one-third of the bed space, mom and dad get the rest.

- To give everyone more space, put a twin bed next to your queen- or king-size bed.

- Take bed sprawling as a sign that it's time to start transitioning baby to his own bed. Dad may be right! (See chapter 7.)

Try this parent's "stay in your own lane" trick from Dr. Jim:

Jonathan used to sleep with us, sprawled across the bed with his arms stretched out forming the letter H. When he was around two years old, I was watching a swimming competition and I noticed the lane dividers that kept the swimmers from swimming on top of each other. That gave me an idea. What if I could keep Jonathan in his own lane in the bed? We had tried pillows, but even though we had a king-size bed, they took up a lot of room, and it was hard to have an entire pillow between him and us. I went downstairs into our garage and noticed that we had some of those swimming noodles, long thin cylinders made of firm foam. Choosing ones that had hollow centers, I slid broom handles in to add some rigidity. After Jonathan fell asleep I placed one on each side of him, each one running the length of the bed. This worked beautifully. If he started to roll over or rotate sideways, the foam was firm enough to keep him from going over it. They were perfectly safe, too. They were rigid enough that he didn't become entangled in them, and light enough that he wouldn't be hurt if he somehow slipped under one. They were also easy to store under the bed when not in use. One additional point: Don't use old noodles that have been sitting in the pool or in the sun. The foam tends to break down and become quite flaky and messy. Go out and get some new ones.

FEAR OF MONSTERS

Our three-year-old wakes up yelling about the "monsters" in his room. I try to tell him that Daddy has chased the monsters away. Is this the best way to deal with this? I don't want him to believe that there really are monsters in his room.

Children's dreams distort reality, and young children have difficulty knowing what's real and what's pretend. Therefore, if they see a monster in their dream, they may believe that the monster is real. There are two schools of thought on monsters and other imaginary creatures. The usual suggestion is to play along and just get rid of the monsters or try to teach your child that monsters are fun and friendly. When your child wakes up frightened about them, you search the bedroom and say things like "No monsters anymore," "Monsters went bye-bye," and "Monsters are nice and cuddly." If he worries at bedtime, you can make a show of ordering the monsters out of the bedroom and reassure your child that they're not coming back. While we are skeptical of this approach, for some children it does work. The problem is it's not true. When you chase monsters away, you're reinforcing your child's concern about monsters, and since you say those monsters are indeed real, they might come back.

Here's a better alternative: Tell your child the truth. Monsters don't exist. They are pretend. If your child is going through a "seeing-monsters-in-his-sleep" stage, avoid scary TV or cartoons that could be distorted into monsters in his dreams. Your child trusts you. If you say there are no monsters, he will believe you. You might also talk about other things besides monsters that are only pretend in order to help your child learn to tell the difference between what's real (a family pet, elephants at the zoo) and what's not (characters in cartoons, storybook animals who talk).

NIGHTTIME ANXIETY

Our three-year-old had been sleeping well on his own for a few months, but now he's waking up and coming into our room at night. He seems really upset. How can I help him get back to sleeping through the night in his own room?

Realize your child has a need. He is growing and developing, and new fears and worries are going to come along. Sometimes they will disturb his sleep, and you are right in thinking that he needs your help to cope with his nighttime anxiety.

Why is your child suddenly feeling insecure about nighttime? There are many possible reasons. Here are just a few:

- Imagination. As kids get older, they develop the ability to imagine that there is a monster in the closet, a giant hand under the bed (that was Dr. Bob's fear as a child), or something looming in the darkness outside. They don't necessarily have to see these things first on TV or hear about them in stories. Kids can create these fears all on their own.

- Separation anxiety. This occurs not only around nine months of age but also again between ages two and three. Your happy sleeper becomes anxious because you are not there. Your child needs your physical presence as reassurance that you aren't going anywhere.

- Life changes. Changes in a child's life, such as starting preschool or day care, moving, or having a new sibling, can trigger some temporary nighttime anxiety. Changes in the family's life, such as in a parent's work schedule, can also affect how well a child sleeps.

WHAT'S ON YOUR CHILD'S MIND?

Do you think that your awake-at-night child is purposely trying to manipulate you? Do you think he is lying in bed thinking, "Hmmm. Mom and Dad are having a relaxing evening. How can I disrupt them? I know! I'll get up and go ask for a drink of water. They hate that!" If your child is really thinking like that at the age of three, then good luck. But we really don't think kids are that devious (at least not until they are older).

When your child gets out of bed at night to come find you, you may be tempted to send him back to his own bed with firm orders to stay there. Instead, put yourself into the mind of your child as he crawls back into his own bed, wide awake, and lies there staring at the wall. "I'm afraid, and my mommy won't help me," he thinks. Or, "I wish my daddy was here with me." Remember that a child's needs are not always rational from an adult's point of view, especially at night.

I don't want her nighttime memories filled with her screaming from her crib. I don't want my memories filled with hearing her scream from her crib.

Here are some ideas you can try to help your child learn to sleep through the night again:

Talk it out during the day. Sit your child down in the afternoon and tell him that you want to help him with his nighttime worries. Decide on a plan together. Perhaps you will go back to his bed with him when he wakes up and lie down with him until he falls asleep again. Or maybe you will decide to put a mattress or a comforter on the floor in your room, where he can sleep if he gets scared during the night. Or maybe you and your child will come up with another idea.

Act quickly at night. When your child wakes up in the night and comes into your room, don't get into a debate with him about going back to his own bed. Just do what you planned to do. Take him back to his room and fall asleep together in his bed. Or get him settled in his little bed in your room. Or let him climb in bed with you. The object here is to get everyone back to sleep as quickly as possible without feeding your child's night-time fears.

Enjoy a peaceful day with active play. As we have said before, minimizing the stress in your child's daytime life will minimize night-time problems, too. If the daytime stress is unavoidable, be prepared to live with a few sleep problems until things settle down. Encourage your child to run, jump, and be active during the day. This will tire him out and also alleviate tension and anxiety.

Wean him back to sleeping alone. As your child starts to feel more secure at night, you can begin to work on getting him back to sleeping alone. If he wakes up, he may decide to join you by climbing into his special bed in your room without waking you. Or you can take him back to his bed, staying with him just until he's nearly asleep. Tell him, "I'll be back in a minute to check on you," and then be sure to come back.

Dim the lighting. A night-light may keep your child from being afraid when he wakes up alone in the dark, but too much light may keep him awake. Leaving the hall light on with the door open is another good option.

WHY NIGHTTIME PARENTING MATTERS

Long-term nighttime stress can lead to long-term sleep insecurities that can create daytime insecurities and problems with self-confidence.

That's a mouthful, but it's important, and we want you to understand it. Picture the following two scenarios:

Four-year-old Aaron had been sleeping well in his own room. Bedtime was a relaxing routine of stories, hugs and kisses, and sweet dreams. Until recently. Now, when his dad tries to put him to bed, he protests that he wants his dad to stay with him. When dad says no, Aaron asks for an extra hug and kiss, a longer story, for the covers to be tucked in better, or whatever else he can think of to keep dad around even for an extra minute or two. Dad leaves his room, and Aaron starts getting out of bed every five minutes to ask for a drink of water, to find out what his parents are watching on TV, to ask what he will be doing tomorrow, or to complain that he's hungry. His parents send him directly back to bed, alone. On some nights, Aaron's tactics

escalate into complaints of tummy aches and headaches. He takes a long time to fall asleep and doesn't seem quite as happy and secure in the daytime anymore. He even starts wetting the bed (something he'd never done before). This goes on for several years, and as he grows through childhood, he feels that bedtime is a time of loss and separation.

Now let's meet the same child, but with different parental responses.

Four-year-old Aaron had been sleeping well in his own room. Bedtime was a relaxing routine of stories, hugs and kisses, and sweet dreams. Until tonight. When his dad tries to put him to bed, he protests that he wants his dad to stay with him. His dad gives him an extra long hug, stays in his room for a few minutes, pretending he's putting some clothes away, lingers in the hallway, and then tells Aaron good night (kiss, hug, and tuck again) and leaves. Aaron is asleep in two minutes. He just needed a little extra something tonight, and his dad gave it to him.

Dad discusses the situation with mom. While they want to keep Aaron's early bedtime routine (they like their evenings uninterrupted and don't want to have to spend an extra hour every night catering to his bedtime fears), they also have been sensitive to his changing needs over the years. They didn't push it when he needed some time getting used to preschool. They didn't leave him crying with a babysitter but took the time to help him feel comfortable and playful. They've yet to go on a vacation without him. Now they realize that their child is trying to tell them he is feeling anxious about being away from them at night. They understand that if they fulfill his needs now for the short term, they won't turn into long-term unfulfilled needs that will leave him feeling insecure over the years. They also know that if they meet those needs without Aaron continuously having to ask (or protest), his needs should diminish faster. Plus, everyone will be happier.

The next night, when Aaron protests as dad turns to leave the room, dad sits on Aaron's bed and says, "I don't mind staying with you for a little while. You rest your eyes, and I'll sit by the bed here for a few minutes." Dad winds up spending the next three weeks lingering in Aaron's room or in the nearby hallway at bedtime. Sometimes he folds laundry while waiting for Aaron to fall asleep. He sits in the rocker and uses a tiny clamp-on book light to read instead of turning on the overhead light. He doesn't interact much with Aaron, he's just there. Sometimes he tells

Aaron that he needs to go into the other room but will be back to check on him in a few minutes. He putters around, making just enough noise for Aaron to know he is close by. It is a very slow weaning process that, while time-consuming now, really pays off in the long run. Eventually Aaron returns to his former easy-to-sleep routine, and his parents get their evenings back.

Bedtime was always a drawn-out affair in our family. The routine took forty-five minutes to an hour, especially with my oldest son, who has always been very tuned in to what's going on around him. Now, many years later, everybody goes to bed on their own. My three children are expert sleepers who rarely have trouble falling asleep at night. I'm the one who needs to stop at my kids' bedroom doors to chat for a few minutes and connect with them before I can fall asleep.

The Facts About Infant Sleep and What They Mean for Parents

THE STEPS AND TIPS on how to get your infant and toddler to sleep that we shared with you in the first two chapters of this book are based on general principles about how babies and toddlers sleep. When you know why babies do the things they do, it is easier to figure out how to respond. Learning more about how babies sleep and why they wake up during the night will help you understand the nighttime parenting strategies we suggest in this book. It will also help you bring a helpful attitude to caring for your baby's nighttime needs.

LEARN THE FACTS OF INFANT SLEEP

Read all about it! We want you to understand why babies sleep the way they do — or don't. First, here are some general facts about sleep.

How Adults Sleep

There are two main states of sleep — REM (rapid-eye-movement) and non-REM sleep.

The term "falling asleep" is biologically correct. As you drift off to sleep, you enter non-REM sleep, and over the next hour and a half, you descend through the levels of this sleep state until you are at level four, the deepest level of sleep. At this level, you may even sleep through a phone ringing, or, here in California, through a mild earthquake. If you are awakened from this deepest level of non-REM sleep — say, by a persistently crying baby — you are more likely to be disoriented and grouchy than when you are awakened from a lighter level of sleep.

After the first ninety minutes of gradually descending into non-REM sleep, your brain begins to arouse and move into a lighter and more active kind of sleep, the state of REM sleep. During REM sleep, the brain is quite active (it's when you dream), although the rest of your body is usually relaxed and relatively quiet. You experience rapid eye movement (hence the term "REM sleep"), even though your eyes are closed. During REM sleep, facial muscles may twitch, producing sleep grins. It's fun to watch for this in babies.

Since REM is the lightest stage of sleep, it is the easiest to waken from.

Adults cycle through REM and non-REM sleep approximately every ninety minutes. Early in the night, the periods of non-REM sleep may last as long as sixty minutes, and REM periods may last from ten to thirty minutes. Toward morning, the proportions of non-REM and REM reverse, so that much of early-morning sleep is REM. The length and pattern of these sleep cycles vary greatly between individuals and at different ages. However, during an average eight-hour sleep, adults may spend two hours in REM, or active (light), sleep, and six hours in non-REM, or quiet (deep), sleep.

Both of these states of sleep are important for a person's overall well-being. Non-REM, or deep, sleep is necessary to help the body rest and recuperate. It is known as the restorative state of sleep. REM sleep is necessary for brain development.

How Babies Sleep

Why do babies wake up so much? This is probably the question new parents ask most. The simple answer: because they're babies, and babies sleep differently than adults do. Their different sleep cycles explain why they awaken so easily and why it may not be wise to fiddle around too much with babies' natural sleep cycles. Read on.

Babies go to sleep differently. Infants take longer (at least twenty minutes) to drift off and enter a state of deep sleep. This is unlike adults and older children, who can "crash" into deep sleep in just a few minutes. The younger the infant, the longer it takes him to drift into deep sleep.

What does this sleep fact mean to parents? Babies awaken easily during this drifting-off period. Parents don't have to be sleep scientists to figure this out. Many parents describe their baby as "difficult to settle," or they say, "She has to be fully asleep before I can put her down." Many parents have had the experience of thinking their baby is asleep, so they carry her to her crib and gently lay her down — only to have her wake up as soon as mom or dad turns to tiptoe out of the room. A baby is not truly asleep until he arrives in the state of deep sleep, twenty to thirty minutes after closing his eyes. Putting baby down too quickly can leave parents feeling very frustrated.

You can see why the advice from sleep trainers to put babies down in their cribs awake doesn't work, especially for babies who are less than three months old. Babies need to be gentled through this first period of REM sleep, so that they can stay asleep until deeper sleep overtakes them. Between three and six months, babies begin to drift more quickly into non-REM sleep. At this time, they can be put down awake, or partially awake, and they will enter deep sleep fairly quickly. *Bottom line: Babies need to be patiently parented to sleep, not just put down to sleep.*

Babies stay asleep differently. While adults cycle from deep to light sleep approximately every hour and a half, infants move through these states every hour or less. The younger the infant, the shorter the sleep cycles. What does this mean for parents? When passing from one state of sleep to another, the brain is more likely to awaken than at other times. We call this the "vulnerable period." If by chance an arousal stimulus (teething pain, loud noise, hunger, separation anxiety, and so on) bothers baby during this vulnerable period, baby is likely to awaken. Because babies have shorter sleep cycles than adults, they have more vulnerable periods — more times during the night when they are likely to wake up. In addition, babies spend more time in REM (light) sleep in the second half of the night. This explains why babies often wake up more during that time. *Bottom line: Minimize arousal stimuli during vulnerable periods for night waking.*

As babies grow, their sleep cycles lengthen and the percentage of deep sleep increases. This means there are fewer vulnerable periods during the night when they can awaken easily. They also sleep more deeply, and they stay asleep longer — a sleep maturity milestone called "settling." The age at which babies settle varies greatly according to the sleep temperament of the baby. The good news is that all babies eventually settle.

Babies' developing sleep patterns change.

Much like their feeding patterns, babies' sleep patterns change as they get older. In the early months, babies take small, frequent feedings and short, frequent naps. About 50 percent of the total sleep of a newborn is REM sleep. This percentage is even higher in premature infants. As babies grow, they learn to sleep and feed more like adults. These five things happen:

- REM (light) sleep decreases.
- Non-REM (deep) sleep increases.
- Sleep cycles lengthen.
- Vulnerable periods for night waking occur less frequently.
- The total number of hours of daily sleep decreases.

Finally they reach a stage of sleep maturity.

Babies are designed this way on purpose.

Why are babies' sleep patterns so different from adults'? Answer: because babies need to sleep this way. How babies sleep is one of many things throughout infancy and childhood that parents can't control, and it may even be unwise and unsafe to try to change it. Keep in mind that babies sleep the way they do — or don't — for both developmental and survival reasons.

Babies sleep smarter. REM sleep is more than an annoyance that keeps parents as well as babies from sleeping more deeply. The fact that babies' developing brains don't turn themselves off as well as adult brains do during sleep has developmental benefits. Sleep researchers believe that REM sleep stimulates the infant brain at a time when it is growing very rapidly. Blood flow to the brain increases during REM sleep. The lower brain centers fire off electrical stimuli toward the higher brain centers. This stimulation works like mental exercise to help the brain centers develop. The mental activity of dreaming helps the brain grow more neurons. This theory that REM sleep stimulates brain growth is supported by the fact that the young of highly intelligent animal species spend more time in REM sleep than the young of less intelligent species. One day as I was explaining the light sleep/better brain correlation to a tired mother of a wakeful infant, she replied with a chuckle, "In that case, my baby is going to be a genius."

Babies sleep healthier and safer. Not only do these immature sleep patterns help babies grow smarter, they help them grow healthier and sleep safer, too. Suppose your baby slept like an adult. Suppose baby slept so deeply that he couldn't signal when he was hungry, cold, had a stuffy nose and was having difficulty breathing, or was just plain scared? Baby's well-being would be threatened. Babies come wired to awaken so that they can let nearby caregivers know what they need in order to thrive and survive. These arousals are thought to be *protective arousals,* and they are beneficial. What does this mean to parents? Training a baby to sleep too deeply for too long at too young an age is not in the best interests of the baby's development and well-being.

Sleep trainers ignore these basic biological facts and insist that babies should be able to put themselves to sleep and to sleep through the night. As you can now see, putting a baby down to sleep alone in a crib and leaving him to cry himself to sleep and go back to sleep

---

BABIES SLEEP DIFFERENTLY

Notice how babies and adults sleep differently. Imagine what could go wrong if they didn't.

Infants
- designed to easily awaken
- designed to sleep less deeply
- need night feedings
- have short sleep cycles (sixty minutes)
- have mostly REM (active) sleep

Adults
- designed to stay asleep
- designed to sleep more deeply
- don't need night feedings
- have long sleep cycles (ninety minutes)
- have mostly non-REM (quiet) sleep

---

when he awakens is both biologically and developmentally wrong. We are passionate about both helping parents understand their babies' basic sleep needs and giving them the tools to cope until their babies reach sleep maturity. We hope you'll keep the biological facts in mind when making all decisions about your baby's sleep.

HOW BABIES SLEEP AT VARIOUS AGES

As with all developmental milestones, the age at which babies wake up less often and start sleeping through the night varies from baby

---

SEARS SLEEP TIP

Now that you understand infant sleep, when people ask, "How does your baby sleep?" you can answer, "Like a baby."

to baby. Here are the general sleep patterns that most babies follow at various stages along the way to sleep maturity:

Newborn period. In the first month, most babies sleep a total of sixteen to seventeen hours a day. They sleep in three- to four-hour stretches with an equal amount of sleep during the daytime and nighttime hours. At this age, babies wake up mainly from hunger.

One to two months. Between six and eight weeks of age, babies begin to "consolidate" their sleep into shorter periods during the day and slightly longer periods at night. They sleep from fifteen to sixteen hours a day. At this age, most babies wake up at least once a night and need a feeding and help to resettle (and many will wake up two or three times). Babies start waking up not only from hunger but also from a need for closeness (being alone is very scary).

Three to six months. Babies sleep a total of around fifteen hours a day, taking two or three two-hour naps during the day and doing the rest of their sleeping at night. By six months, most babies begin to sleep four- to five-hour stretches at night. At this age, babies also begin having shorter REM periods of sleep and longer non-REM.

Six to nine months. Babies sleep around fourteen hours a day and may drop one of their naps. Most babies between six and nine months take one morning and one afternoon nap. They may start sleeping seven-hour stretches at night. Most continue to wake up

several times a night, and some can self-soothe back to sleep. Developmental changes start triggering night waking at this stage. Babies practice their motor development, such as sitting up, while still half asleep. Add teething pain to this list and you have a recipe for night waking even in babies who were previously "good sleepers."

Nine to twelve months. Most babies sleep between thirteen and fourteen hours a day, still with two naps. Some babies may sleep ten hours at night, occasionally even twelve hours (often interrupted by one or two feedings). While babies still need a morning and afternoon nap, the morning nap is usually shorter.

One to two years. Babies sleep from twelve to thirteen hours a day, with ten to twelve hours at night and two shorter naps. Around (or even before) eighteen months of age, some infants will begin to relinquish the morning nap, but they still need the afternoon nap. Some need two naps one day and one nap the next. Between twelve and eighteen months, babies often start waking up because of separation anxiety. From eighteen months to two years, the concept of *person permanence* clicks in, enabling babies to fall asleep on their own more easily because they can understand that their parents are nearby in another room, even though they can't see them.

Two to three years. Toddlers sleep between eleven and thirteen hours a day and by now give up the morning nap. Nightmares and

SLEEP NEEDS

Age	Total Hours of Sleep	Number of Naps	Total Nap-Time Hours
newborn	16–17	3	6
1–3 months	15–16	3	4–5
3–6 months	14–15	2–3	3–4
6–9 months	14–14½	2	3
9–12 months	13–14	2	3
12–24 months	12–13	1–2	2
2–3 years	11–13	1	1–1 ½
3–4 years	11–12	0–1	½–1

sleep terrors may begin, as well as sleep fears and fear of the dark. Previously "good sleepers" may become fretful sleepers at this age. Most toddlers graduate from crib to bed between ages two and three.

Three to four years. Finally, by this stage most children's sleep patterns become like those of adults. By four years, many children no longer nap during the day. They still need eleven to twelve hours of sleep at night.

WHY BABIES WAKE UP

Understanding all the things that can go on in your baby's little body and mind when you put her down to sleep at night may help you understand why she wakes up so often. It may also help you develop some creative tips to help her sleep and above all sympathize with her. Here are the main reasons that babies awaken frequently:

1. They're babies! As discussed above, babies have shorter sleep cycles than adults do. Every hour or so, as they pass from the state of deep sleep into light sleep, they go through a vulnerable period for night waking. If they sense any upset or discomfort during this vulnerable period, they cry for assistance. For safety's sake, babies' sleep patterns are defined by an easy arousability, which means that if anything threatens babies' well-being (such as being too warm or too cold), they wake up more easily than do adults. Exhausting as it may be to their caregivers to respond to them, there are survival and developmental reasons for why babies are prone to night waking.

2. They're hungry. Tiny babies have tiny tummies and fast metabolisms. They can't go as long without food as adults can. And breast milk moves through baby's stomach faster than formula. Many infants don't drop night feedings for at least six months, and most breastfeeding babies continue to need a night feeding for quite a while longer. While some books say infants don't need night feedings after a certain age, try telling that to a baby with an empty tummy.

3. They're thirsty. Since your baby was used to nursing or getting a bottle several times at night, now that he has learned to sleep without this (thankfully!), he may start to feel the lack of fluids at night. This becomes more true during the toddler and preschool years. If you find your child is waking up and feeling thirsty, have a handy sippy cup or water bottle nearby that your child can drink from before he fully wakes up. Also be sure to provide a good-size drink of water before bedtime (unless, of course, you are potty training at night).

Our third child used to wake up between eighteen months and two years asking for water (even though he was still breastfeeding). He wouldn't even open his eyes. He'd just lie there asking for water, and when we gave him a drink, he'd fall right back to sleep.

4. They're growing. Growth-hormone levels are much higher during sleep (hence, the saying "he seemed to outgrow his baby clothes overnight"). Growth hormones also stimulate hunger. Waking to feed frequently is the baby's way of making sure he has enough fuel to do the growing. Babies typically experience growth spurts around three weeks, six weeks, three months, and six months. During these stretches, your baby will go on feeding marathons day and night. Don't worry. If your baby is generally a long

sleeper, things should go back to normal within a few days. If your baby has been a night waker all along, then you probably won't even notice the difference. Growth spurts are just another way that Mother Nature robs us of sleep (when we say "us," what we really mean is you moms out there, and you dads who are noble enough to share the nighttime duty).

Don't fall into the trap of thinking that you don't have enough milk. Your body responds to baby's increased nursing by producing more milk. Your baby is nursing more at night during this growth spurt because he needs more "grow milk" at night. These normal, but tiring, phases of breastfeeding and infant growth are dubbed "frequency nights" or "marathon nursing." This is not a time to discourage night nursing.

When younger babies increase their night feedings, mothers need to decrease their daytime commitments so they can accommodate them. Temporarily shelve all energy-draining activities that can be put on hold for a while so you can conserve your energy for extra feedings. Enjoy nap nursing so that you can sleep when the baby sleeps. Housework can be put off or delegated. Realize no one's growth is going to be affected if the housework doesn't get done for a few days. Go to sleep when baby does in the evening. Explain these growth spurts to your husband and enlist his help for more father nursing during nonfeeding times.

5. They're developing. During major motor achievements, baby may start waking up at night to practice what he's learned. Typical times for this are four months for rolling over, six months for sitting up, between seven and nine months for crawling, and between nine and fifteen months for walking. These milestones are adorable during the day but not your idea of a good time at night. Night "practices" usually go on for several nights, and then baby may go back to his normal sleep patterns.

6. They're teething. Baby's first four months are often termed "the honeymoon" when it comes to sleep. Baby may wake up once, twice, or not at all, and life is good. Enter the fifth month, and your worst nighttime opponent enters the game — teeth. Babies begin to feel teething pain as early as three months of age, even though the teeth may not break through for another two months or more. Teething phases sometimes last for only a week, and just when you begin to get really frustrated, baby starts to sleep well again. You'll usually get a couple months' break between teething cycles. However, some teeth will seem to take forever to come in, and you may be in (or up) for a rough month or two. This is also a common problem for toddlers. The infamous two-year molars can surprise you, and your toddler may need more of you during this month or two. Fortunately, that's the last of the teeth until age six.

7. They hurt. Many irritating things go on in that growing little body that can wake baby up. See chapter 11, Hidden Medical and Physical Causes of Night Waking.

8. They're lonesome. Let's step into your baby's mind for a moment. Your baby just spent the last nine months being carried around inside your body, and as baby grew, so did her awareness of your warmth, heartbeat, body sounds, and your motion as you walked. Now that baby is born, where does she spend much of her day? She is cuddled in your arms to feed, carried in a soft carrier, lovingly caressed during baths and while being dressed, passed back and forth between caring friends and relatives, and rocked to sleep. If baby is experiencing so much of you during the day, why wouldn't she want some of you at night? Some babies wake simply because they miss you and want a bit of mom or dad (once again, usually mom) to get back to sleep.

I think he wakes up to check that I'm still there.

9. They're anxious. Closeness, not separateness, is a normal psychological and emotional state for a baby, especially during the first year or two. Just as babies feel incomplete if separated from their mothers during the day, they can feel the same at night. To a baby, separateness doesn't start just because the sun goes down. Many infant development specialists believe, and we agree, that separation anxiety (during the day and night) is a built-in survival mechanism for babies, since naturally it is safer for them to be close to a caregiver. So, when baby wakes up alone, he feels out of touch. Separateness and aloneness are not normal states for a baby. When a baby wakes up alone in a dark, quiet room — sometimes even behind bars — a sort of "what's wrong with this picture?" anxious thought process goes on. More mild-tempered babies will sometimes simply accept nighttime aloneness and go back to sleep. Those with more persistent personalities will cry out in the night, as if summoning their caregivers, "Something is not right here! Please make it right!"

10. They're afraid. You will find that your toddler and preschooler may begin to develop some nighttime fears as his imagination sets in and he begins to contemplate what may be lurking in the dark. Your two-year-old may be dreaming about a giant pacifier chasing him through the sandbox. We discuss nightmares and sleep terrors in chapter 12.

11. They're conditioned to. In our medical practice we have noticed a phenomenon we call "conditioned night waking," which is most frequent in babies who are privileged to breastfeed and co-sleep. Baby awakens, mother presents breast, baby feels comforted, and baby goes back to sleep. He gets to like this immediate gratification. And, of course, any smart baby is literally going to "milk" this nighttime perk for all he can get. "Ah, nightlife is good!" he imagines. And, since babies instinctively do what brings them pleasure and helps them thrive, they are reluctant to give up the very relationship that they not only want but believe they need. A good habit can become a need. Once babies realize that they thrive on night nursing (even at the expense of mom), they are unlikely to give it up without a protest. We believe it is a need rather than a habit. Habits are easy to break, needs are not. In chapter 6 we'll show you how to make night nursing easier.

NORMAL NIGHT NOISES SLEEPING BABIES MAKE

Babies are not soundless sleepers. They sigh, snort, gurgle, coo, snore, sputter, squeak, squeal, hoot, toot, cough, and even whimper and mumble a bit. Your baby's night noises are as unique as her personality, and most of them are not signs of distress. These normal sleep sounds, which often occur as babies are transitioning from one state of sleep to another, may be lovingly misinterpreted as, "Oh, he's about to wake up. I'd better get to him before he does." Sometimes, if you wait out these sounds, you realize that these are not bids for attention. They're just normal sounds, and you don't need to rush in to pick up and comfort baby. He may not even wake up. He may put himself back to sleep without your help if he does wake. If baby's noises escalate into cries, something is "not right" and he needs something from you to make it right. It might be food, it might be holding, it might be a few soothing words, but you can't go wrong by paying attention to the more insistent nighttime noises.

Our son sometimes cries out for a few moments and then goes right back to sleep. We don't go to him unless it's obvious he's awake.

ADOPT A NIGHTTIME PARENTING ATTITUDE

Helping a baby learn healthy sleep habits is not like housebreaking a puppy, and it involves more than simply following a set of instructions. There's a little human being who needs to be taught how to fall asleep comfortably and fearlessly and how to go back to sleep after awakening at night. Teaching these lessons in a nurturing way will also teach your baby to trust you.

You'll notice throughout this book that we use the term "nighttime parenting" rather than "getting your baby to sleep" or, worse, "sleep training." Calling what you do with your baby nighttime parenting reminds you that it is part of the whole parenting package. You want your baby to feel that she can rely on you and trust you to help her feel good during the night as well as during the day. Your attachment to her is something that she can always count on. You show this attachment differently at night, because you need to sleep, but the relationship you have with your baby continues. Once you approach baby's sleep time with a nighttime parenting attitude, you will naturally view the time you spend helping your baby sleep as an opportunity to build your relationship. To get your baby to sleep better, you will rely more on yourself and your own intuition than on a bunch of gadgets and insensitive techniques to "break" baby of night waking.

Having said that you are going to be parenting your baby at night as well as during the day, we have to add that *it's important not to neglect your own nighttime needs.* Many a first-time mother, in her zeal to be a good mother, ends up becoming a martyr mother at night: "My baby needs me so much at night that I don't get the sleep I need. But that's okay. Baby comes first." While some sleep disruption inevitably goes with the territory of being a parent (with children of all ages), neglecting your own need for sleep is not okay. Sleep

---

HELPING OTHERS SLEEP!

Share your wisdom and nighttime experience with others. In our pediatric practice we encourage veteran mothers and fathers who have survived and thrived while helping their own children sleep better to share their experiences with new parents. As a perk, you'll get a "helper's high" — that warm, fuzzy feeling of knowing that some parents and babies are sleeping better because of the advice you gave them. (Truthfully, that high is what keeps us writing books.)

---

deprivation can compromise your emotional and physical health, and it is neither a necessary nor a normal part of nighttime parenting. Your baby needs parents who are well rested enough to be responsive and fun during the day. Babies need sleep in order to thrive, and so do mothers and fathers. It helps to have the attitude "I'm going to keep working at getting *all* of us the best sleep possible."

Some say easy sleepers are born, not made. There is some truth to this. Sleep is not a state you can force a baby into, but some babies have temperaments that allow them to fall asleep easily and to go back to sleep without much help. How you parent your baby also affects how well your baby sleeps. Some parents are more careful to create an environment that allows sleep to overtake baby. Some are more persistent about sensitively teaching their babies how to put themselves back to sleep. How your baby sleeps will depend on both your baby's individual temperament and how you parent at night.

A realistic long-term goal is to help your baby develop a healthy attitude about sleep: that sleep is a pleasant state to enter and a secure state to remain in. Many sleep problems in older children and adults stem from growing up with fears and anxiety about falling asleep. Just as daytime parenting is a long-term investment, so is nighttime parenting. Your short-term goal may be to teach your baby sleep habits that help you get more sleep yourself, but you want to do this in a way that will also accomplish your long-term goal. Teach your baby to have a healthy attitude toward sleep in the first year, and both you and your baby will sleep better in the years that follow.

Some of the parents in our neighborhood adopted the cry-it-out method of getting their children to go to sleep. In the first couple years, they used to boast about how their children would sleep through the night, while I would often doze off during the neighborhood meeting because I was up nursing at night. Now that their kids are older, they wake up with nightmares, see monsters in their room, and seem to be afraid of sleep. Now these mothers are the ones nodding off during the day and losing sleep while my child sleeps happily through the night, as do I.

UNCLUTTER THE DAYTIME LIFE OF A NIGHTTIME PARENT

It's hard to cultivate a positive attitude toward nighttime parenting at 4 a.m. At that hour, you do what you have to do to survive and get back to sleep. The real work of helping the whole family sleep better begins in the daytime, as you adjust your lifestyle to accommodate the changes a baby brings to your family's life.

New mothers often fail to anticipate the toll a baby will take on their energy, especially at night. They believe they'll continue their previous busy lifestyle and baby will somehow fit in. Not so! Tired mothers of new babies often ask, "When will my life get back to normal?" I respond, "This is a new kind of normal. Life won't ever again be the way it was before."

Evaluate your lifestyle. Take inventory of all the things that drain away your energy but don't necessarily have to be done by you. You want to spend your energy where it matters — on your baby and on your own well-being. Consider the following:

- What jobs can you delegate?
- What commitments can you get out of or put off?
- How can you change your daytime schedule to sneak in extra naps? (See napping tips in chapter 9.)
- What changes can you make during the day to help yourself sleep better at night?

I had to redefine my daytime priorities. I had to realize that I couldn't be Supermom and do everything! Once I discontinued almost all outside commitments and gave myself the freedom to have a not-so-perfect house, I felt less resentment about getting up at night and was able to be more accepting. And, after a while, I think I just got used to it.

SLEEPY MOMS ADVISE . . .

Mothers who have survived, and thrived, through many years of nighttime parenting offer these attitude helpers:

I look at it like an investment that will pay off. It's what I signed up for.

◆

Our daytime and general life is so hectic that I actually look forward to those special times of night nursing.

◆

We have good nights and bad nights, but we make a point of celebrating the good ones rather than bemoaning the bad.

◆

We tried everything to get our baby to sleep through the night, and nothing was working. So I tried changing my attitude. Expecting my baby to sleep through the night when it wasn't happening was making me angry, and that kept me awake even more. Once I changed my attitude and reminded myself that it's normal, natural, and expected for babies to wake up at night, I slept better. It's much more difficult to get angry about something you expect and perceive as normal.

◆

When my baby woke during the night, I was careful not to look at the clock, not to count the feedings. Keeping track of how much sleep I was missing made it much harder to get back to sleep and harder to function the next day.

◆

How good a parent you are is not demonstrated by how long your child sleeps. I mention this because someone is bound to ask you the magic question "Is he/she sleeping through the night?" or "Is he/she a good baby?" You will dread those questions and have to learn to ignore them.

◆

Don't make sleep a control issue. You'll both probably lose.

◆

Every mother goes through a period when she is sleep-deprived. We just cope by saying, "This is only for a short time." Before you know it, you'll be sleep-deprived because you're waiting for your teenager to get home after a date.

◆

Sometimes the best way to get over sleep problems is to redefine "good sleeper." Oftentimes, there really isn't a problem, except that people have been told that kids should sleep a certain way.

Have a restful day. Babies — and adults — sleep better at night if they have enjoyed a restful day. Think about especially stressful days in your past and the restless nights that followed. When you go to sleep with a bloodstream full of stress hormones, you set yourself up for a restless night. Daytime stress (from too much running around, mother returning to work, or an illness) is one of the reasons infants have difficulty settling at night. When daytime stress can't be avoided, at least have a restful evening as a prelude to better sleep.

Have a peaceful house. Computers, TVs, loud music, noisy guests, and loud conversations make the atmosphere in your home supercharged. Turn off the TV, the radio, and other noisemakers, and turn down the bright lights to make your home a quiet, peaceful place. Your baby will sleep better, and so will you.

Strive for a daily routine. Newborns come disorganized. All of their physiological functions are irregular. They don't follow a predictable routine. If mom and dad's life is also unpredictable, baby will have a much harder time settling into regular routines for sleeping and eating. Notice we use the term "routine" rather than "schedule." Your pre-baby life may have been run by your Palm Pilot, but babies need some flexibility. They change from week to week. Don't expect to have a "day planner baby." You will get more joy out of parenting if you create a routine that fits your baby rather than trying to make your baby fit the routine. Babies are creatures of

habit, and the more predictable their day, the more restful the night is likely to be.

Get some exercise. You will sleep better at night if you are active during the day. Put your baby in the baby sling or stroller and go out for a walk. Run and play with your toddler at the park. Stretch the kinks out of your back and shoulders with yoga or other forms of exercise. Can't get to the gym? Buy some exercise equipment for the home.

Take naps. Adult lifestyles don't often allow for the luxury of napping, but parents of babies who are awake at night are entitled to sleep during the day. Don't use your baby's nap time to get the housework done. Use this downtime to rest or to do things that rejuvenate your tired spirit.

Don't compare, don't complain. When parents of babies get together, they inevitably talk about sleep. Sometimes this is helpful, sometimes it's not. It all depends on whom you're with. Don't be discouraged by parents who brag about their own babies sleeping through the night at an early age. Seek out experienced parents who share your parenting values and who have helpful, positive ideas to share.

Have reasonable expectations. If you expect your baby to sleep for twelve hours straight, or even half that amount, every single night, you are bound to end up frustrated. This is not the way babies are made. If you understand why your baby wakes up at night and expect it, it will be easier to live with.

GET CONNECTED

The concept of nighttime parenting that we have described above is part of *attachment parenting,* a style of parenting that we advocate. We summarize this style of parenting briefly in this chapter. Other chapters in this book apply the ideas of attachment parenting to various nighttime challenges. If you want to learn more about attachment parenting, read some of our other books, including *The Baby Book, The Attachment Parenting Book,* and *The Discipline Book.*

Even though we started using this term in 1980, attachment parenting (AP) is not a new way of raising children that we and others have dreamed up. It's what mothers and fathers would do instinctively if they were raising their baby on a desert island without the advice of sleep books, in-laws, and psychologists. It is a high-touch, highly responsive style of infant care. Parents invest a lot of time and energy in their relationship with their baby, and they get a high return on this investment. They learn to know and understand their child, and their children respond with trust and respect. Attachment parenting is what many parents naturally do without even realizing it has a name.

AP helps parent and child get to know and trust each other by using the connecting tools we call the eight Baby B's:

1. *Birth bonding.* Start the connection as soon as possible after birth.
2. *Breastfeeding.* When you breastfeed, you learn to read your baby's cues — both day and night. The physical closeness of breastfeeding rewards both mother and baby with good feelings.
3. *Babywearing.* Wear your baby in a carrier several hours a day. Babies who are held are calmer and more fun to be with. A baby who is happy and peaceful during the day will sleep better at night.
4. *Bedding close to baby.* Sleeping within an easy distance for touching and nursing lessens nighttime separation anxiety, both in baby and in mother.
5. *Belief in the language value of baby's cry.* Babies cry to communicate, not to manipulate. When parents respond to babies' cries, babies learn to trust their moms and dads and their own ability to communicate.
6. *Beware of baby trainers.* Putting your baby on a schedule or letting your baby "cry it out" to sleep puts a distance between you and your baby. (See chapter 10 for how rigid baby training can sabotage your parent-child relationship.)
7. *Balance.* Use your knowledge of your baby to decide when to say yes and when to say no to your baby. Also, have the wisdom to say yes to caring for your own needs, too.
8. *Both.* Babies need both parents to share in their care, day and night. For single parents, a relative or close friend who bonds with and shares in the parenting of a baby is helpful.

AP is flexible. The Baby B's are not a set of rules for parents to follow. They are tools that you use to accomplish your goals of knowing and enjoying your baby. These tools are based on biology — how your baby and you are "wired" to respond to one another. There may be medical or family circumstances that prevent you from being able to practice all of these Baby B's all of the time, and some will work better for you than others. Do the best you can with the resources you have. The most important thing is to get connected to your baby. As you and your baby learn to fit together, you can adapt and modify the Baby B's to suit your circumstances.

AP is not indulgent or permissive parenting. A frequent criticism of attachment parenting is that it puts baby, rather than parents, in control. But can parents actually control their babies anyway? Parenting your baby at night forces you to come to terms with the realistic fact that you *can't* control your child's behavior. Parenting, by day and by night, should not become a control issue. Parenting depends on trust. Because AP allows mutual trust to develop between you and your child, you learn to respond to your child's needs appropriately, knowing when to say yes, when to say no, when to intervene, and when to back off and let your child work through a problem on his own.

Instead of controlling their children, AP parents shape their children's behavior, like gardeners tending their plants and flowers. While there are plenty of things in a garden that you can't control, such as how many buds are on a plant or when those buds open up into flowers, there are also plenty of things that you can do: you can pull the weeds and you can water and prune the plant so that the plant blooms more beautifully. Over our

many years of experience as parents and as pediatricians, we have noticed that the Baby B's of infancy often lead to the childhood C's. These children are more likely to become cuddly, caring, compassionate, considerate, confident, and cooperative.

AP shines at night. Using the Baby B's to help you get connected to your child during the day will give you an important advantage in working out the best plan for nighttime parenting. When you know your child well and are confident in your parenting, you can work out a sleeping plan that is custom-made for your baby. You don't have to flounder around in the dark, following someone else's ideas about how your baby should sleep. You'll think about your baby and the problem you are trying to solve, and a light will go on. AP helps turn on those switches.

AP parents do not buy into the cry-it-out approach for getting babies to sleep and feed according to a rigid schedule. Nor are they big fans of sleep-inducing gadgets that fill in for parents on night duty. The sensitivity AP parents develop toward their babies tells them that what babies need most is a parent's presence. Leaving a baby to cry feels wrong to these parents, because they know that baby trusts them to respond to crying.

AP offers high-touch parenting in a high-tech world. This style of parenting encourages you to take time and smell the roses. Busy lifestyles have made this a stressed nation, and less responsive styles of parenting may only make it worse. Could there be any correlation over the last decade between

CONNECTED KIDS SLEEP BETTER

In our practice, we have noticed that parents who use the Baby B's have babies and children with fewer sleep problems, especially as they get older. Investing in this style of nighttime parenting when your baby is small will bring dividends of restful nights in the years to come.

- Connected kids tend to be less afraid of the dark and have fewer nightmares and episodes of sleep terrors. They tend to sleep better as older children. One reason for this is that these children have lower levels of stress hormones, by day and by night, so that they sleep less anxiously than less connected children.

- AP allows you to be so intimately in touch with your baby and young child's needs that when you are faced with parenting challenges at night, you are able to create an action plan that works for you and your child. If AP parents reach a point where they feel that the family would be better off if baby learned to sleep more independently, they find sensitive ways to help baby learn to do this, ways that do not violate the trusting relationship between child and parents.

- Children who are products of insensitive cry-it-out sleep-training methods do appear to "sleep through the night" at an earlier age. But they are sleeping more anxiously (see Sleep Anxiety, page 104), and as a result, they tend to have more sleep problems as toddlers and preschoolers. (See chapter 10 for what science says about the cry-it-out method of sleep training.)

the flurry of sleep-training books and the fact that sleep-disorder clinics for children have sprung up in nearly every major city? The current epidemic of sleeplessness could be compared with the epidemic of child-hood obesity. When children grow up with junk food, they become fat. When children begin life with stressed sleep, they grow up anxious. Connected kids sleep better as older children because they slept less anxiously as infants.

Keep working at it. No single approach to nighttime parenting will work with all babies all the time, or even all the time with the same baby. Babies have different nighttime temperaments, and families have varied lifestyles. Develop a style of nighttime parenting that fits the temperament of your baby and your own lifestyle. If it's working, stick with it. But if your sleep program isn't working for your family, don't persist with a bad experiment. Be open to trying other night-time parenting styles, especially as your child enters new developmental stages. Follow your heart rather than some stranger's sleep-training advice, and you and your baby will eventually work out the right nighttime parenting style for your family.

GET TO KNOW YOUR BABY'S SLEEP PERSONALITY

You probably entered parenthood with some definite ideas about what type of parent you wanted to be and with some plans for how your new baby would fit into your life. Some of your plans probably are working out just fine, but some other things — say, nighttime — might not be going so well, because your baby seems to have plans of her own. She has a personality, which may not have figured into your original plans.

Your baby's sleep habits are in large part determined by your baby's temperament, which is not something you can change. Temperament is the part of a person's personality that is inborn and genetically determined. For example, people are naturally calm or sociable or high-strung. This is true even of tiny babies. When your baby is born, you spend the first few months just getting to know your newborn. You are finding out what kind of baby you have been blessed with. Your baby's temperament will be an important factor in how you parent baby at night.

Easy babies. Of course, easy babies aren't "easy"— no baby is. But some babies are easier to care for than others. They need less of

your time and energy to be content. Sure, they love to be held and played with, but they will also be happy to sit in an infant seat or lie in the crib and entertain themselves for a little while. These babies also tend to need less of you at night. They fall asleep more easily and stay asleep longer. (We prefer the term "long sleeper" rather than "good" or "bad sleepers.") If your friend's baby is "sleeping through the night" at three weeks, she probably has this type of baby. (Or she's not giving you the whole story.)

Even though parents may report that their infants sleep through the night, videotape studies show that most older infants still wake up at least once at night. Some infants (called "settlers") are able to put themselves back to sleep, so parents don't ever know they woke up. The main issue is not night waking but self-settling. The goal of most sleep books is for an infant to learn to be a self-settler. To some extent, our book has that goal also, but with the caveat that different children attain this goal at different ages and that the parents' job is to sensitively help babies learn to sleep, not to just stand back and let babies teach themselves.

High-need babies. Babies who ask more of their parents can be just as pleasant and just as much fun as easy babies, but they need more input from you to stay that way. (In chapter 5, you will meet "Miss More," our first high-need baby, daughter Hayden.) Some will term these babies "fussy babies." We find that they are more outgoing, energetic, and anxious than easy babies. A high-need baby likes to be held much of the day. In fact, high-need babies *need* to be held much of the day. They just aren't content to be put down for more than a few minutes. Tiringly, the high-need label holds true for nighttime as well. These babies need more attention from mom and dad when they fall asleep, and they wake up more often because they need a "dose" of mom or dad (okay, usually mom) to stay asleep.

I feel that our one-year-old is a very good sleeper. I usually get a full eight hours of sleep each night. I think I was able to achieve this because I followed my instincts and cared about what my son wanted rather than going with the socially acceptable "let him cry it out" method. I feel good as a parent that I met my son's needs rather than forcing him into the misery of lonely nights for my convenience. Besides, when I cuddle him to sleep at night, I remember that these are moments that last a relatively short time. In my son's entire life, how many years will he want to be at mommy's side? I feel that by working with my son's temperament, I am making the most of my mother-son relationship, teaching him trust, and ultimately self-reliance; he will realize that he is a person of worth because I've shown him that he is.

How Does Your Baby's Personality Type Predict Her Nighttime Needs?

If you are reading this book because your baby is having sleep problems, you have probably just now decided that you have a needy baby. Some high-need babies are just not fans of sleep in general. And if you are

parents just getting to know your newborn, you are probably thinking, "Oh, please be the easy kind of baby, please, please, pleeeeeease!"

The truth is all babies have nighttime needs. Easy babies will make these needs known less often, and parents may find it easier to teach easy babies to sleep longer at night. High-need babies are a different story. Here's why:

Need to touch. High-need babies thrive on touch. They've been inside mom for the past nine months, and they aren't ready to give up that feeling of being enclosed and held. They've grown used to mom's movements and heart sounds. Now that they are out in the world, they can experience this closeness just as intensely, but in different ways. They hear you, smell you, see you, feel you, and even taste you (during nursing). When mom isn't near, high-need babies feel unsettled and incomplete. They sense that something is missing even if they are sound asleep. They may sleep for hours on end when sleeping next to someone, but they wake up every half hour if sleeping solo.

Need to suck. High-need babies usually have a great need to suck for comfort. Whether it's with your breast or finger or a bottle or pacifier, comfort sucking is almost as important as food for these babies. They won't easily fall asleep without it, and when they stir during the night, their "suck alarm" goes off and they start looking for whatever they can get their mouth on. If you're not there, your baby will let you know loud and clear that she needs you.

Need to move. You probably know by now whether your baby is one of those "always needs to be rocked or bounced" babies. High-need babies are not content to simply be put down to fall asleep in a crib or bed that doesn't move. There is something soothing about the gentle rocking of a parent's arms, a baby swing, or a cradle, and your baby knows it. It's almost as if your baby needs to be "coached" into falling asleep — as long as you keep moving, baby won't notice that sleep is sneaking up on him.

Balancing Baby's Nighttime Needs with Yours

Are your baby's needs unreasonable? Is your baby really hungry every two hours at night? Does your baby really need to sleep near you, or does she just want to sleep near you? Do you sleep close to baby because baby wakes up frequently? Or is baby waking up at night because you are close? And where does *your* need for sleep fit into the picture?

The art of nighttime parenting is about making choices that get everyone's needs met most, if not all, of the time. The choices you make for your family will depend on both your baby's sleep temperament and your own sleep needs. Keep in mind that how you parent your baby at night may change as your baby matures. A two-month-old high-need baby may need to nurse every two hours at night, but a fourteen-month-old high-need toddler may be ready to cut back on nighttime nursing, with some firm but loving guidance from parents. Some babies need more help than others in learning to fall asleep and stay asleep. There are different ways to provide this help,

and in this book, we try to give you lots of options. We won't tell you exactly what to do with your baby in every situation, but we will help you understand your baby so that you can sensitively meet his needs and get enough sleep yourself. You don't have to be a sleep-walking zombie during the day just because you are meeting your baby's needs at night.

MATCHING YOURSELF, YOUR BABY, AND YOUR SLEEP PLAN

Now that you have more insight into your baby's temperament, how does it affect your baby's sleep habits, and how will it affect your nighttime parenting approach? Here are some ideas to keep in mind as you continue to work through your sleep plan:

Easy babies and independent sleep. Babies with mild, easygoing temperaments are often the best sleepers. They have a low level of need at night. They will therefore easily learn self-soothing techniques, accept independent sleep associations (see page 20), and probably learn to sleep through the night relatively quickly. For parents who are hoping that baby will go to sleep fairly easily, sleep well in his own bed, and not wake too often during the night, this is a realistic hope if baby is generally easygoing.

Easy babies and attachment-based nighttime parenting. Like more demanding babies, easy babies also thrive when parents choose a closer nighttime arrangement, such as nursing to sleep and co-sleeping. Because such babies are mild mannered, they may not demand such closeness at night, but they will certainly welcome it!

High-need babies and independent sleep. Parents who are hoping their baby will learn to sleep well in a crib in another room with minimal night waking but who are blessed with a high-need baby are in for a big surprise. Its very unlikely that such a baby will learn to fall asleep unassisted in a crib in her own room and then sleep through the night. When a high-need baby is subjected to the cry-it-out method of sleep training, a very long and unfortunate battle of wills ensues. It is important for parents to understand what their baby's nighttime needs are in this type of situation and to listen to their own instincts. A high-need baby will thrive and blossom into a self-confident and independent child if his needs are met in the early months and years. Read chapter 5 for more insights into raising a high-need baby.

High-need babies and attachment-based nighttime parenting. It is a wonderful mix when a baby with many needs has parents who are open to meeting those intense needs at night by night-nursing and co-sleeping. However, *both* parents must team up and share night duty (and day duty), because a high-need baby is very demanding. In chapter 5, we detail how parents with a high-need baby can team up to thrive as a family unit and avoid mother burnout.

As you work through your sleep plan, keep your baby's needs and temperament in mind. Always run any advice you get (from us or from anyone else) through your own parenting-instinct filter. Go with your gut feelings. You will be right 99.9 percent of the time.

SLEEP SAFETY

Here are practical ways to help your baby sleep comfortably and safely at nap time and nighttime.

Sleepwear — How to Dress Your Baby Safely and Comfortably for Sleep

The more comfortably you dress your baby for sleeping, the better she is likely to sleep. Try these suggestions:

Sleep cool. Get used to feeling your baby's forehead for clues that she's too hot. A hot, sweaty head may indicate a need for a cooler room or less clothing. Other signs of overheating include damp hair, rapid breathing, a prickly heat rash, and restlessness. If you are worried that your baby is too cold, check her hands and feet. While it is normal for the extremities to be slightly cooler than the body, if your baby's toes and fingers are truly cold, she may need an extra layer of clothing. If your baby was born premature, your doctor may advise you to cover your baby's head with a cap for the first month or two, since babies lose a lot of heat through their heads. After the first night or two, term babies should not wear a cap or hood while sleeping, since this may lead to overheating. Babies who co-sleep should not be dressed as warmly at night as babies who sleep solo (see page 77).

> ## SEARS SLEEP TIP
>
> As a general guide, babies sleep most comfortably covered like mother, *plus* one more layer.

After an entire winter of being completely sleep-deprived, I decided one night to take my nine-month-old out of her long-sleeve outfit and dress her in a short-sleeve onesie at bed-time. It worked like magic! She is now sleeping much better, only waking up once. When she sleeps with only her diapers on, she sleeps even better.

Cotton is cool. Cotton absorbs body moisture and allows air to circulate more freely. Also, the occasional infant may be sensitive to synthetic sleepwear, and the itching may keep her awake. Flame-retardant cotton sleepwear is available.

Sleep loose. Most babies prefer to sleep loose. Buy your baby's sleepwear to fit loosely enough to allow free and comfortable movements. There are two types of sleepwear for tiny infants: loose, tie-at-the-bottom sacques, and footed sleepers. Warm sleepwear is more practical than blankets, since babies often kick off their blankets. Sacques tend to be looser fitting, better fitting for a longer time, and easier for changing diapers. It's harder to get a good fit in footed sleepers for the rapidly growing baby. Some babies sleep well in sleepers that cover the feet. Others prefer to have their feet uncovered or covered with booties instead. Remove labels if they are rough, scratchy, or irritating to baby's skin.

I found that when my toddler was able to choose his own number of blankets, he chose none and slept better. I wonder if I kept him too warm when he was younger.

Sleep safe. To avoid the danger of baby strangling, do not dress your baby in sleepwear with dangling ribbons, strings, or ties longer than seven inches. If baby co-sleeps, she needs less clothing than if solo sleeping, since she gets extra heat from the warm body next to her. Babies who are too warm at night may be at greater risk of SIDS, since overheating diminishes the protective arousals from sleep. If you choose to swaddle your baby to help her sleep longer, avoid overheating by using fewer covers. Arms-free swaddling is the least restrictive and allows baby more freedom of movement. Use a single cotton blanket and avoid heavy comforters. To keep the crib-sleeping baby from sliding under the covers, tuck the bottom portion of the blankets snugly beneath the end and each side of the crib mattress but not so tightly as to restrict baby's freedom of movement. (For more information about safe co-sleeping and safe crib sleeping, see below and page 80.)

Safe Co-sleeping

Co-sleeping is safe when you follow some simple, sensible precautions. Here's what you need to know to safely share sleep with your baby:

- Place baby to sleep on his back. Back sleeping is associated with a lowered risk of Sudden Infant Death Syndrome (SIDS).

- Take precautions to prevent baby from rolling out of bed. It's unlikely that a small baby sleeping next to mother will roll out of bed, since, like a heat-seeking missile, a baby automatically gravitates toward mother's warm body. But to be safe, use a guardrail when baby sleeps between mother and the edge of the bed. Guardrails made of plastic mesh are safer than those with slats, which can entrap baby's limbs or head. Be sure there are no crevices that baby could sink into between the mattress and the guardrail, the mattress and the headboard, or the mattress and the wall. Push the mattress flush against these structures and fill in any gaps with folded towels or blankets tucked down firmly.

Trust your mother radar. Baby will be okay in bed with you.

- Place baby adjacent to mother rather than between mother and father. Mothers we have interviewed on the subject of sharing sleep feel they are so physically and mentally aware of their baby's presence, even while sleeping, that they would be extremely unlikely to roll over onto their baby. Some fathers, on the other hand, may not enjoy this same sensitivity to baby's presence while asleep, so it is possible they may roll over or throw out an arm onto baby. After a few months of sleep sharing, most dads seem to develop a keen awareness of their baby's presence.

- Use a large bed, preferably a king-size. ("California Kings" are the widest.)

- Do not sleep with your baby if you are under the influence of any drug (such as alcohol or tranquilizing medications) that could diminish your sensitivity to your baby's presence.

- Do not allow older siblings to sleep with a baby under one year of age. Sleeping children do not have the same awareness of babies that parents have. Ditto this precaution for substitute caregivers.

- Avoid overheating from overbundling. Because baby is sleeping next to a warm body, a co-sleeping infant needs to be dressed less warmly than a baby who is solo sleeping. If you bring your baby from crib to bed, you may need to remove a layer of his clothing. (Overheating can diminish baby's natural arousability from sleep.)

- Don't fall asleep with baby on a couch, beanbag chair, or any other sinky surface that could cause baby to suffocate. One of the dangers of sleeping on a couch is that baby can get wedged between the back of the couch and the larger person's body, or baby's head can become buried in cushion crevices or soft cushions.

- It's safest not to lie down and breastfeed your baby on a cushiony surface, such as a couch, since if you are tired, you could fall asleep breastfeeding and roll over onto your baby.

- Recliners are a favorite for dads falling asleep with babies. Be cautious about this practice. Baby can slip sideways from your chest and become wedged between you and the sides or arms of the chair.

- Do not sleep with baby on a free-floating, wavy water bed (those without internal baffles), as a sleeping infant's face can get trapped in the depression formed by the weight of the head and the body. "Waveless" water beds are safer for sharing sleep. As an added safety measure, baby could sleep on a firm sleep mat rolled out on top of the firm water bed.

- Don't wear dangling jewelry or lingerie with string ties longer than seven inches. Baby may get caught in these.

- Avoid pungent hair sprays, deodorants, and perfumes. Not only may these camouflage the natural maternal smells that baby is used to and attracted to, but foreign odors may irritate and clog baby's tiny nasal passages. Reserve these enticements for sleeping alone with your spouse.

- No smoking when baby sleeps. Smoking greatly increases a baby's risk of SIDS. Even the odor of smoke in your hair or clothing or on your breath is a risk.

- Put away your bed frame and place your mattress and box spring directly on the floor. Assume that your baby will crawl or roll out of bed at some point, and this will shorten the fall and eliminate the chances of injury.

- If your mattress or bed is on a hard floor, soften baby's landing by placing rugs, futons, or pillows on the floor around your bed.

- Do not use an egg-crate mattress pad or other extra-soft padding on your mattress. This can make baby's sleeping surface too soft and may block baby's breathing if baby's face sinks into the soft padding. A pillow-top mattress may also be too soft. If you feel that your mattress surface is too soft, place a waterproof mattress pad under the sheet on baby's side. This will provide a firmer surface for baby. It will also protect your mattress when baby's wet diaper leaks during the night.

- Remove pictures or any other hanging decorations from the wall near the bed. Such objects can come loose and fall onto baby. An active older baby may pull them down.

- Blinds and drapery cords near the bed are potentially dangerous. Keep them out of baby's and children's reach. Cut blind cords and use safety tassels and inner cord stops to prevent strangulation.

- If you are extremely obese, your infant could be at greater risk of smothering when snuggled close to you. Consider an alternative to co-sleeping, such as an Arm's Reach Co-Sleeper.

- It's safest and easiest when breastfeeding to place baby's head at the level of your breast. Your blanket will then end up around your rib cage. Choose sleepwear that keeps your neck and shoulders warm, so that you don't need to pull the covers up and over baby's head.

For an in-depth analysis of the science of safe co-sleeping, see chapter 5.

When baby sleeps alone on an adult bed, in addition to observing the same precautions as above, be sure to do the following:

- Use a baby monitor so you can hear when baby stirs. Immediately check on baby when you hear rustling to make sure baby isn't crawling or rolling off the bed.

- Cover baby with a small baby blanket only. Pull the bed sheets and blankets down to the foot of the bed.

- Once baby starts scooting on her tummy or crawling, teach her how to safely crawl backward down off the bed. Practice this technique over and over during daytime play. If you have placed your bed close to the floor (off the bed frame), baby can safely climb down. A futon on the floor will provide a soft landing pad.

- Place bed rails on both sides of the bed.

Safe Crib Sleeping

To keep your crib sleeper safe, go through this list:

- Place baby to sleep on his back. Back sleeping is associated with a lowered risk of Sudden Infant Death Syndrome (SIDS).

- Use a crib that has a Consumer Product Safety Commission (CPSC) or Juvenile Products Manufacturers Association (JPMA) label stating that the crib conforms to government safety standards.

- Be sure the mattress fits the crib perfectly. An undersize mattress will leave a gap along the side or end of the crib where an infant's head can get stuck. There should be no more than a one-and-one-half-inch (four-centimeter) gap between the mattress and the side or end of the crib. No more than two fingers should fit in the gap.

- The firmer the mattress, the safer.

- Many safety experts believe crib bumpers should not be used because they may be a suffocation hazard.

- If using a crib bumper, make sure it fits snugly around the entire perimeter of the crib and is secured by at least six ties or snaps. To prevent your baby from chewing on the ties and becoming entangled in them, trim off excess length. Remove bumpers and toys from the crib as soon as your child begins to pull up on the crib rails.

- Place the crib in a safe area in the room, preferably near your bed. Don't place a crib near a heater, against a window, near any dangling cords from blinds or draperies, or close to any furniture that the baby could use to climb out of the crib.

- Don't attach crib toys between side rails or hang them over the crib after baby is old enough to push up on her hands and knees (usually about five months). Be sure pacifiers and mobiles do not have strings longer than seven inches.

- Don't place breathing blockers in baby's crib (or wherever baby sleeps). Breathing hazards include pillows, fuzzy stuffed animals and toys, string toys, and tiny chokable toys.

- Spread sheets and undersheets smoothly and tuck them in tightly beneath the mattress. This lessens the chance of looseness on the bedding that could obstruct baby's breathing.

- Check the crib railing and hardware for splinters, sharp joints, or cracks where baby's fingers could get pinched or stuck. Frequently check the mattress support system to be sure it is secure.

- Be particularly vigilant when traveling, since baby will be sleeping in an unfamiliar and potentially unsafe environment. Bring along a firm roll-out safe-sleeping mat, since the beds and cribs in hotels may not be up to the same safety standards you have at home.

- No smoking in baby's bedroom. Smoking greatly increases baby's risk of SIDS. Even the odor of smoke in your hair and clothing or on your breath is a risk.

- Avoid pillows until an infant is around two years of age. As a general guide, when a child is ready to graduate from a crib to a toddler bed, he's old enough to use a pillow. Be sure the pillow is not too squishy. Foam pillows are safer than feather pillows.

- To check updates on crib safety, consult the Consumer Products Safety Commission website, www.cpsc.gov.

PREFERS TUMMY SLEEPING

My three-month-old sleeps soundly on her tummy but wakes up every hour when I make her sleep on her back. I know that sleeping on the back is important to reduce the risk of SIDS. What should I do?

"Back-to-Sleep" campaigns have been the biggest breakthrough in lowering the risk of SIDS. In most countries, back-sleeping campaigns have lowered the rate of SIDS by around 50 percent. Always put your baby to sleep on her back, at least for the first six to nine months.

There are several reasons why back sleeping lowers the SIDS risk. We believe that the main reason is that back sleepers rouse from sleep more easily and sleep less deeply than tummy sleepers. Easy arousability from sleep is an important protective mechanism. Another reason why back sleeping is safer is that babies lying on their backs are less likely to become overheated, because back sleeping leaves the internal organs more exposed, so they radiate heat more easily. Another possibility is that when sleeping facedown, a baby may press her face into a soft surface and suffocate.

If you do allow baby to sleep on her tummy, consider the numbers. The tummy-sleeping SIDS connection is a statistical correlation only. It does not mean that if your baby sleeps on her tummy, she is going to die of SIDS. Current SIDS rates in the United States are around one in two thousand babies, meaning that there is a much greater than 99.9 percent chance that your child will sleep just fine, regardless of her position. Having

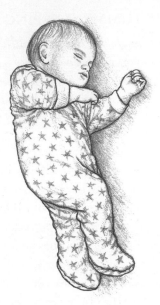

side, as shown in the illustration. With the outstretched-arm technique, a side-sleeping baby is then more likely to flip over onto her back than onto her tummy.

We never tell parents of a reluctant back-sleeper, "Okay, go ahead and let baby sleep on her tummy. She'll probably be just fine, and you can all sleep better." Parents whose babies don't sleep well on their backs must decide for themselves what the best choice is for them.

A safe and effective option for restless back sleepers is the Amby Baby Motion Bed. Its gentle rocking motion and soft contoured bottom help baby sleep comfortably on her back. See it on page 25.

ROLLS OVER ONTO TUMMY DURING SLEEP

My five-month-old rolls onto her tummy during the night. Is it safe to let her stay asleep in this position?

Many SIDS researchers believe that babies will naturally assume the sleep position that allows them to breathe more comfortably during the night. If your older baby habitually flips over to sleep on her tummy after you've put her down to sleep on her back, this may be the right sleeping position for her. If you want to be completely safe, however, you might want to turn her onto her back when she is in a deep sleep and put her to sleep on her back any time she wakens during the night.

Also, SIDS is less likely to occur if baby sleeps in the same room as the parent. This is a good option for any baby who prefers tummy sleeping.

said that, we still do not recommend tummy sleeping for infants.

One option is to encourage side sleeping. To lessen the chances of a side-sleeping baby rolling onto her tummy, stretch her underneath arm forward as shown in the illustration above. This arm can act as a stabilizer to keep baby from rolling onto her tummy. If the baby's arm stays closely tucked into her side, it will be easier for her to roll onto her tummy. Wedges to keep babies positioned on their back have never been proven to be either safe or effective and are generally discouraged by the Academy of Pediatrics.

Because of medical conditions, some babies sleep more safely on their tummies, such as babies who suffer from gastroesophageal reflux (see page 215) and infants with small jawbones or other structural abnormalities of the airway. For babies with GER, an alternative to tummy sleeping is sleeping on the left

Meet Different Families with Different Sleep Plans

IN THE FIRST TWO CHAPTERS you learned general tools to help your infant and toddler sleep happier and stay asleep longer. In chapter 3 you learned some general facts about sleep, which were necessary to help you understand why babies sleep the way they do. Now we're going to put the information you learned into practice by relating the most common night-life situations that we encounter in our pediatric practice and helping you put your baby's individual sleep plan (ISP) into practice. We will give you step-by-step instructions on how to bring together the many sleep tools listed in this book and help you formulate your baby's own ISP. As we journey through these real situations, we will refer you to the appropriate pages in the book that deal with particular situations in detail.

Working out your baby's ISP will take time. The longer your baby has had tiring sleep habits, the longer it's going to take to reshape them. Your baby may be unwilling (or unable if there is a medical problem causing the night waking) to "get with the plan,"

but be patient and persistent, and keep modifying the plan. Don't expect an overnight cure, or an every-night cure. There are no quick fixes in daytime or nighttime parenting situations. Any sleep plan that will last and is sensitive to your baby's nighttime needs and your individual lifestyle will take time. Hopefully, you can identify with some of the following nighttime challenges and apply some of the advice to your family.

NEWLY BORN OR SOON TO BE

We're expecting our first baby. How can we help her learn to sleep well right from the start?

Meet the Newborners. Neil and Nancy were first-time, dual-career parents. They both had Ph.D.'s and worked in the field of scientific research. In fact, when I saw them for prenatal counseling, they opened the discussion with, "Doctor, this is a well-researched baby." Neil went on to say, "We have done a lot of reading, and we've decided that the attachment style of parenting is best for our baby." Nancy added, "It's amazing how much research there is out there showing that babies of responsive parents grow up to be happier, healthier, and smarter."

We frequently see parents like this in our pediatric practice. We dub them "high investors." They realize that investing early in a high-touch attachment style of parenting will bring great rewards down the road. Here's how we worked with this family through the early years with their baby.

When Neil and Nancy brought baby Naomi in for her one-week checkup, they told us how glad they were to have studied up on sleep tools before their baby was born, since they didn't have much time to read now. They didn't regard sleep as a problem. Nancy said, "We're sleeping with our baby, since naturally breastfeeding and co-sleeping go together."

At little Naomi's one-month checkup, Nancy told us that co-sleeping was working well for her. "It just makes sense to have her sleep next to me and breastfeed. It would disturb my sleep a lot more if I had to get out of bed in the middle of the night, pick up a crying baby out of a crib, and sit up and nurse her. It would take both of us a long time to resettle. With her next to me at night, I don't even wake up completely. I just instinctively nurse her, and we both quickly drift back to sleep. Sometimes in the morning I don't even know how often she fed during the night." She added, "I am going to be working part-time out of our home, so I'm glad that co-sleeping is helping me to get a reasonably good night's sleep."

This mother and baby had discovered nighttime harmony. Their sleep cycles were in sync, and both got their nighttime needs met. Nancy got enough sleep, and Naomi got enough milk, along with the closeness she needed. She was growing well and was alert and calm during her checkup.

Neil agreed that co-sleeping was working well for the family. "Frankly," he half joked, "I like it because I don't have to get up and feed the baby in the middle of the night." He continued more seriously, "I may not be able to breastfeed Naomi, but I try to be involved in every other part of her care. I do baths and diapers. The other night, Nancy handed her to me after she had nursed her, and I walked her around the house until she fell asleep on my shoulder. While breastfeeding is Naomi's favorite thing in the whole world, it's nice to know that she feels safe and trusts me to take care of her, too."

As the months went by, Nancy and Neil encountered some challenges. Naomi went through a couple high-need periods when she nursed several times during the night, but Nancy was prepared for these growth spurts, and Neil stepped in to comfort Naomi when he could, and to take care of Nancy when he couldn't do much with Naomi. Neil spent a lot of time with Naomi on weekend mornings, allowing Nancy to escape to the university library and concentrate on her work.

When Naomi became a toddler, night nursing became more challenging for Nancy. Naomi sometimes wanted to nurse all night long as she slept, and Nancy often found this tiring. She wanted to continue to meet her baby's needs at night, and she realized that continuing to have positive feelings about nursing was also important. So when she nursed Naomi during the night, she would carefully ease her off the breast, roll over, and drift off to sleep, facing away to discourage Naomi from latching on every time she stirred. If Naomi fussed a bit, Neil or Nancy gently rubbed her back and soothed her. This didn't work all the time, but it worked enough. When Naomi turned two, Neil and Nancy got her a "big girl" bed, and over the course of the next year, Naomi learned to sleep by herself, although Nancy continued to nurse her to sleep in her own bed. If Naomi woke up during the night, one or the other parent went in to comfort her. Sometimes dad ended up sleeping in Naomi's bed.

When her parents brought Naomi into our office for a two-year checkup, Nancy and Neil reflected on how far they had come since Naomi's baby days. Naomi still nursed to sleep at bedtime, but some nights she fell asleep during her bedtime story or while her mother rubbed her back. Nancy said, "I never thought I'd see the day when Naomi would fall asleep without nursing. But she's getting there. Someday I know she won't need me at all at bedtime, and I will miss snuggling with her."

As we follow families like this over the years, we find that one word describes them best: "thriving!" These babies and children not only get bigger, they thrive, which means growing optimally — physically, emotionally, and intellectually. The parents thrive, too. They become astute and sensitive disciplinarians, and they truly enjoy being with their children. A deep trust and mutual respect between parents and child grow out of this early investment in nighttime parenting.

If you have a newborn or you are expecting a baby soon and would like to give your baby a healthy sleep start by studying baby sleep like the Newborners did, try these six steps:

1. Choose your parenting style. Read about the attachment-parenting style of baby care on pages 70 to 73 and see how many of the Baby B's you want to practice. If your baby is not yet born, you will not be able to decide fully. Begin your parenting career with as many of these eight attachment tools as you can, and modify them to fit your baby's individual temperament and your lifestyle. Once you "get connected," you will naturally use all the other sleep strategies in ways that best fit your baby.

2. Get dad involved early. Read chapter 8, Twenty-three Nighttime Fathering Tips. The high-touch style of attachment parenting can lead to mother burnout unless dad shares some of the nighttime parenting.

3. Make the bed and bedroom safe and sleep-friendly for youselves and for baby:
• Start your nighttime parenting career off in the right bed. A king-size bed is a must, since, whether you expect it or not, nearly all infants, even toddlers, need to spend some time in their parents' bed during their journey toward nighttime independence.
• Turn on sounds to sleep by (see page 23).
• Darken the bedroom (see page 11).

- Dress your baby safely and comfortably for sleep (see page 76).
- Create a comfortable bedroom temperature (see page 12).

4. Try a variety of bedtime rituals. It's important to get your baby used to a variety of ways of going to sleep — and back to sleep — early on so you won't suffer from mother burnout. Study the bedtime rituals listed on pages 13 and 37.

5. Teach baby how to sleep for longer stretches. Early on, your baby will need you to parent him to sleep. As he grows into sleep maturity, teach him self-help tools to peacefully go to sleep — and back to sleep — without always needing your help. Especially in the early months, don't expect to put an awake baby down in a crib, pat him "night-night," and expect him to go to sleep. If your baby could talk, he would say, "No one has yet taught me how to go to sleep on my own. I'm just a baby." Study the stay-asleep-longer tools listed on page 30.

6. Make night feedings easier. For tips to both meet your baby's nighttime nutritional needs and get enough sleep yourself, study the night-feeding suggestions on page 137.

DOING IT DIFFERENTLY WITH THE NEXT BABY!

We're expecting our second baby. Now that we have an active toddler in the house, I want to find ways to sleep with our new baby but not have to nurse so much at night.

Let's meet the Doitdifferentlys. Don and Dana are expecting their second baby. Their first child, Daniel, is now three years old. The three have enjoyed the family bed from day one. Daniel is now weaned and sleeps in his "big boy" toddler bed on the floor next to mom and dad's bed. Don snuggles Daniel down to sleep every night.

As these parents sought counseling on sleeping better with the next baby, Dana confided, "Sleeping close to Daniel, and even the frequent night nursing, was a wonderful bonding experience. I wouldn't change it for the world. We are so close, and he is such a secure child. However, I do remember that his frequent night waking sometimes made me sleep-deprived, and I'd be cranky and resentful the next day. I don't want to be one of those moms who fall asleep at the wheel when driving the car pool. I need help figuring out a way to get more sleep with our next baby than I did with Daniel."

We praised Dana for having the wisdom to know her limitations and for planning ahead to prevent resentment before it occurred. She realized that she had to figure out a way to get more sleep at night in order to care for two children during the day.

During the first month, Don and Dana got to know their new baby. Dana naturally nursed Darcy whenever she wanted to be fed. Toward the end of the first month, with Darcy's first growth spurt and consequent marathon day-and-night nursing, Dana started thinking, "I'm going down the same road I did before. It wasn't a bad road with Daniel, but it was tiring."

With the new baby, can Dana breastfeed,

co-sleep, and get a better night's sleep herself? Yes she can, but right from the start, she will need to teach Darcy other ways of falling asleep, in addition to breastfeeding. To avoid going down the same tiring road as before, Dana and Don started using the following list of ways of helping baby thrive, while they also got Darcy used to other "nursings" to sleep. Here's what we advised:

Get dad involved early. Read chapter 8, Twenty-three Nighttime Fathering Tips. After reading these tips, Don learned not only how to "father-nurse" his baby but also how to help Dana get more rest so she could night-nurse more easily. In the first few months, Don's role was mainly to free Dana from many of the non-baby-care chores that would drain her energy away from the children. As Darcy got more used to accepting father's "nursings" at night, she stepped up her daytime feedings but did not demand to be breastfed so often at night.

> ## SEARS SLEEP TIP
>
> Don't tinker too much with the supply-and-demand recipe for successful breastfeeding. By being too forceful at scheduling too soon, you run the risk of not giving your baby enough milk.

Find ways to make nursing easier. Read the sections Fifteen Ways to Make Night Nursing Easier, pages 137 to 144, and Twelve Tips for Getting Baby to Nurse Less at Night, pages 149 to 155. If you teach baby how to cluster her feedings more during the day, her need to nurse at night will lessen, yet she'll still get enough nourishment to thrive.

When Dana nursed Darcy down to sleep and back to sleep when she awakened, she didn't nurse her completely to sleep. As Darcy was just about to fall asleep after nursing, Dana would do the "hand-off" to dad, who added the finishing touch by walking baby down in the neck nestle position (see page 177) and experimenting with a variety of "finishing touches" (see page 179). Don also took his nighttime fathering role seriously and found creative and effective ways to put Darcy down to sleep so she wouldn't get hooked on just breastfeeding to sleep.

Over the next few months when we saw the family for Darcy's regular checkups, they were happy to report that the above tips were working. Dana confided, "It's really not that we're giving Darcy less quality care than we gave Daniel, it's just that now we've learned some strategies to both meet her needs and get more rest ourselves."

BABY TRAINING

We went to a class that listed ways of getting baby on a predictable feeding schedule so she would sleep through the night. I'm tired, and this method sounded very convincing. Is it okay to put our baby on a set feeding schedule so she doesn't need to be fed so often, especially at night?

Let's now meet the Babytrainers, well-meaning, yet vulnerable, new parents who let themselves be convinced that scheduling was convenient and suitable.

One day new parents Bob and Betty brought in their three-month-old baby, Billy, for his routine checkup. When I talked with this family during previous exams, parents and baby seemed to be thriving, though the parents occasionally voiced their desire that Billy would sleep longer. At this visit I noticed several differences in the way the parents cared for baby Billy. First, they carried him in a plastic infant seat rather than wearing him in the baby sling as they had done at previous exams (Cry-It-Out clue number 1). Second, they put their baby down a few feet away from them and started talking to me without looking at their baby (CIO clue number 2). Then father proudly piped up, "We've got him trained to sleep through the night, and he's such a good baby. He rarely cries" (CIO clue number 3).

As I began examining this "good baby," I became concerned. There was no sparkle in his eyes. He didn't connect with me. His muscle tone was weak, and when I weighed him, I found that he had gained only a few ounces during the past month. I asked the parents what they were doing differently. They mentioned that they had gone to a baby-training class where, the father reported, "We learned how to get him to sleep through the night by letting him cry it out, and how to get him on a feeding schedule during the day so that he wouldn't control us." Mom added, "It was initially hard on me, but now I get more rest." Alarm bells went off in my head. This baby probably was not getting enough to eat. In addition, the baby had de-veloped what I call "shutdown syndrome," or failure to thrive. His basic biological cues were not being listened to, and his needs were not being met. So he had given up trying to connect with his caregivers.

Bob and Betty were caring, yet misled, parents. When I explained to them what was going on, they were wise enough to realize that their baby-training plan was not working for baby Billy. I asked them to go back to feeding their infant more frequently and wearing him in a baby sling like they used to. I advised them that sleeping through the night was not a reasonable expectation for a three-month-old. Basically, I asked them to soften and follow their hearts like they had done before they got sabotaged by the CIO crowd. We worked out a more sensitive way to help their baby sleep longer at night, using the tips described in chapter 1. When they returned a couple weeks later for a recheck, Billy's muscle tone had improved, he had gained weight, there was sparkle in his eyes, and the family seemed reconnected, though the father half jokingly admitted, "He's no longer such a 'good baby.'"

Be discerning about baby training. Observe these precautions:

- Baby training forces baby to sleep rather than teaching baby to sleep, just the opposite of our sleep-training philosophy.

- Neither a book nor a class should tell *you* when *your* baby needs to be fed. Only a hungry baby knows when he needs to be fed. Baby training teaches you to follow a book rather than learning on your own how to read your baby.

- Don't start too early. If you decide to do baby training or hire a "baby trainer," it's best to wait until baby is at least four months old. By that time, you will know your baby's individual sleep temperament. Also, if you undertake sleep training when baby is too young or if you do it too fast, baby runs the risk of not having enough feedings to thrive.

- Do your homework. Read Ages and Stages of Nursing at Night, page 134, to understand why babies, especially those who are breastfed, need to be fed frequently.

- Most baby-training methods are variations of the tired old cry-it-out theme. Be aware of the possible health consequences of scheduling a baby's feedings by the cry-it-out method (see chapter 10). Scheduling feedings too rigidly when baby is too young is risky. One of the most common causes of the failure-to-thrive syndrome is the parents' failure to listen to and respond to their baby's feeding cues. When babies are not listened to, they quit cueing their needs. As a result, baby gets less milk, mom therefore produces less milk, neither mother nor baby thrives.

Are all babies who go through CIO going to suffer a severe shutdown? Of course not. However, we have seen it often enough in our office, and research warns about enough negative effects of CIO that we strongly urge parents to find more sensitive alternatives. See chapter 10 for more suggestions.

BABY FIGHTS SLEEP

Our baby fights going to sleep. By 10 p.m. we're exhausted, but he's still awake. Help!

Meet the Sleepfighters. Steve and Sylvia came to our office for help with five-month-old Sammy. Steve and Sylvia's main concern with Sammy was that he wouldn't settle down easily at bedtime. They spent hours trying to get him down, but he fussed, squirmed, and just wouldn't give in to sleep. Here is how we helped them make bedtime easier.

1. Learn baby's tired time. As we discussed in chapter 1, taking advantage of baby's natural tired time to put him down to sleep makes the whole routine much easier. Sylvia wrote down Sammy's tired times every night for one week (the times he showed signs of being tired, not the times he ended up falling asleep). Sylvia wasn't surprised to find that these tired times varied from as early as 7:30 to as late as 10 p.m. There was no predictability to Sammy's evening tired times. We shared with Sylvia our ideas about scheduling baby's nap times to create a predictable bedtime (see chapter 9). Sylvia wasn't sure about this idea. She said, "I didn't really want to schedule Sammy's naps. I'm more of a play-it-by-ear kind of parent. I'm used to letting him nap whenever he wants. Nap scheduling sounds like a lot of work."

2. Focus on the timing of naps. Sylvia kept a journal of baby's naps for a week and found an obvious pattern. On the days that Sammy had a late-afternoon nap, he wasn't tired until ten that night. When an early-afternoon nap occurred, he was tired earlier in the evening. We asked Sylvia to take the next two weeks and do whatever it took to make sure Sammy napped around 2:30 each afternoon. Sylvia put her afternoon activities on hold for these two weeks as she got that nap time consistent. This also necessitated making sure the morning nap was consistent.

Some days when Sammy didn't seem likely to go down for a nap, Sylvia "tricked" him into napping, using our ideas in chapter 9, especially co-napping. Baby Sammy couldn't resist snuggling next to mom for some special high-touch time in the early afternoon. She tried her best to make sure he napped for at least an hour in the afternoon so that he was happy through the evening. Sylvia happily reported to us at the end of two weeks that Sammy started showing tired signs around 8 p.m. almost every night. We explained to her that once she learned what his tired time was, she could begin the bedtime routine about a half hour before this time so that when tired time hit, he would more easily fall asleep.

3. Create an environment conducive to sleep. Another key step for Steve and Sylvia to focus on was setting the stage for sleep very thoroughly. By using many of our ideas in chapter 1, they began to get Sammy used to this soothing environment as a prelude to sleep. When the tired signs came, Sammy would already be relaxed and ready for sleep before he could begin to fight it.

4. Try a variety of sleep routines. Steve and Sylvia used to take turns rocking, walking, and bouncing baby while he fought his way to sleep. They wished Sammy would learn to fall asleep on his own (an independent-based primary sleep association), but they were willing to use attachment-based associations if necessary. We suggested they spend the next week or two trying a number of different ways to lull baby to sleep (see pages 15 to 27). They would never know what would work best until they had tried them all. They borrowed a friend's baby swing to try and a cradle for a month. They laid him in the crib and shushed him down. They carried him around. They snuggled with him in bed. They made sure he was well fed, burped, and changed before they began the ritual. Many of these things they had already been doing, but now they were doing them at Sammy's natural tired time. Sylvia was thrilled to tell us, "Some of these rituals get him to sleep fairly quickly, especially when we use motion. He will even settle down and go to sleep in his crib, although it takes a bit longer."

They decided to take advantage of Sammy's love of motion and try the Amby Baby Motion Bed (see page 25). It worked like a charm. He now went to sleep fairly quickly and consistently every night around the same time. He usually awoke once each night, but Sylvia accepted this as a normal part of parenting.

HIGH-NEED SLEEPLESS BABY

Our baby is wired, day and night. She's calm as long as we hold her during the day and sleep close to her at night. We're exhausted! How can we get her to sleep for longer stretches?

Now let's meet the Highneeders. This family has been blessed with what we call a high-need baby (see page 76 for a discussion of baby personalities and sleep temperaments). Hugh and Harriet shared with us in the first month how much work their baby was both day and night. Now that baby Hannah is two months of age, they are looking to make nighttime easier. Here is how we worked out a plan with them:

1. Be realistic about baby's nighttime needs. We helped Hugh and Harriet understand Hannah's high need level. We suggested that she would be unlikely to sleep through the night in a crib in the next room at an early age. She would need more daytime and nighttime touch.

2. Find out where you and baby sleep best. Hugh and Harriet had Hannah's nursery all painted and furnished weeks before her birth, but baby wanted nothing to do with it. She wouldn't sleep for more than fifteen minutes in her crib. They bought a bassinet and let baby sleep right next to their bed, but she still awakened just as much. We suggested they try the one thing they'd been reluctant to do: let Hannah sleep with them in their bed. They didn't like this idea. They had envisioned an easy baby who would easily learn to sleep alone, but our explanation of what a high-need baby is made sense to them, so they were willing to give it a try. Hannah slept better in their bed but still woke every one and one-half to two hours, and the only way she would go back to sleep was to nurse. Hugh and Harriet tried her in

her crib again, with the mattress slightly upright at our suggestion (in case her waking was caused by reflux, or heartburn, as illustrated in our next story). Hannah didn't buy it. She demanded to sleep snuggled close. Like many dads, Hugh couldn't sleep in a bed with a baby that tossed and turned all night, so he set up a mattress on the floor of baby's nursery (ironic, isn't it?), where he got a full night's sleep. (We don't advocate dads sleeping separately, yet in the early months many dads choose an occasional solo sleep night if they anticipate a busy workday.)

3. Learn baby's tired times. Hugh and Harriet knew that Hannah routinely got tired and would nurse to sleep around 10 p.m. They tried changing her nap times so that she'd go to sleep earlier, but she seemed innately wired to stay awake through the evening. They decided just to go with what worked and not to try to force an earlier bedtime.

4. Get baby to accept more than one way to fall asleep. When Hannah was three months old, Harriet gave us an update: "Honestly, the baby sleeps very well. As long as she is in my arms or the baby sling for naps, or snuggled up in bed next to me at night, she's happy. She wakes every hour or two to nurse, and as long as I respond quickly, she nurses right back to sleep."

Harriet looked tired but was happily adjusting to her role as a very involved mother. She seemed willing to give whatever it took to help Hannah thrive with her high-need personality. She admitted to us that there were drawbacks: "It would be nice to sleep in the same bed as my husband. It would be nice to have twenty minutes to myself once a day. It would be nice to sleep more than two hours straight without having her attached to my breast."

We assured Harriet that her investment would pay off. She was helping a very energetic and intelligent baby thrive into a self-confident, outgoing, head-of-the-class type of child. Yet we shared with her two very important pieces of advice for parents of a high-need baby:

- Avoid mother burnout.
- Share the daytime and nighttime parenting with dad.

Because high-need babies turn into high-need toddlers who then turn into high-need preschoolers who finally mature into confident, outgoing older children, it was critical that Hannah learn to be equally bonded to both parents. She needed to feel comfortable being parented by Hugh so that Harriet could take a break and avoid eventual burnout. We made a few suggestions that have worked with many high-need families:

- Try to get baby comfortable falling asleep in dad's arms or in the baby sling with dad. (See chapter 8, Twenty-three Nighttime Fathering Tips.)
- See if baby can learn to fall asleep without always nursing, but with rocking and walking instead. (See Fifteen Ways to Make Night Nursing Easier, page 137.)

- Have dad hold baby as much as possible, and especially get baby used to being worn in the baby sling.

Hugh confided that he was tempted to urge Harriet to just let the baby cry it out. We shared with him our concerns about crying it out (see chapter 10) and the simple fact that crying it out is not for high-need babies. A baby as persistent as Hannah will just keep crying harder.

Hugh and Hannah spent a few weeks focusing on the nighttime (and daytime) fathering techniques we present in chapter 8. Instead of feeling shut out of the parenting relationship, Hugh decided to jump right in and take on a more sensitive and supportive role. Hugh tried to give Hannah a bottle of pumped milk one night, but she rejected it. He took on more nap-time and nighttime duty on the weekend, often wearing Hannah in the sling so Harriet wouldn't need to. Some fathering techniques worked well and kept Hannah happy, but sometimes she demanded mom, no matter what. At least Harriet did get a break from time to time.

The one thing that they couldn't change, however, was Hannah's need to snuggle close to a parent during sleep and to nurse several times during the night. Hugh still often sleeps in the next room, and he continues to take on some nighttime fathering duties when Harriet burns out. When friends jokingly ask, "So when are you having a second baby?" Hugh and Harriet always laugh the loudest.

5. Help baby stay asleep longer. Harriet used every technique we suggested, but still

Hannah would go to sleep and back to sleep at night only by nursing. But by three years of age, Hannah learned to fall asleep and stay asleep without nursing, and all family members finally slept through the night. Years later, after sharing glowing reports about Hannah's school progress, both parents told us, "It was a long, hard road, but we're seeing the rewards of our investment!"

PAINFUL NIGHT WAKING

Our baby wakes up a lot shrieking, not just crying. I just know something is wrong with him. Help!

Let's meet the Refluxer family. We met them when their baby was two months old. He had been waking up every hour since three weeks of age, and he wouldn't nap for more than thirty minutes when lying down. Rawly is a thriving breastfed baby who is easygoing and happy most of the day. He just won't sleep long without waking up crying, unless his mom or dad is holding him. Then he'll sleep for hours.

First, instead of immediately pigeonholing this baby into the category of "bad sleep habits" or "conditioned night waker," we listened carefully to the clues his astute parents, Rhonda and Ralph, provided.

The Refluxers' story immediately set off an alarm in our heads that suggested gastroesophageal reflux (GER). GER occurs when milk and stomach acid move up into the esophagus and throat and cause painful burning, and therefore night waking. Baby Rawly had some classic signs:

- He woke up frequently when lying down but slept well when held upright in a parent's arms (in the upright position, gravity keeps food and acid in the stomach).
- He cried when laid down flat but would sit happily for long periods of time when upright in an infant seat.
- His parents knew instinctively that their baby awoke because he hurt somewhere.

Ralph and Rhonda shared with us that their friends had told them to let Rawly cry it out, to stop tending to him at night, and to stop spoiling him. Their previous doctor called the problem "colic" and didn't mention GER. Rawly didn't have some of the other classic signs of GER (see chapter 11 for a fuller discussion). His type of GER is called "silent GER," and is often missed. Thankfully, Ralph and Rhonda listened to their intuition and came looking for answers. We went over the clues that can indicate a medical cause of night waking (see page 214), such as GER and intolerances to particular foods in a breastfeeding mother's diet (oftentimes these two causes are both present). After a few weeks of trying all the treatments listed on pages 217 to 221, they found that Rawly slept best in the Amby Baby Motion Bed (see page 25). Its upright position and gentle rocking motion helped to minimize his reflux and easily soothed him back to sleep.

WON'T SLEEP WELL IN A CRIB

Our three-month-old is still waking up every few hours, and we're tired of stum-

bling down the hallway to get him back to sleep. How can we get more sleep?

Welcome our new patients, the Sleepaloners. Sam and Susan have been trying to get a good night's sleep ever since baby Sal was born three months ago, and it's just not happening. He has been sleeping in his crib in the nursery, and Sam and Susan had hoped he would be like some of her friends' babies — sleeping through the night by now. Three months of stumbling down the hallway several times each night to put him back to sleep have left Susan tired and cranky during the day. She wants him to stop waking up so much.

We shared with Sam and Susan that each baby has unique nighttime needs and that Sal might need a different nighttime parenting style than her friends' easy sleepers needed. We also reminded them of the many normal reasons that babies wake up at night (page 62). We suggested they start over at square one with baby and take our sleep plan step by step. Here's how we helped them get more sleep.

1. Rule out a medical cause of night waking. We asked Susan several questions to make sure Sal didn't have a hidden medical cause of night waking (see chapter 11). We determined he probably did not.

2. Create an environment conducive to sleep. Sam really wanted Sal to stay in his own room and crib, so Susan and he followed all our recommendations on pages 76 to 77 and 80 to 81 to make the sleeping environment both comfortable and safe.

3. Be wary about replacing breast milk with formula at night. Sam surprised Susan by volunteering to give Sal a middle-of-the-night bottle. "Because he's in part-time day care, he gets one or two bottles of formula on those days," he said. "Why not give him one at night, too? His tummy will stay full and he might sleep longer." Susan had been breastfeeding Sal every time he woke up because he seemed hungry and she found it much easier to give him the breast than to mix a bottle during the night.

We offered a word of caution: Nursing at night helps maintain mom's milk supply, especially since she works away from home some days. The more formula you give, the less breast milk mom will make. We explained that Sal was doing what any smart baby would do: breastfeeding more at night to make up for the feeding he missed during the day. We advised Susan to tank him up with more "cluster feeds" before bedtime (see tips on how to cluster feed, page 139) and increase the frequency and duration of nursing on days she didn't go to work. We went through the night-nursing-made-easier tips on pages 137 to 144.

4. Open your box of sleep tools. One week later, Susan reported that Sal was still waking up every two to three hours. We went through the many sleep tools that they could use to help Sal stay asleep longer (see pages 20 to 26). Susan and Sam tried them all and found that using white noise and leaving a used nursing pad in the crib helped some.

Then teething pain began at four months, and Sal began waking up even more. We offered ways to treat Sal's teething pain (see page 228), and they helped, but not enough. Susan told us she was burning out and was worried that Sal wasn't learning to be a good sleeper.

Step 5. Determine where baby sleeps best. We offered advice that seemed drastic to Sam but made good sense to Susan. We suggested that it was likely their baby was stressed by sleeping alone. We explained that long-term sleep stress is very unhealthy for babies. We posed the question, Would Sal sleep longer and happier if he were closer to his favorite people in the world? Susan confided, "I've always wondered if he'd sleep better in our room, and maybe even in our bed. Sam has resisted this suggestion because he doesn't want to get stuck with the baby in our bed for years. But I'm the one who usually gets up with Sal during the night. I need more sleep!"

We asked Sam if he'd rather have a baby who sleeps very well in their room or bed or a baby who keeps waking up stressed. We shared with him the many advantages of sleep sharing (see chapter 5). He saw our point but worried that letting Sal sleep near them would create a long-term bad habit. We agreed that it would create a long-term "habit," but not necessarily a bad one. We reassured Sam that many babies sleep close to their parents, and all these babies eventually do move out of their parents' bed.

We explained the various co-sleeping options (see pages 5 to 8), and Susan decided to bring Sal right into their bed. We advised them how to do this safely (see page 77). After a few nights in bed with mom and dad,

Sal woke up less often and fell back to sleep more easily because mom tended to him more quickly. More important, mom's sleep was less disrupted because she didn't have to get up.

Sam, however, wasn't happy. Sal's squirming, grunting, and breathing kept him awake much of the night. He hung in there for a week because he saw Susan was getting more rest, but then he had had enough. He needed sleep in order to function well at work, so he ended up sleeping on a futon in Sal's room for a few nights. He was not happy about that either. Susan was torn between her need for sleep and Sam's and her need for a close marriage. She decided to try another sleep option with Sal nearby.

They tried the Arm's Reach Co-Sleeper, which we have seen work very well for many families (see page 127). Sam was able to sleep a lot better back in bed with Susan, since he didn't feel Sal's squirming.

Now Susan reports that in the co-sleeper he still wakes up twice each night. She breastfeeds him at each waking, but she feels more rested, Sam is more relaxed, and things are overall much better than before. They think this may be because baby is sleeping closer but not too close. They still wish that Sal would wake up at night only once, or, even better, not at all — that's what their neighbor's baby does.

NURSING ALL NIGHT

I love nursing our baby to sleep, but she still wakes up every two to three hours at night and won't go back to sleep without

nursing. I'm burning out! What I don't know is just how long this night-waking pattern is going to last. I don't mind a couple more months of this, but I'll go crazy if she's still doing this at nine months or fifteen months.

Meet the Nightnursers. Six-month-old Nicole has been sleeping with Nathan and Nancy since birth. They found this arrangement natural for them, and Nancy knew there would be some night nursing involved. Nancy knows sometimes Nicole is hungry and needs to be fed, but baby Nicole has developed a habit of waking more often than Nancy can cope with.

Babies who night-nurse seem to follow one of two courses: They either naturally begin to sleep longer stretches and wake only once or twice to feed (and mom gets enough sleep), or they develop a habit of waking up more frequently because they know they get to, and love to, nurse. And mom *may* get burned out. In the early months of breast-feeding, when babies need to feed at night, it's impossible to know which babies will gradually nurse less as they get older and which ones will continue to wake up because they are conditioned to expect the comfort of nursing.

So what can Nathan and Nancy do right now with their six-month-old that will ensure less night waking down the road? The main thing they are going to do is help baby Nicole learn to fall asleep and go back to sleep without breastfeeding. By changing her association between sleep and feeding, they hope she will wake less at night because she knows she

won't always get to nurse. Here's how we helped them work through their individual sleep plan:

Step 1. Decide if night nursing is a problem for you. We counseled Nathan and Nancy that many breastfed babies need one or two night feedings during the first six months of life. Baby Nicole has been demanding three or four feeds, and she showed no signs of letting up. We knew that someday she would sleep longer, but Nancy confided in us that she wasn't one of those moms who can just hang in there and wait it out. She needed a change now!

Step 2. Evaluate where baby is sleeping. It helps to try various arrangements if baby isn't sleeping well in your current setting. Some families find putting baby to sleep a short distance away, such as in a co-sleeper or a crib next to the bed, will help baby wake less often. Other babies will sleep more soundly in a different room altogether.

Nathan and Nancy were happy having baby Nicole sleep in their bed. They wanted to work through the rest of the plan without changing their sleeping arrangement.

3. Create an environment conducive to sleep. Nathan and Nancy knew that if Nicole was going to fall back to sleep at night easily, she would need a soothing setting to fall asleep in. By reading through the options on pages 10 through 13, they gained several new ideas they could use to make Nicole's nighttime environment more sleepy.

4. Evaluate the bedtime ritual. Nancy told us that she always nursed Nicole to sleep. We shared our thoughts about sleep associations (see page 16) and explained that this was a very natural choice for a breastfeeding pair. However, if she now wanted to decrease night feedings, she needed to change Nicole's association between breastfeeding and sleeping. She could gradually and sensitively help her learn other ways to fall asleep. Nancy and Nathan both felt they wanted Nicole to learn attachment-based sleep associations, but they wanted to see if this could occur without always breastfeeding.

They spent two weeks trying many of our sleep-association rituals (see pages 13 to 26), writing down what worked best in their journal. They found that Nicole fell asleep the fastest when being carried around or rocked (no surprise!). Nancy told us that this routine actually took more work than simply sitting down and breastfeeding her to sleep, and we advised that she could choose to go back to breastfeeding. But Nancy really wanted to help Nicole learn other sleep associations and was willing to keep trying. Nathan and Nancy hoped that once Nicole got used to falling asleep without feeding, she would wake up to feed less at night.

We made sure Nathan and Nancy were equipped with ways to lay baby down once she was asleep (see page 208).

5. Learn baby's tired time. Since Nathan and Nancy chose to get baby Nicole to sleep at bedtime without breastfeeding, they took some time to learn her consistent tired times (see page 8) and used this information to their advantage.

6. Take measures to lessen night nursing. Now that Nathan and Nancy had considered making some changes to Nicole's bedtime ritual, we focused on their main concern — her frequent night waking to breastfeed. We knew that when moms get burned out on night nursing, they are tempted to let baby cry it out. As an alternative, we offered Nancy twelve tips to lessen night nursing (see page 149) that don't involve excessive crying.

She and Nathan worked on these methods for a month and came back to discuss their progress. "She's still waking up every few hours and won't go back to sleep unless I breastfeed her," Nancy told us. "I tried a pacifier, rocking, walking, a water bottle — everything! She fusses until I give her the breast. I followed your suggestions on nap nursing to catch up on my sleep, and I tanked her up with more frequent feedings during the day, but she's still waking up to feed."

We noticed she said "I" did all this, so we asked Nathan how he was involved in the nighttime parenting. "What can I do?" he said. "I don't have breasts, and that's all the baby wants at night."

It was time to get dad involved. We discussed with Nathan our ideas on nighttime fathering in chapter 8. Nathan spent the next few weekends following many of our ideas to get baby Nicole to accept him as a substitute when falling asleep for daytime naps. He sometimes got up at night and "father-nursed" Nicole back to sleep. As expected, she took longer to get back to sleep without nursing and often spent several minutes fussing in dad's arms. This understandably led to frustration on Nathan's part. "At three in the morning, I hand her back to Nancy and say, "Just nurse her back to sleep, please!" he said.

We encouraged Nathan to hang in there. Eventually Nicole would learn that she had two parents and come to accept either one to comfort her back to sleep. After a while Nathan found that he could successfully get Nicole back to sleep about half the time. Nancy felt that at least once a night Nicole truly seemed hungry, and she couldn't imagine withholding food from her in the name of getting better sleep. Nancy decided to get out of bed with baby and nurse in the rocking chair (so baby would learn that nursing didn't occur in bed) once each night. She also started giving her baby food (Nicole was seven months old now) and hoped this would help keep her tummy full through the night. Nathan also kept a sippy cup with water or pumped breast milk handy to see if this would get her back to sleep without waking mom.

Step 7. Help baby stay asleep longer.
Nancy shared with us that Nicole at eight months was only waking up twice each night. Because she had learned that breastfeeding no longer happened while lying in bed, Nancy and Nathan could often get her back to sleep using our suggestions on pages 27 to 30, such as gentle shushing, laying on of hands, and offering a pacifier on occasion. Nancy was able to cope with the one long breastfeeding

each night in the rocking chair. As expected, Nicole gradually woke up less often to nurse once Nathan and Nancy taught her other ways to go to sleep and back to sleep.

READY TO LET BABY CRY IT OUT

Our whole family is falling apart because of sleep deprivation. I'm depressed, and our marriage is suffering. We have tried everything we can think of to get our night-nursing baby to sleep more. Is it okay to use the cry-it-out approach as a last resort? Is there a sensitive way to do this?

Say hello to the Burnouters. I recently saw tired parents Ben and Barbara and their son, Brian, for sleep counseling. Ben is an obstetrician, and Barbara is a full-time mother, and they had driven an hour and a half to talk with me about Brian's frequent night nursing. At eighteen months he was still waking up every two hours during the night to nurse, and this was keeping Barbara from getting the sleep she needed. When the family came into my office, I observed that the baby was thriving but the parents looked absolutely wiped out. I realized how serious the family's sleep deprivation was when Barbara revealed that she had almost fallen asleep at the wheel the other day. They needed a solution to their toddler's night waking, and they needed it NOW!

I was happy that Ben had come along for this consultation. In my experience, mothers tend to downplay the impact of baby's sleep patterns on the family's health. Dads tend to be more honest about the situation.

First I observed the family dynamics. Barbara was a very nurturing, yet supersensitive mother. If Brian made so much as a peep, she would scoop him up in a millisecond and nurse him. She told me, "It's just easier for me to comfort him before he gets so worked up. I refuse to let him cry. I just can't." Ben told me that Barbara was so tired that she was becoming depressed and was considering taking antidepressant medication. He, too, was tired at work, and their marriage was suffering. Basically, the whole family was falling apart because of lack of sleep. Many kids ago we learned an important survival principle: IF YOU RESENT IT, CHANGE IT! When the whole family is falling apart, it's time to take some action.

Ben was proposing that they just let Brian cry. Barbara didn't want to do this. I found myself in a dilemma. On the one hand, I couldn't agree with dad's remedy of putting the baby in his crib, closing the door, and letting him cry. (The first day in medical school I learned "First, do no harm!") On the other hand, things couldn't continue the way they were. I had seen Ben and Barbara once before and had given them some sleep advice, but apparently this approach had not helped. The situation had reached a point where mom's need for sleep had to take priority. So, these are the steps we went through:

1. Understand the problem. I explained to Barbara and Ben that Brian had become a conditioned night nurser. He was so accustomed to nursing to sleep and nursing back to sleep when he woke up in the middle of the night that he didn't know any other way

to relax and go to sleep. So he stayed attached to mom's breast for much of the night. (In reviewing baby's early history, I suspected that Brian had had GER in the early months and that this had taught him that sleep was a painful state. He had outgrown the GER, but the anxiety about falling asleep remained. See page 163 for explanation of post-GER conditioning.)

2. Realize when a change needs to be made. It took a while to gently convince Barbara that what her baby needed most was a happy and rested mother and that she couldn't be the good mother she wanted to be if she didn't get some sleep. Barbara and Ben were aware of the saying "If Mom ain't happy, ain't nobody happy!" but Barbara had been willing to set aside her own need for sleep to keep her baby content at night. With her husband's support, she finally agreed that her need to sleep was the priority here. I reassured her that turning over nighttime parenting responsibilities to dad didn't mean that she was an uncaring or insensitive mother. On the contrary, she was ultimately doing what was best for her baby.

3. Work out a plan. I first reassured Barbara that the plan I was suggesting was not the standard cry-it-out program of nighttime neglect. We would like to call this the "no-fuss sleep plan," but let's be honest. Of course a high-need baby with a persistent personality is going to protest when his favorite all-night diner shortens its hours and his favorite waiter takes a break. The critical difference with our plan was that Brian would not be left to cry *alone*. I was also careful not to offer these tired parents a quick fix. I explained to them that this problem could not be solved overnight and that it might take a month or two before Brian learned to sleep in five- or six-hour stretches. Here is what I suggested Ben and Barbara do to help Brian learn to sleep better:

Barbara would continue nursing Brian frequently during the day. She would continue wearing him in the baby sling and doing all the other things she had been doing that had built their close attachment. Ben would start putting Brian to sleep at night. At first Barbara and Ben would use the "finishing touch" technique described on page 179. Barbara would nurse Brian until he was *almost asleep* and then hand him off to Ben to complete the process with rocking, shushing, and whatever else it took. When Ben was home, he would also take care of getting Brian down for naps.

When Brian woke and cried at night, Ben would be in charge of helping him go back to sleep. He would be the "father nurser." Fortunately, Ben was ready and willing to do this. He planned to take a week off from work so that he wouldn't have to worry about getting enough sleep. Barbara would sleep in a room away from baby.

I could see that this part of the plan made Barbara uneasy. She did not want Brian to cry at night. I explained to her, "Allowing a baby to cry in someone's arms is vastly different from leaving a baby alone to cry in a crib. Crying in the arms of someone he knows and trusts is not the same as crying it out alone." It could be called CIDA — crying in dad's arms. (If there is no dad in the house, some-

one else whom baby is close to could step in.) I prepared Barbara that because she had been sensitively responsive to Brian, it would be hard for her to hear Brian crying, even though she'd know he was with his dad. Ben and I reassured her that if he saw that Brian was "over the edge," he would come get her. (Fortunately, Ben was a nurturing dad.)

In a follow-up conversation a month later, the parents happily reported that Brian was sleeping longer and that Barbara was getting more rest. The whole family was now thriving. Barbara reported that allowing Ben to struggle with comforting Brian at night was one of the hardest things she had ever done, but she had come to see that there was more than one way to comfort Brian at night. She had moved beyond the unrealistic ideal that she had to be the only night nurser and had found a practical solution to Brian's sleep problem.

Ben confided that it had been hard for him, too. "It was so hard to hold a crying, arching baby when I knew that if Barbara just nursed him, he would go right to sleep. But now Brian and I are closer than we ever have been, and I have a lot more confidence in my ability to calm him."

Depending on your baby, your family situation, and your own gut feeling as a parent, you might choose to try letting your baby fuss — but in a way that respects his need to be responded to. Here are some guidelines to follow:

- Try other approaches first — and give them time to work. Go through our step-by-step approach in chapters 1 and 2. Realize that teaching your child to sleep better by any method will take time and dedication on your part.

- Check the causes of night waking in chapter 11 before trying the crying-in-dad's-arms approach. You need to be sure that your baby's night waking is not caused by a medical problem.

- Don't try the CIDA approach unless you believe that in your particular family situation it is necessary for you and your baby. The older your baby is when you do this, the better. A baby under eighteen months will have trouble handling this kind of frustration. If you try it with a baby younger than that, be very careful to watch for the warning signs we describe on page 211. Don't persist with a failing experiment. Be alert for changes in your baby's behavior during the day. If your observations and your "parent gut" tell you this is too hard on your baby (and only you can tell), try something else. Experiment with other alternatives. If they don't work, try this approach again when baby is more mature and accepting.

- Don't leave baby to cry alone in a room. With our approach, baby cries in the arms of a nurturing caregiver. Even if baby can't have mom, he needs *someone*.

- Increase your nurturing and attachment during the daytime.

- Remember, it takes time. Do not follow anyone else's preset schedule. Your baby has unique needs, and you have a unique sensitivity to those needs. One top-selling sleep-training book answers the question "How long can I let my baby cry?" with "one hour"! The book doesn't know the effects of an hour of crying on a particular baby. An hour, even five minutes for a younger baby, is like a hopeless eternity. If, when, and how long to let your baby cry in dad's arms is a cry-by-cry call. Again, only the people who know the baby very well can make the right call.

- Focus on night-to-night progress, not on the achievement of a fixed goal, such as "sleeping through the night within a week." Expect to take two steps forward and one step back. If baby gets a cold or a tummy ache, is teething hard, or is being weaned from the breast, or even if you take a trip or have visitors, expect that her nighttime needs will increase for a time.

Remember, parenting is a long-term investment. Listen to your babies when they are young, and they will listen to you when they are older.

THE FADE-AWAY STRATEGY: AN ALTERNATIVE TO THE CRY-IT-OUT METHOD

My baby wakes up too much at night, and I really need him to learn to sleep more independently. I just can't function on so little sleep.

Meet Sara Sleepdeprived. Her baby was eight months old and slept fairly well in a crib in the early months, but then his night waking became too much for Sara to manage. She didn't want to turn to her husband, Steve, for help, because he worked long hours and was often away on business. Sara was a responsive parent, and she had never felt the cry-it-out approach was for her. We helped her work through the various suggestions in chapters 1 and 2 and excluded medical causes of night waking by going through the topics in chapter 11. Yet, after another month, Sara was running out of steam, and she felt she needed a faster solution. We helped her work through the fade-away technique in a sensitive way that didn't involve intense crying alone.

Sara laid her baby, Sam, in his crib just before tired time. She soothed him with a gentle massage, lullabies, soft music, and other methods she had learned in steps 3 and 4 of the sleep plan in chapter 1. As baby's sleepy signs set in, she continued whatever soothing measures were needed (such as rhythmic patting, humming, and laying on of hands) to keep baby relaxed. When Sam began to fuss, she continued comforting him but did not pick him up for a minute or two during the mild fussy phase. Sometimes he would calm down and fall asleep, but often he wouldn't.

If Sam's fussing escalated, she picked him up because she took this as a sure sign that he wasn't going to easily settle. She walked around the room with him to calm him, then laid him back down in the crib and continued her soothing techniques. The goal was for Sam to fall asleep while lying in the crib, not in mom's arms. Sometimes he needed to be picked back up several times before finally settling. On the nights when this seemed to

go on forever, Sara gave in and comforted Sam to sleep by walking around or rocking him in her arms until he was in a deep sleep. Sometimes she fed Sam, because with all that fussing, he had worked up an appetite.

Sara found over time that she didn't need to pick Sam up as often, as he learned to fall asleep in the crib with only gentle patting and soothing. Once Sam was used to falling asleep easily on a routine basis, Sara began to lessen the amount of physical contact she gave him, and he gradually learned to fall asleep with less hands-on comforting. The nights when fussing escalated and she had to pick him up became fewer. Once Sam was used to this, Sara began moving herself away from the crib. She sat in a chair, and every night she moved the chair farther away from the crib while she sang lullabies or talked softly to Sam. Soon she was able to quietly slip out of the room after Sam's tired signs set in and she'd tucked him in. She did need to quietly step back into the room from time to time, and sometimes she needed to hum or talk in the hallway so that Sam would know she was there.

Once Sam learned to easily fall asleep in the crib, Sara used this same technique to teach him to settle himself back to sleep in the middle of the night when he awoke. She gradually lessened her level of interaction with him, and he gradually learned to wake up less often.

She carefully observed Sam for any warning signs that he was not handling this transition well emotionally. By ten months of age, Sam slept through the night (and so did Sara), and he continues to thrive physically and emotionally. (See page 161 for more fade-away strategies.)

The Joys of Sleeping with Your Baby

AH, THE SIMPLE PLEASURES of nestling next to mommy!" If babies could talk, this is what they would say about the oldest sleeping arrangement in the world — co-sleeping. When we are asked "Where should baby sleep?" our usual reply is "Baby should sleep where all family members sleep the best." But where would babies themselves prefer sleeping? Suppose you were a baby. Would you rather sleep alone behind bars in a dark room or snuggled close to your favorite person in the whole wide world? The choice is obvious.

Not only do babies give the family bed the thumbs-up, so do mothers. Most mothers cherish the special closeness of sharing sleep with baby. At international parenting meetings we asked mothers from other countries what they thought about sleeping with their baby. They found this question as odd as should they breastfeed their baby. Mothers whose opinions are not skewed by American sleep books and "sleep experts" do not regard co-sleeping (or breastfeeding) as optional. They believe it's the only natural thing to do.

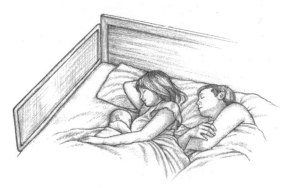

Even in Western cultures, many mothers we have interviewed feel the same way. As one mother volunteered, "Just because it's night-time, that doesn't mean my baby needs me any less."

It's not only mothers who instinctively feel that their babies belong near them at night. Many fathers feel likewise:

When my husband entered our bedroom and saw our newborn lying alone in the bassinet next to our bed, he said, "Our son is sleeping in THAT? He will get cold, and how will we know that he's breathing?" My husband took our son out of the bassinet and brought him into our bed.

Even sleep experts believe that babies belong with their parents. In a conversation with Dr. James McKenna, director of the Mother-Baby Behaviorial Sleep Laboratory at the University of Notre Dame, and a leading expert on mother-infant co-sleeping, I voiced my amazement that in some circles co-sleeping is considered weird, even unsafe. Dr. McKenna replied that crib sleeping is what should be considered abnormal and unsafe. We believe he is right, and later in this chapter we tell you why.

Sleeping with your baby is a natural part of the whole parenting package, and it fits in well with modern lifestyles. Co-sleeping is becoming more popular in today's society, partly because more mothers are breastfeeding, and co-sleeping makes nighttime breastfeeding much easier. Employed mothers who are away from their babies for long hours during the day have also made co-sleeping popular.

You may choose not to sleep with your baby, but no Sears book would be complete without the message of this chapter. If you want to know how we have parented our babies at night, this chapter will tell you. We practice what we preach in these pages.

Though we are known for being advocates of parent-infant co-sleeping, we haven't been so "preachy" about co-sleeping in the other chapters of this book. We have written *The Baby Sleep Book* to help all kinds of parents with sleep problems, no matter what parenting style they use. We understand that where your baby sleeps is a very personal choice. We want to help everybody be more sensitive to their baby's nighttime needs. And we want everyone to get a good night's sleep, too.

SLEEP ANXIETY

The deeper we get into our sleep counseling, the more we see a condition we call "sleep anxiety" — in babies and mothers. Recent studies have shown that sleeping alone may not be in the best physiological or emotional interest of a baby, especially in the early months. In experiments, infant animals separated from their mothers exhibit a higher level of stress hormones (see page 111). Could a baby sleeping alone become an anxious sleeper? Dr. James McKenna has videotaped infants and mothers sleeping in various arrangements. His solo sleepers are often fitful sleepers, even though they may not always completely awaken.

Sleeping apart from her baby could cause a mother to become an anxious sleeper because, either consciously or subconsciously, she feels uneasy with this arrangement. Intuitively, mother feels baby belongs close to her at night. Yet, due to the dire warnings of sleep-training books and societal norms, she may join the separate-sleeping set. Could this feeling of unease, in both mother and baby, be one of the causes of sleep problems?

Honestly, there is nothing better than having my baby in bed with me in the morning and waking up with slobbery "raspberries" (his favorite thing to do in the whole world), or hearing him babble "da da da" over and over. I know it won't last, so I'm trying to soak up as much "touch time" as I can.

We know that some of you love sleeping with your babies and wouldn't trade it for the world. If you have read other books we've written, you have found only encouragement and support for this style of nighttime parenting. This particular book, however, is also written for parents who may not be sharing sleep with their baby, so we offer a broader range of approaches. We would ask you to notice, though, that nowhere do we encourage parents to try the cry-it-out-alone method of getting their baby to sleep. While we feel that there are other ways to meet babies' needs at night, our hearts (and our brains) tell us that this is not one of them.

We are going to say things in this chapter that support co-sleeping to the fullest. We are going to report on what research has shown about the benefits of co-sleeping. If you are undecided about co-sleeping, then read this chapter and consider what we have to say. You may still decide not to co-sleep. In other parts of this book, we'll show you how to sleep separately from your baby in a way that still recognizes and meets your baby's needs. Those of you who are already sure that you don't want to sleep with your baby, consider yourselves warned: Read this chapter at your own risk. It may change your mind and convince you to start sleeping with your baby.

OUR CO-SLEEPING EXPERIENCES

Our first three babies were easy sleepers. There was really no demand for them to share our bed, except for the occasional early-morning snuggle when they were awake before we were ready to get up. Then along came our fourth child, Hayden, in 1978. Right from the start, we knew she had a different temperament. She slept fine for six months in her cradle right next to Martha, waking two (now and then three) times a night to nurse. Then she graduated to a crib across the room. Hayden hated her crib and woke more and more often. Finally, one night, out of sheer exhaustion from being up every hour, Martha brought Hayden into our bed, and they both slept. All Hayden needed was to be close to Martha, and from that night on, we all slept much better — together. We slept so happily together that we did it for four years, until our next baby was born.

Even as we ventured into this "daring" sleeping arrangement, we were aware of what the baby books said. They all preached the same old tired theme: Don't take your baby into your bed. Martha said, "I don't care what the books say, I'm tired and I need some sleep!" We had to get past all those worries and warnings about our baby manipulating us and about terminal nighttime dependency. You're probably familiar with the long litany of "you'll-be-sorry" reasons. Well, we were not sorry; we were happy. As we write this book, Hayden and her husband, Jason, are sharing sleep with our one-year-old granddaughter, Ashton.

Here's what Hayden wrote just after the birth of her daughter:

Our first night together outside my womb was very tender. She slept so peacefully nestled up against me in our bed. She was only inches away from where she had spent the last nine months. Maybe her peaceful demeanor came from the familiarity of my body movements, breathing, heartbeat, smell, voice, and touch.

Sleeping with Hayden opened our hearts and minds to a nighttime parenting style that is as old as the human race but that was new to us. We learned that there is more than one way to care for babies at night and that tired parents need to be flexible and use whatever arrangement gets all family members the best night's sleep. Over the next fifteen years, we slept with four more of our babies (one at a time). While it's nice now to have the bed to ourselves, our minds are full of beautiful nighttime memories of sharing that bed with our children.

We must have made sleeping with our young ones look not only normal but pleasant, because our other grandchildren's parents, Dr. Bob and Dr. Jim and their wives, Cheryl and Diane, have also enjoyed sleep sharing in their families. Here is Bob's story:

When Cheryl and I first got married, she thought my parents were crazy. "I'm not going to have a baby in our bed," she stated firmly. I didn't co-sleep with my parents when I was a baby, but I'd seen them do this with my younger brothers and sisters. I wasn't sure what I wanted to do with my own kids. I just figured we'd wait and see.

When child number one came along, he spent the first night in his cradle next to our bed. Well, at least that was the plan. After Andrew woke up six times in the first five hours, I

finally said, "Why don't you just keep him next to you and let me sleep?" (Yes, I was a compassionate, self-sacrificing, I'm-right-there-with-you-honey type of husband even back then.) She kept Andrew in bed next to her, and I slept the rest of the night. So did she. So did baby Andrew. The two of them slept until ten o'clock the next morning. And we all slept wonderfully for the next two years, though we were a little squished in our queen-size bed. (Note: Get a king! It's worth it!) Oh, and Cheryl doesn't say that my parents are crazy anymore (at least not with regard to co-sleeping).

The crib ended up being used as a nice laundry basket in "Andrew's room." I put Andrew's room in quotes because I don't think he ever went in there. It ended up being the extra room where we folded laundry, stacked books and boxes, and stashed anything else we didn't know what to do with. We ended up selling the crib when we moved.

THE TRUTH ABOUT CO-SLEEPING

At least once a year we are guests on some TV show that poses the question "Should babies sleep with their parents?" First, let's take the confusion and controversy out of this normal and healthy sleeping arrangement.

Co-sleeping is not an unusual custom. At first we (Bill and Martha) thought we were doing something very unusual when we slept with our babies, but we soon discovered that other parents slept with their babies, too. They just didn't tell their doctors or in-laws about it. In social settings, when the subject of sleep came up, we would admit that we slept with our babies, and then other parents would confess that they did, too. We wondered why parents thought they had to be so hush-hush about this nighttime parenting practice. Why did they feel as if co-sleeping* were unnatural? Most of the world's parents sleep with their young ones. Why is this natural human parenting behavior somewhat taboo in our society? How could a culture have made so much progress in other areas, yet be so misguided about sleep?

In 1989, renowned anthropologist Dr. Melvin Connor reported on a study of sleeping practices in 173 developing societies around the world. In seventy-six of these societies (44 percent), mother and infant shared a bed. In another 44 percent of the societies, mother and infant at least shared a room. Dr. Connor also found that parents in "primitive" societies considered solo sleeping for babies barbaric and abusive. After listening to Dr. Connor read a passage on the dangers of spoiling baby from a famous baby book, one African mother said, "Doesn't he understand it's only a baby? That's why it cries. You pick it up. Later,

---

*The term "co-sleeping" does not mean that baby must sleep immediately next to mother in an adult bed, although for physiological reasons, this is ideal. Co-sleeping really has a broad array of options, such as baby in a co-sleeper or in a hammock, crib, cradle, or bassinet next to parents' bed. Sleep researchers broadly define co-sleeping as any arrangement in which the child is in seeing distance of a caregiver. Naturally, one would add the other senses, too: hearing, smelling, tasting, and touching. We define co-sleeping as a sleeping arrangement in which baby and mother are close enough to be mutually influenced by each other's nighttime physiology and sleep cycles, and close enough that the infant is able to effectively cue the mother to his nighttime needs and the mother is in close enough proximity to easily respond with a minimum disruption to her sleep.

> ## CO-SLEEPING — EVERYONE'S DOING IT!
>
> A National Center for Health Statistics survey from 1991 to 1999 showed that 25 percent of American families always (or almost always) slept with their baby in their bed, 42 percent slept with their baby sometimes, and only 32 percent of families said they never co-slept with their baby. For those of you who co-sleep or are thinking about co-sleeping, you're in good company.

when it's older, it will have the sense and it won't cry anymore."

What to call it. Sleeping with babies has various names: The earthy term "family bed," while appealing to many, is a turnoff to parents who imagine mom and several kids squeezing into one bed, along with dad and the family dog. "Bed sharing" is a term frequently used in medical writings. We like the term "sleep sharing" because, as you will learn, parents and babies share more than just bed space. Infants and mothers sleeping side by side share lots of interactions even when they are sound asleep. Co-sleeping is the newest term. The prefix "co-" means "together," so co-sleeping sums it up pretty well. It's the word we use most often in this book.

With Ashton asleep next to me, I feel like I am mothering her in my sleep.

Co-sleeping is a mind-set. Sharing sleep involves more than a decision about where your baby sleeps. It is a mind-set, an attitude of acceptance that acknowledges that your baby is a little person with big needs. You understand that your infant trusts you, his parents, to be continually available during the night, just as you are during the day. In our culture, co-sleeping also means that parents trust their own intuition about parenting their baby, instead of unquestionably accepting the norms of the neighborhood. When you accept and respect your baby's needs, you don't worry that you are spoiling your baby or letting him "manipulate" you when you welcome him into your bed. Co-sleeping parents are flexible and adapt their nighttime parenting style to their baby's changing needs.

Observations of a Co-sleeping Pair

Healthy things happen. In the early years of sleeping with our babies, I turned sleep sharing into an informal research project. Whenever I observed Martha and the baby cuddled up together, I noticed a special connection between them. Was it brain waves, motion, or just something mysterious in the air that made them seem to be so closely in touch?

I noticed that when Martha and baby slept alongside each other, even if they started out not touching, the baby, like a heat-seeking missile, naturally gravitated toward Martha. Sometimes they faced each other, only a breath away. Martha and baby seemed to share even the air as they slept face-to-face, almost nose-to-nose. I wondered if the carbon dioxide that mother was exhaling might

> ## CUTE QUOTES FROM CO-SLEEPERS
>
> Some memorable moments from co-sleeping families:
>
> *Whenever I try to put my daughter, twenty months old, back in her crib after she wakes at night, she just looks up at me very pitifully and says, "Bed, Mama," wanting to come into our bed. How can I resist?*
>
> ◆
>
> *One of our joys is the way our child wakes up. He wakes up smiling, and we wake up to this precious bundle lying next to us, and we smile, too.*
>
> ◆
>
> *My daughter would ask me to sing the Barney "I love you" song when she woke in the middle of the night between her dad and me. I would sing it, though these were not exactly the sentiments foremost in my mind at the time.*
>
> ◆
>
> *One morning I woke up to find my two-year-old kneeling over me trying to pull my eyelids open.*
>
> ◆
>
> *When I nurse her off to sleep, her sleep grins fill me with such joy that all the worries of the day just melt away, and I can rest, knowing my daughter is happy.*

be influencing baby's breathing. In fact, sleep researchers have shown that the carbon dioxide mother exhales does help trigger baby's normal breathing patterns.

As I watched the sleeping pair, I was intrigued by the harmony in their breathing. Sometimes when Martha took a deep breath, baby would take a deep breath, too. It was as if her breath were a sort of "magic breath" that shaped the baby's breathing.

The sleep-sharing pair frequently seemed to be tuned in to each other. Martha and baby would often enter a state of light sleep together. They would move around a bit, gravitating toward each other. Martha would turn toward baby and nurse or touch her, and the pair would peacefully continue to sleep, often without either one awakening. Also, they seemed to stir at the same time. If one moved, the other would also move. After watching this "sleep dance," I became certain that something biologically healthy was going on besides just sharing space on the mattress.

Then there was the "reach out and touch someone" phenomenon. The baby would extend an arm, touch Martha, take a deep breath, and resettle. Martha, without waking up, would reach out and touch the baby, who would move a bit in response to her touch. Martha would semi-awaken from time to time to check on the baby or rearrange the covers and then drift easily back to sleep. I was amazed by how much interaction went on between Martha and baby when they shared sleep. It seemed that baby and mother spent a lot of time during the night checking on each other.

With Ashton right next to me, I am always aware of her temperature. If I wake up a little chilly, then I know she must be cold and I cover her up more. If I feel myself getting a little too

warm or wake up sweating, then I know to check her to see if she needs less cover.

I also noticed that the baby nursed at least a couple of times during the night, usually without Martha or baby completely awakening. The next morning, if I asked Martha how often our baby nursed, she would reply, "I don't know, as often as he needed to, I guess." (I later learned why frequent night nursings are so physiologically healthy for mother and baby.)

Most of the sleep-sharing mothers I have interviewed tell me that they spend most of their night naturally sleeping on their backs or sides, as do their babies. Not only is back sleeping the safest for baby, but this position gives mother and baby easy access to each other for breastfeeding.

All of these observations taught me to reevaluate the nighttime parenting advice I was giving medical students and the parents in my pediatric practice.

SAILING ASLEEP

Dr. Jim, an avid sailor, offers a father's viewpoint on sleep-sharing sensitivity: "People often ask me how a sailor gets any sleep when ocean-racing solo. While sleeping, the lone sailor puts the boat on autopilot. Because the sailor is so in tune with his boat, if the wind shifts, the sailor will wake up. A co-sleeping mother seems to have the same kind of awareness of changes in her baby."

OUR CO-SLEEPING EXPERIMENTS

To study the physiological effects of co-sleeping in a real-life environment rather than in an artificial sleep laboratory, in 1992 we set up equipment in our bedroom to monitor eight-week-old Lauren's breathing while she slept in two different arrangements. One night Lauren and Martha slept together in our bed, as they were used to doing. The next night, Lauren slept alone in our bed, and Martha slept in an adjacent room. Martha nursed Lauren down to sleep in both arrangements and sensitively responded to her nighttime needs. Lauren was wired to a computer that recorded her electrocardiogram, her breathing movements, the air flow from her nose, and her blood oxygen level. The instrumentation was painless and didn't appear to disturb her sleep. The equipment detected only Lauren's physiological changes during sleep. It did not monitor Martha's changes. A technician and I observed and recorded the information as Lauren slept. The data was then analyzed by computer and interpreted by a pediatric pulmonologist who was blind to the situation — that is, he didn't know whether the data he was analyzing came from the shared-sleeping or the solo-sleeping arrangement.

Our study revealed that Lauren breathed better when sleeping next to Martha than when sleeping alone. Her breathing and heart rate were more regular during shared sleep, and she experienced fewer "dips" — low points in respiration and blood oxygen from slower-breathing episodes. On the night Lau-ren slept with Martha, there were no dips in her blood oxygen, whereas on the night Lauren slept alone, there were 132 dips. We obtained simlar results when we studied a second infant.

Since this was the first study of sleep sharing in the natural home environment, in 1993 I was invited to present our sleep-sharing research at the eleventh International Apnea of Infancy Conference. Our studies would not stand up to scientific scrutiny — and we didn't expect them to — because we studied only two babies. It would be wrong to draw sweeping conclusions from studies of only two babies. We meant our experiments to be only a pilot study. But we showed that with the availability of new technology and in-home nonintrusive monitoring, our belief about the protective effects of sharing sleep was a testable hypothesis. We hoped this preliminary study would stimulate SIDS researchers to scientifically study the physiological effects of sharing sleep in a natural home environment.

My observations of Martha and our babies and our experiments led me to conclude that co-sleeping mothers and babies seem to enjoy a mutual awareness without a mutual disturbance. As a pediatrician, I learned that co-sleeping and night nursing was a recipe for health. Over the past decade, studies in sleep laboratories have confirmed our observation that when mothers and babies share sleep, their movements and arousals are synchronized. Scientific research is validating what human beings have known instinctively for millennia: Something good and healthful happens when parents sleep with their babies.

SCIENCE SAYS: CO-SLEEPING IS HEALTHFUL

Infant-development specialists all agree: Togetherness, not separateness, is the healthiest state for babies. Mother and baby are both biochemically better off when they co-sleep. Here's a summary of what science says about sleeping with your baby:

Stress hormones are lower. Studies in both animals and humans have shown that an infant's attachment to his mother affects the infant's cortisol balance. A baby's body needs just the right amount of cortisol at the right times. Too much or too little, and the body is not in tune, sort of like an engine trying to run with the wrong mix of gasoline and air. Separation anxiety causes prolonged elevation of the stress hormone cortisol, which may diminish growth and suppress the immune system. Cortisol balance contributes to thriving.

Studies in animals have shown that separation from the mother affects the infant's physiology. For example, the longer the infant animals were separated from their mothers, the higher their cortisol levels were, suggesting that frequently separated babies could be chronically stressed. The mothers also experienced elevated cortisol levels when separated from their babies.[6, 15, 16, 17*]

When we consider all the evidence for the beneficial effects of babies and mothers sleeping together, the cry-it-out sleep-training advice begins to look downright unscientific.

References can be found in Appendix C.

Talk about high stress hormone levels! We can't imagine a more stressful situation for a baby than being left alone in a dark room to cry herself to sleep. This baby has stress hormones surging through her body, and she gets a booster shot of stress hormones every time she wakes up. This can't be of any biochemical benefit to baby — or to mother. When a mother says, "It just doesn't feel right for my baby to sleep in another room," she may be responding to more than just her emotions. Her body may be telling her to keep her baby close.

Growth hormones are higher. Growth hormones are secreted during sleep so babies will grow while they are sleeping. Growth hormones not only make your baby grow, they also stimulate hunger. Waking up to feed is a baby's way of getting the fuel needed to pack on the pounds. Endocrinologists have discovered that human infants who are deprived of sufficient closeness to their mothers have lower levels of growth hormones. In studies with experimental animals, those infants that stayed close to their mothers had higher levels of growth hormones and enzymes essential for brain and heart growth. Separation from their mothers, or lack of interaction with their mothers when they were close by, caused the levels of these growth-promoting substances to fall.[4, 22]

Sleep is more peaceful. Research shows that co-sleeping infants seldom startle during sleep and rarely cry during the night. Solo sleepers startle frequently throughout the night and cry four times more than co-sleepers. When babies who routinely slept solo were moved to a co-sleeping arrangement, they cried less. When babies who routinely co-slept were studied sleeping alone, they cried more. Startling and crying release stress hormones, which increase heart rate and blood pressure, interfere with restful sleep and can lead to long-term sleep anxiety.[27]

Physiology is more stable. Studies show that infants who sleep nearer to their parents have more stable temperatures, more regular heart rhythms, and fewer long pauses in breathing than babies who sleep alone. This means baby sleeps physiologically safer.[11, 33, 35, 40]

The risk of Sudden Infant Death Syndrome is lower. The SIDS rate is lowest in countries where co-sleeping is the norm. Babies who sleep either in or next to their parents' bed have a fourfold decrease in their likelihood of dying from SIDS. Co-sleeping babies actually spend more time sleeping on their backs or sides, which also decreases the risk of SIDS. Research has shown that the carbon dioxide exhaled by a parent actually works to stimulate baby's breathing.[2, 8, 10, 13, 23, 28, 30, 31, 36] When infants are separated from their mothers, there is a decrease in REM sleep, the state of sleep that seems to be most influential in brain growth, and the state of sleep in which protective arousals (see page 60) occur.[38, 39]

Sleep researchers, including Dr. James McKenna, professor of anthropology and director of the Mother-Baby Behavioral Sleep Laboratory at the University of Notre Dame, have shown that when mothers and babies co-sleep and night-nurse, they have similar patterns of movement and arousals. We believe that these protective arousals reduce a baby's risk of Sudden Infant Death Syndrome. One explanation for SIDS is that it is caused by a defect in baby's arousability from sleep. Babies need this arousability when their regular breathing patterns are interrupted due to the immaturity of their brains. Nearly all babies wake up and start breathing again when this happens, but having mother close by helps them wake up more easily. Babies who sleep alone may be at greater risk of not waking up when there is a problem with their breathing.[28]

Current sleep research validates the hypothesis that we first proposed in 1985 in our book *Nighttime Parenting:* "Co-sleeping and breastfeeding can lower the risk of SIDS." We believe that mother's presence during the night helps regulate baby's breathing, which can reduce the risk of SIDS. Studies of co-sleeping mother-baby pairs have shown that they share many interactions during the night. Recent studies in Japan have shown a further decrease in SIDS as the rates of co-sleeping have increased in an already co-sleeping culture. Mothers in Asian countries that enjoy some of the lowest SIDS rates in the world say, "If you are sleeping with your baby, you always sleep lightly. You notice if baby's breathing changes. Babies should not be left alone. Babies are too important to be left alone with nobody watching them."

Co-sleeping is safer than crib sleeping. A recent major study concluded that bed sharing does not increase the risk of SIDS unless the mom is a smoker or abuses alcohol.[5] In addition, even though the Consumer Products Safety Commission published data on non-SIDS fatalities to infants who sleep in adult beds, this same data actually showed more than three times as many non-SIDS crib-related infant fatalities.[9] (For more on the CPSC study, see page 120.)

Co-sleeping promotes long-term emotional health. In a long-term follow-up of infants who co-slept with their parents and those who slept alone, the children who co-slept were generally happier and less anxious, had higher self-esteem, were less likely to be afraid of sleep, showed fewer behavioral problems, tended to be more comfortable with intimacy and their own sexual identity, and were generally more independent as adults.[7, 12, 14, 21, 25, 29] These long-term behavioral benefits may, of course, be attributed to more than just co-sleeping. Co-sleeping is part of an overall increased parental-nurturing package, so it's difficult to separate the effects of co-sleeping from other nurturing attachment tools.

NINE BENEFITS OF CO-SLEEPING

Remember, the goal of this book is to help you and your baby get more restful sleep. If practiced safely and with the right attitude and strategies, sleeping with your baby can be a wonderfully simple way to accomplish this. Here are nine reasons why:

1. Babies sleep better. When we sleep, we move from light sleep to deep sleep and back again a number of times during the night. As babies go from one sleep state to the next, they go through a transition period in which they are vulnerable to waking. Babies with easy temperaments, or "settlers," are sometimes able to soothe themselves through this restless period and move on into the next sleep cycle. Others, the "wakers," feel more anxious during this sleep-state transition and are not able to put themselves back to sleep — especially if sleeping alone. However, the presence of a parent can ease baby through this transition. Your warmth, closeness, heartbeat, and breathing all convey the message "It's okay, you're not alone, you can go back to sleep. . . ." Reassured by your presence, baby resettles and goes back to sleep. A co-sleeping mother often senses when her baby needs a little help in going back to sleep, and she intuitively offers a reassuring and familiar touch or a short feed. Often neither one totally awakens, and they both drift back to sleep easily. In a way, co-sleeping is a type of sleep training, because it trains the baby to do what the parents do — sleep. Babies get the message that when they lie down in the bed, they're expected to sleep.

Whether it is during the day or at night, Ashton sleeps much better when she is next to me. This could be lying in bed or in the sling. I also see a difference if I am in the room while she sleeps. Noise or commotion does not bother her then. But if I put her in another room and leave, she often won't stay asleep as long.

Many parents have been led to believe that babies sleep better when sleeping alone. Science says otherwise. Studies at the University of California, Irvine, comparing co-sleepers with solo sleepers revealed that co-sleepers enjoy calmer and less restless sleep. In these studies, the infants who slept alone exhibited many signs of nighttime separation anxiety. Even though they appeared to be asleep, they startled frequently, went through periods of irregular breathing, and made more unpleasant sounds, such as squeaks and moans, which were interpreted by the observing researchers as signs that the infants were unhappy. The researchers noted that the physiological responses they observed in the solo sleepers probably reflected an increase in production of stress hormones, especially in infants who cried themselves back to sleep. In our sleep-counseling practice, we use the term "anxious sleepers" to describe these babies. (In contrast, just look at the face of a co-sleeping baby, and you'll see how happy he is.)

Another interesting observation that came out of the same study was that when the co-sleeping babies woke up, their mothers seemed to engage more instinctively in nurturing behaviors to get their babies back to sleep. The mothers of solo sleepers showed more annoyance at their babies' night waking. They perceived it as a problem and were not as naturally nurturing.

Not only do co-sleeping babies sleep less anxiously, they go to sleep more easily. They learn to associate familiar, enjoyable scenes and activities with sleep, so they relax and fall asleep easily when the simple, familiar pattern is repeated. Imagine that you are your baby. At the first hint that you are tired, Mom picks you up and lies down beside you. You nurse and drift off to sleep. What baby could resist that!

Our two-year-old tells us when she's ready for bed ("Night-night, Mama"). She and I have a wonderful routine: We go upstairs and get into bed together and read a few books. Then she climbs down from the bed and turns off the light. She then quickly falls asleep engaged in a wonderful nighttime hug. This gives her a positive association with sleep, and we avoid evening battles.

2. Mothers sleep better. It's not just co-sleeping babies who go to sleep more easily and sleep more peacefully. So do mothers. In general, what's good for babies is good for mothers, and vice versa. Here's where sleep sharing shines. When mother nurses her baby off to sleep, hormones at work in her body help both of them sleep better — in a kind of biochemical mutual giving. Mother gives baby her milk, which studies have shown contains natural sleep-inducing substances. Baby's sucking triggers the release of lactation hormones in the mother's body that, as a perk, help her relax. In effect, mommy puts baby to sleep, and baby puts mommy to sleep. Both members of the nursing pair sleep more easily when they do what comes naturally.

I regard sleeping with my baby as a "lazy mom" option. I like my sleep. Since she sleeps right next to me, I don't worry, and I don't have to get out of bed and wander down the hall when she wakes up to nurse. Besides, she likes nestling next to me. That makes me happy.

◆

Nursing my youngest child in the late afternoon is like having someone inject a relaxing drug into my arm. After half a minute of nursing, this wonderful warm relaxed feeling flows through my veins. I often fall asleep.

Many co-sleeping mothers and babies share what we call "nighttime harmony"— their sleep cycles are in sync. Mother partially awakens as baby is going through the vulnerable period of night waking, but because baby is just inches away, she can comfort or nurse baby back to sleep without fully awakening. Because her sleep cycles follow a pattern similar to that of her baby's, mother is seldom awakened from a deep sleep to attend to baby. It can be harder to get back to sleep when you are jolted out of a deep sleep state.

I awaken seconds before my baby. When the baby starts to squirm, I lay on a comforting hand, and she drifts back to sleep. Sometimes I do this automatically and don't even wake up.

With a welcoming attitude about co-sleeping and a little practice, most mothers achieve this nighttime harmony, and get a restful night's sleep while being there for their babies. Achieving nighttime harmony may depend on a mother's ability to let go of her preconceived ideas about infant sleep. In fact, studies show that parents who have more rigid expectations about how their baby is supposed to sleep often have children with more sleep problems. The parents' expectation becomes a self-fulfilling prophecy: When their child's sleep pattern deviates from how the parents believe their child should sleep, they perceive it as a problem.

When Ashton needs to nurse in the middle of the night, I look next to me and see her rooting around like a little birdie. She is only half awake. Because I can start nursing her before she starts crying, she usually doesn't ever have to fully wake up. Her sleep is not disturbed, nor is mine as much. I find that at seven months she sleeps longer stretches between feeding when she is curled up against me. Maybe my body presence allows her to stay asleep longer.

Another perk of co-sleeping is that it helps make child spacing easier. In fact, night nursing is essential if you are relying on breastfeeding alone for natural child spacing. Frequent breastfeeding delays the return of ovulation and menstrual cycles, so, since co-sleeping and breastfeeding babies nurse more often, co-sleeping mothers are less likely to have another baby in the bed soon. (There's much more to natural child spacing than just co-sleeping and breastfeeding, of course. You must breastfeed exclusively — and frequently — day and night, not use pacifiers or bottles, delay starting solids, and so on. Please read the whole story on breastfeeding as a natural method of birth control in *The Baby Book* [Little, Brown, 2003].)

3. Babies grow better. In my three decades as a pediatrician and baby watcher, I have noticed that co-sleeping babies grow better. They thrive. Babies who are trained to sleep through the night at too early an age often show slower weight gain and lag behind in their development. They don't thrive, because their need for closeness and security is not being met. We call this condition the "shutdown syndrome." (For an explanation of this condition, see page 88.)

THE HORMONAL HELPERS OF CO-SLEEPING

As you have learned in this chapter, something biochemically healthful happens to mothers and babies when they co-sleep. It's those hormones again! Besides stress hormones being lower and growth hormones being higher in babies who co-sleep, here are some other hormonal perks for mothers.

Feel-good hormones are higher. When the body is biochemically right, the mind is more likely to feel emotionally right. Studies on the neurochemical basis of mother-infant attachment suggest that being close to mother can stimulate the infant brain to produce feel-good hormones called endorphins. Frequent nursing and lots of contact with baby, as happens while co-sleeping, stimulate the release of hormones that help mothers feel more relaxed. Prolactin and oxytocin, the hormones released in the mother when baby sucks at the breast, not only help mother's body to make more milk, they also help her feel more relaxed and nurturing.

As I nursed her off to sleep, I would feel those great sleepy hormones kick in, and we would both drift off to sleep.

There is an interesting biochemical quirk about these mothering hormones that tells us a lot about co-sleeping. Most of these hormones have a short half-life. In simple terms, this means they don't last very long in the bloodstream. They enter the bloodstream, do their job, and quickly exit. This suggests that babies and mothers need frequent doses of attachment to keep these hormones active. Co-sleeping gives mothers and babies frequent booster shots of these hormones, and that helps them stay in tune with each other. As an added hormonal perk, the increased hormonal levels that co-sleeping mothers enjoy suppress ovulation and promote child spacing.

There are several reasons co-sleeping helps babies grow and develop better:

- Co-sleeping is an energy saver not only for mother but also for baby. Instead of wasting energy crying at night, baby can use that energy to grow.
- As has been known for decades, extra touch stimulates brain growth. Co-sleeping babies get lots of touching at night.

- Co-sleeping makes breastfeeding easier. Babies who sleep with their mothers get more milk at night. They are also likely to enjoy a longer duration of breastfeeding. This is good not only for baby's body but also for baby's brain. Recent research has shown that breastfeeding babies grow up to be not only healthier but also smarter. This may be because of the extra brain-building fats in mother's milk.

Co-sleeping is particularly therapeutic for babies and mothers who were separated for the first few weeks after the birth because of a medical situation such as prematurity. Co-sleeping provides extra touch time and extra opportunities to nurse. Premature babies and those who have struggled with other health problems naturally benefit from enjoying a "womb environment" of closeness with mother a little longer — both day and night. If we notice a distance developing between a mother and baby who were separated in the first days after birth because of a medical situation, or if we see that a baby is not developing optimally, one of our prescriptions is "Take your baby to bed and nurse."

4. Mothers "grow" better. What's good for babies is good for mothers. As the extra milk helps your baby thrive, the extra nursing helps you thrive and grow as a mother. A co-sleeping mother is literally "in touch" with her baby for eight more hours than if they slept separately. Co-sleeping, night-nursing mothers enjoy higher levels of prolactin, one of the hormones that not only make milk but also make mothering easier.

Co-sleeping, like breastfeeding, teaches a mother to read her baby. Co-sleeping mothers learn to know their babies very well. The many extra interactions with their baby that they enjoy while falling asleep, during the night, and when awakening boost their intuition. If baby fusses or has difficulty falling asleep at night, co-sleeping mothers are able to figure out why and what to do about it. They instinctively know when a baby can comfort himself and when they need to step

in. Also, because bed sharing helps parents feel so close to their baby, their daytime parenting style is likely to be one that is very responsive to baby's needs. They will want to do the other Baby B's that are part of the whole attachment-parenting package, such as babywearing and breastfeeding. Because they are intuitive parents, they are able to adjust to their baby's changing needs.

Ashton is the happiest when she first wakes up in the morning. After some big stretches and yawns, she starts smiling, chattering, and squealing. It's almost as if she is trying to describe the great dreams she had. This tells me that she had a good, restful sleep. Plus, we are there to enjoy her morning enthusiasm. If I were not there when she woke up, who would she tell? Coffee is nothing compared with the effects of Ashton in the morning. No matter how tired I am, I can't help but catch her enthusiasm, and we both end up cuddling and laughing. My husband, who loves to sleep like no one else, is often the first one to reach out and hold her. I look over, and there she is in the air above him as they both squeal with joy.

5. Fathers "grow" better. Many fathers do not have a lot of time with their children during the day. Co-sleeping gives dads extra hours of closeness at night.

I think that being a dad in the family bed is in some ways akin to being a breastfeeding mother. There is an intimacy that comes from sleeping with your children that is about as close as a dad can get to what a mother experiences through the nursing relationship. I work long hours, and having our children in our bed helps

MYTHS ABOUT CO-SLEEPING

How many of these erroneous admonitions have you heard about sleeping with your baby?

Myth: Your child will become too dependent!
Fact: Both experience and research have shown that co-sleeping children tend to grow up to become more secure and independent.

Myth: Co-sleeping is unsafe!
Fact: As long as you follow the sensible precautions for safe sleep sharing (see page 77), co-sleeping may actually be safer than solo sleeping (see pages 120 to 122).

Myth: Co-sleeping children have more sleep problems!
Fact: Children who co-sleep as infants and toddlers have fewer sleep problems as they get older.

Myth: They'll never get out of your bed!
Fact: Yes, they will. So what if it takes a while? How many parents have you ever talked to who wished they had spent less time with their children when they were young?

me spend quality time with them, even though we're all asleep.

6. Night feedings are easier. Breastfeeding and co-sleeping naturally go together. Because breast milk is digested more rapidly

than formula, breastfed babies need more frequent feedings. They are not able to sleep as long at night without feeling hungry. When co-sleeping, a breastfeeding mother's sleep cycles are more likely to be in sync with her baby's, so she can partially awaken just in time for a feeding and easily drift back to sleep. If the baby is sleeping alone, mother may be awakened from a deep sleep for feedings, which is a lot more jarring. Getting back to sleep then is harder, too.

Just before my baby wakes up for a feeding, my sleep seems to lighten and I almost wake up. By being able to anticipate his hunger, I usually can start breastfeeding him just as he begins to squirm and reach for the nipple. Getting him to suck immediately keeps him from fully waking up, and then we both drift back into a deep sleep right after the feeding.

Co-sleeping often helps breastfeeding work better. When we counsel mothers who feel they don't have enough milk or who seem anxious about breastfeeding, we find one of the most effective "treatments" is again the time-honored "take your baby to bed and nurse." Mother and baby are more relaxed while lying down at nap time and nighttime. Baby settles in for a long, comfortable feeding, and the milk seems to flow better. (For more information on how to make night feedings easier, see chapters 6 and 8.)

7. Co-sleeping is contemporary. For the many mothers who work outside the home and are therefore separated from their babies during the day, co-sleeping is even more necessary. Breastfeeding at night helps to perk up

CO-SLEEPING FOR BOTTLEFEEDERS

Co-sleeping also makes bottlefeeding easier. When baby wakes up or is about to wake up, you can quickly reach for a bedside bottle and help baby feed back to sleep before both of you are too revved up. Or, you can quickly send your husband for the bottle while you and baby stay snuggled in bed.

a mother's milk supply, which can dwindle if she is pumping rather than nursing during the workday. Sleeping with your baby at night allows you to reconnect and make up for the missed touch time during the day. Babies of working and nursing moms often breastfeed a lot at night to make up for not being able to nurse during the day. (See the co-sleeping advice for working moms on page 232.)

8. Co-sleeping babies tend to be better behaved. We have noticed, and long-term studies have confirmed, that co-sleepers tend to be easier to discipline. In fact, co-sleeping could be considered part of discipline. "What?" you say. "Letting your child sleep in your bed is good discipline?" Yes, it is, but first you have to understand what we mean by "discipline."

Traditionally, discipline has been equated with being in control of your child. To have well-behaved children, parents felt they had to be strict about enforcing rules and careful

not to spoil their infants and young children. The idea was that if they did not indulge a child, that child would soon learn to be more independent and to have more self-control. Better insights into children's emotional development have shown that this idea is wrong. When children are forced to become independent too soon, they end up being more needy instead of less. When parents do not respond to their child's need for closeness and comfort, they increase the chances of the child's becoming angry and difficult to discipline.

In the journey to nighttime independence, infants need to go through an early stage of dependence on their caregivers — which usually means some form of co-sleeping. When their needs are met during this dependent stage, children learn to feel secure, and in the long run they become more independent and even better-behaved children.

Co-sleeping parents need to understand that this independence may not emerge as soon as they would like it to. The friends who said "You'll never get him out of your bed" are probably now saying "We told you so." Realize that your baby is not going to suddenly decide that he's ready to sleep in a crib at six months — or even two years — of age. When you decide to co-sleep with your baby, you are making a commitment to allow your child to reach nighttime independence on his own timetable. When children feel secure and self-confident in their relationship with their parents, they gradually learn to sleep alone. As they mature, they learn to use the sense of security they experience in their parents' bed to help them sleep in their own beds. This same inner security helps them behave better in the daytime, too. They obey their parents because they trust them, not because they are afraid of being punished.

9. Co-sleeping is safer. In recent years stories in the media claiming that co-sleeping is dangerous have confused and unnecessarily alarmed parents. Certainly, your infant's safety while sleeping is the top priority. For this reason, we have personally researched the issue of infant safety while co-sleeping, and we have also consulted with experts on infant sleep.

Why do so many people who advise new parents warn them that co-sleeping is dangerous for their babies? And how is it that these advisers claim to have science on their side when so much of what behavioral scientists and parents know about infant needs and how mothers can best meet those needs suggests that co-sleeping is the norm for the human species?

When there is a conflict between scientific studies, or between science and common sense, suspect that somewhere there's a fault in the science. This is the case with the U. S. Consumer Products Safety Commission (CPSC) study that is cited by the "experts" who scare parents away from sharing sleep with their babies.

The CPSC study entitled "Hazards Associated with Children Placed in Adult Beds" was first published in the October 1999 issue of the *Archives of Pediatrics and Adolescent Medicine,* a professional journal for physicians, and it was widely and prominently reported in the popular press. Front-page headlines in newspapers warned that babies should not sleep in the same bed as adults, and television news programs across the country played up the story and alarmed viewers. In response, sleep researchers such as Dr. James McKenna and breastfeeding advocates spoke out against the study. As a well-known advocate of co-sleeping, I was interviewed by the *New York Times,* the *Washington Post,* CNN, and ABC's news program *20/20.* I made a strong case against the results of the CPSC study and the commission's recommendations, but rebuttals never have as much impact on readers and viewers as breaking news. I fear that, without questioning the study or knowing anything about the benefits of sharing sleep, many, many people — parents, soon-to-be parents, and health professionals — absorbed only the alarming message about the risks of co-sleeping.

Here's a summary of the study: Researchers looked at death certificates in the United States for the years 1990 through 1997 and found 515 cases in which a child under two had died in an adult bed. Of these deaths, 394 were caused by entrapment in the bed structure (for example, wedging of the child between the mattress and side rail or wall, suffocation in a water bed, or the infant's head becoming trapped in the bed railings). The other 121 deaths were reported to be due to overlying of the child by the parent, another adult, or a sibling sleeping in the bed with the child. Most of these deaths occurred in infants under three months. Based on a review of the death certificates, the CPSC issued a recommendation that parents should not sleep with babies under two years of age.

They stated that the only safe place for an infant to sleep was in a crib that met the CPSC's regulations.

The CPSC study certainly highlighted the need for safety precautions when infants are put down to sleep in adult beds. (Read more about the safe co-sleeping on page 77.) The study estimated that in the United States, sixty-four deaths per year occur in infants sleeping with an adult, but there is no way to determine the actual risk of co-sleeping, since the study did not determine the total number of infants who sleep with their parents some or all of the time. Nor did the study examine how many infants each year die while sleeping alone in cribs. While the researchers were quick to raise the alarm about co-sleeping, the study did not actually demonstrate that co-sleeping was more dangerous than solo sleeping. The gold standard of science is to do matched controls — in this case, to also examine the cases of infants dying in cribs over the same period of time. The CPSC study failed to use matched controls. *The fact is that many more infants die when sleeping alone in a crib than when sleeping in their parents' bed.* This number includes approximately twenty-five hundred babies who die of SIDS annually in the United States, most of them while sleeping alone. A different study, one that would also have examined death certificates of infants dying alone in cribs, might well have produced headlines such as "Hazards Associated with Infants Sleeping Alone in Cribs." Instead of making parents afraid to sleep with their babies, a more valid approach would be to teach parents who choose to co-sleep how to do it safely.

The truth is that babies have slept with their mothers for thousands of years, and they have slept in cribs for only a century or two — and then only in certain "civilized" parts of the world, in families well-off enough to buy cribs and furnish nurseries. Wise mothers and fathers should not go against their instincts and their knowledge of what works for their families because of a single faulty study. As anthropologists, sleep researchers, and behavioral scientists continue to study mothers and infants who sleep together, they are certain to show that this practical and responsive approach to nighttime parenting is, on the whole, good for everyone involved.

During the first six months of Leah's life, I noticed some dramatic differences in her sleeping when I wasn't sleeping next to her. In the morning I would often get up while she was still sleeping. With the baby monitor turned on, I could hear loud and irregular breathing rather than the quiet and regular breathing she had when we slept together. There was a definite change in her breathing patterns after I got out of bed. I think that I actually helped her breathe. Maybe I was her "pacemaker." I also noticed that when she was five months old, after I got out of bed, she would roll over onto her belly after a while. She never rolled onto her belly when I slept next to her. She was always on her side or back.

One of the experts I talked with about the study was Dr. James McKenna, who said "The CPSC's conclusion is backward. The question that should be asked is 'Is solo sleeping safe?'" Dr. McKenna went on to explain

TRUTHFUL CONFESSIONS

Okay, so co-sleeping is wonderful and healthy for parents and babies. But is it always so peaceful and magical every single night? Of course not. Co-sleeping is not problem-free, and it's not always "easier" than solo sleeping. Having slept with many of our babies and having counseled thousands of co-sleeping families in our pediatric practice, we have learned that there are challenges associated with every sleeping arrangement, and co-sleeping is no exception. Sometimes the bed gets a little crowded; sometimes baby disrupts the parents' sleep. Read about what was happening with Dr. Bob's two-year-old Joshua during the writing of this book:

Of course we wouldn't give up co-sleeping for the world. But for the last two weeks straight, *the little guy (now not so little) has started turning sideways in our bed with his head toward me. You'd think his head would gravitate toward his favorite food source, but no. Every morning around 6 a.m. I feel his little fingers gently stroking my chest, or his big head squished up against my tummy. I wouldn't mind at all if this occurred at 6:30 or 7:00, when I normally get up. But 6 a.m. is too early, and it's tough to go back to sleep on the narrow piece of real estate that's left to me. If I scoot Joshua over toward Cheryl, he wakes up (and that's a big minus for me on the good-husband rating scale). Of course, this little annoyance is minor compared with the joy Cheryl and I share in having Joshua sleep with us. We know it will change all too soon.*

that he had come to the same conclusions that we had: "If you look thoroughly at all the studies about sleep safety, it's impossible not to conclude that solo sleeping is the most dangerous of all sleeping arrangements." Dr. McKenna and others have questioned the CPSC's interpretation of the data in their study. A critical look at the CPSC's report shows that the data in their study simply do not support the headline-grabbing claim that co-sleeping is dangerous. When parents pay proper attention to their infant's sleep safety, co-sleeping is as safe as, or safer than, crib sleeping.

NINE WAYS TO MAKE CO-SLEEPING EASIER

Many things happen while baby is in your bed. Some are funny (well, maybe not so funny in the middle of the night, when you'd rather be sleeping, but they're funny later). Some things make wonderful memories. Others are nuisances that come with the territory of nighttime parenting. Here are some co-sleeping tips that will help everyone in the family sleep better.

1. Be sure both parents agree. Whatever nighttime parenting style you choose, it should bring husband and wife closer together, not divide them. Many modern fathers are proponents of co-sleeping, yet others may hesitate to jump into this nighttime parenting style. If you want to co-sleep but your husband doesn't, read together the benefits of co-sleeping in the beginning of this chapter. Suggest to him that you give co-sleeping a "30-day free trial." Many initially skeptical husbands get hooked on co-sleeping and find it brings them closer to baby. If your husband is concerned about sex, tell him that you'll do what you can to keep your sex life alive and healthy (see suggestions, page 183). Oftentimes, it's just a matter of getting your husband to trust your intuition, to trust that here mother knows best. You could also point out to him that his sleep is less likely to be interrupted if baby is in your bed rather than in a crib down the hall — especially if it's his job to get out of bed and bring the baby to you for breastfeeding.

My husband initiated sleeping with our baby because he was tired of getting up to get our baby out of the crib to bring him to me for breastfeeding.

2. Start early, be happy. Attitude is everything, in life and in night life. We have noticed that parents who embrace co-sleeping as a natural part of the whole parenting package and begin co-sleeping with their baby from baby's birth on usually come to regard it as not a big issue. And co-sleeping seems to work better for them than for parents who don't really want their baby in their bed but give co-sleeping a try because they sure aren't

---

SLEEP SCIENCE SAYS: BE HAPPY WHERE BABY SLEEPS

Researchers at the University of California, Irvine,[21] compared two groups of co-sleepers: "early co-sleepers," families in which the parents brought their baby into their bed right after baby's birth and regarded co-sleeping as a natural part of parenting; and "reactive co-sleepers," families in which the parents reluctantly took their child into their bed only after night waking became a problem. In contrast to the early co-sleepers, reactive co-sleepers perceived co-sleeping as a solution to a problem rather than as a natural extension of their daytime parenting. We wonder if the reason co-sleeping sometimes doesn't work as well with reactive co-sleepers is that the babies perceive that the parents don't really want them there but have them in their bed as the last resort.

---

getting enough sleep with baby in the crib. Parents who co-sleep for sheer survival often regard nighttime parenting as a chore rather than a bonding experience. Everything about co-sleeping becomes a big issue for them.

If you are a parent who is sleeping with your baby mainly so that you can survive and get some rest, try to get past the feeling that co-sleeping is a big imposition that you are putting up with for the sake of your sleep. See if you can find reasons to enjoy co-sleeping with your baby. Look upon it as a joyful experience

OBSERVATIONS FROM OUR PEDIATRIC PRACTICE

Co-sleeping is not always romantic and problem-free. Over our combined forty years in pediatric practice, we have cared for thousands of co-sleeping families. We have seen co-sleeping work, and we have seen it not work. In the overwhelming majority of co-sleeping families, we've noticed the following outcomes:

- The infants thrive. They grow optimally physically, emotionally, and intellectually.

- The parents are closer to their children. They are better able to read and appropriately discipline their children.

- The parents are more confident in giving intuitive and appropriate care to their children and need to rely less on outside advice (even *our* advice!).

- The children tend to be happier and healthier.

- The children grow up to be appropriately independent, or, more accurately, *interdependent.* This may be a new term to you. Interdependence is the most mature stage of independence; an interdependent child learns that he can do something by himself, but he can do it better in cooperation with another person. People who are interdependent strive to cooperate with others. Relationships, not just personal power, are what matter most to them.

(Mastering interdependence is one of the hallmarks of successful CEO's.)

A phrase we commonly use during a checkup when describing attachment-parented kids is "He/she seems nurtured." Throughout my years in pediatric practice, I have noticed a remarkable difference between children who are co-sleeping and night-nursing and those who are not. More often than not, the co-sleeping children radiate happiness. Oftentimes while examining a baby, I will notice that there is something unique about that baby. He's happy, not anxious, and seems connected. I'll sometimes say, "I bet you co-sleep and night-nurse!" Mothers will usually respond, "How did you guess?" The baby makes it obvious.

On the other hand, co-sleeping problems, if not addressed early and appropriately, can lead to mother burnout. The most common problem we see is the conditioned night nurser, whom we dub the "all-night sucker." Some mothers simply cannot get enough rest when their babies nurse every hour or two all night long. They end up feeling sleep-deprived, and this affects not only mother but the whole family. In the next chapter you will learn sensitive, appropriate ways to prevent a baby from becoming a conditioned night nurser, as well as ways to correct the problem if a mother is on her way to burnout because of lack of sleep.

that will soon pass. Take a few minutes at night and in the morning to gaze at your sleeping baby, who is so content and secure when nestled next to you. You make everything right with his world just by being close. Besides, grumbling about your baby's presence in your bed won't make anyone sleep better.

3. Forget the "what ifs . . ." "What if he becomes dependent on sleeping with me and never sleeps in his own bed?" you may wonder. Don't worry about next month or next year. Parent in the present. Enjoy each night and solve problems as they occur. Of course your baby will come to enjoy sleeping close to the people he loves. What smart baby wouldn't? Once babies settle into a sleeping arrangement that feels so right to them, they're not going to suddenly one day wake up and say, "Let's go crib shopping." But babies change and grow. As newborns, their days and nights are mixed up and their brains are immature. As that first year goes by, they learn to sleep at night and play during the day. In the second year, they become more confident in their ability to handle the world. As they acquire new self-settling skills, they won't need to co-sleep anymore. Someday, with a little creative marketing, you will be able to ease your child out of your bed and into his own, and he will take a healthy attitude toward sleep into his new life as an independent sleeper. We can't tell you exactly when this will happen. Every child is different. Yet we can promise you that your baby will not be in your bed forever (just like we can promise you that your baby will stop breastfeeding — someday). You don't

need to worry that you'll be buying your child his own bed as a high school graduation present.

The "authorities" dispensing sleep advice need to lay off the timelines.

◆

Dr. Bob relates: *I often wonder why my older kids sleep so well (they are now nine and twelve). Starting from when they were about the age of six, we have been able to tuck them into bed, turn off the light, and be done with our parenting duties for the night (except, that is, for putting their younger brother to bed). They never try to procrastinate by asking for water. They never come get us to tuck them in again. They seldom complain that it's bedtime. They never have nightmares or sleep terrors. They never wet their bed. They simply fall asleep quickly and peacefully, every single night. I don't know, maybe they're just genetically perfect kids, and it has nothing to do with how they have been parented to sleep at night. But honestly I think growing up in a stress-free sleeping environment has everything to do with it.*

If you like to think in the future, consider this. One of the most precious memories you can give your child is of being parented to sleep and of waking up each morning and seeing the people he loved. Isn't this a memory you would like your child to have? Or do you want your child to remember waking up in his room in a wooden cage, peering out through bars. We still remember waking up next to those beautiful faces and imagining that if babies could talk, they would say, "Thanks, Mom and Dad, for sleeping so close to me."

> **SEARS SLEEP TIP**
>
> If you begin co-sleeping when your baby is a bit older, be prepared to go through a warm-up period before you start experiencing the biological benefits mentioned earlier. Eventually, you and your baby will get used to this new closeness at night.

4. Use a king-size bed. When you co-sleep, a big bed is not a luxury, it's a necessity. Take the money you would ordinarily have spent on a fancy crib and all that cute bedding and buy a king-size bed. That tiny bundle snuggled next to you in a tiny space doesn't stay tiny very long. As baby grows, the nighttime gymnastics may begin. If you have a small bed, your baby will soon outgrow his allotted space. Bed sharing is more comfortable when there is a big bed to share.

5. Try different sleeping spaces. Some parents and babies sleep best with baby in the middle, while others prefer to have baby sleep between mom and a side rail. The baby-on-the-outside position is usually less disruptive, especially to dad, since baby can nurse without waking him up. Babies sleeping between mom and dad have been known to wake and try to nurse from dad — which is a little disconcerting for both of them. On the other hand, some moms feel "penned in" being in the middle. It's also awkward for the middle sleeper to get out of bed without disturbing the other two co-sleepers.

I don't know if other mothers feel this way, but I hated sleeping between my husband and the baby, and especially between my husband and the toddler. Too confining. Too claustrophobic. Too many people needing a piece of me.

6. Make night nursing easier. Breastfeeding and co-sleeping go together, so be prepared for extra nighttime nursing. Read the tips for easier night nursing in chapter 6.

7. Try a co-sleeper. Some mothers believe they will feel too anxious to sleep well with their baby right next to them. These mothers do better with baby sleeping in an Arm's Reach Bedside Co-Sleeper, a baby bed that connects to the parent's bed and gives baby his own sleeping space. Some babies also sleep better in a bedside co-sleeper than in their parents' bed, where they may wake up every time mom or dad stirs. With a co-sleeper, both you and your baby have your own separate sleeping spaces, but baby is within arm's reach for easy nursing and comforting. As an extra perk when using the co-sleeper, you don't have to worry about keeping your pillows and covers away from your baby's face.

Our co-sleeping toddler sometimes seems too stimulated by having mom and his "yum-yums" so close.

For some parents the term "co-sleeping" means not sharing the same bed but having their baby next to their bed or just in the same bedroom, such as in a crib next to their bed. Even though there may be bars between you and baby, this arrangement may work for you. Here's what mothers noticed after mov-

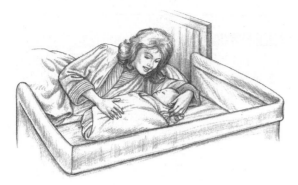

ing baby's crib from a separate room to alongside their bed:

He used to stand up in his crib when he woke up and couldn't see me. Now he sees me and goes right back to sleep.

◆

I wake up less frequently to check on her because I can hear her, since she's in our room and so close to us.

8. Try a mattress or futon on the floor. There comes a time in the nightlife of every co-sleeper when you still want to sleep close to your baby, but not so close. It may be that she's squirming and keeping you awake, or you may worry that she'll crawl away when you're not there and fall off the bed. In this case, try putting a futon or toddler-size mattress at the foot of your bed and co-sleep there with her briefly to get her to sleep and sometimes back to sleep. Here is an arrangement that our daughter, Hayden, and her husband, Jason, tried with their baby.

At nine months, Ashton could crawl off our bed, so we took our mattress off the box spring and put it on the floor. We placed it in the corner of the room so that two sides of the bed would be

against walls. We put her in that corner, where she would be safe.

9. Try part-time co-sleeping. Co-sleeping doesn't have to be an all-or-nothing arrangement. As baby gets older and willingly accepts sleeping alone, try putting your baby down to sleep first in his crib (or on a futon) and then take him into your bed the first time he wakes up. This arrangement gives you some privacy at the beginning of the night and also means you don't have to worry about your baby crawling off your big bed in the hours before you retire.

Sometimes part-time co-sleeping means that baby sleeps most of the night in the crib and comes into the parents' bed in the early morning after dad awakens. Mom and baby then enjoy co-sleeping for a few hours in the morning. This works well in situations where dad does not sleep well with baby in the bed, but he doesn't want to sleep alone in another room. This approach may keep an active toddler from wanting to get up and play at dawn.

COMMON QUESTIONS ABOUT CO-SLEEPING

CO-SLEEPING WHEN SICK

Our two-year-old went through a period when he had lots of ear infections. He would wake up often during the night, so we took him into our bed so we all could sleep better. Now we can't get him out. Help!

Nighttime is scary for little people, especially when they are hurting. A child wakes up in physical pain, and being in a dark room alone

CO-SLEEPING MADE EASIER FOR DAD

Co-sleeping is often easier for moms than for dads. Fathers don't enjoy the relaxing biological effects of breastfeeding, and their sleep cycles are not in sync with baby's, like mom's are. This biological fact of parenting nightlife may naturally make dads less enthusiastic about sharing the bed with baby. To keep dad from having to move into the guest room to get enough sleep, try these alternatives:

Get a big bed. For co-sleeping, a king-size bed is not a luxury, it's a necessity.

Try a co-sleeper for baby. A co-sleeper lets mother and baby sleep close to each other, yet it still leaves plenty of room for dad (see page 127).

Get a "co-sleeper" for dad. Leave mother and baby in the big bed and have dad sleep in an adjacent twin bed.

Make sure you get your "couple time." Try putting baby to sleep earlier, or take advantage of the time you spend putting baby down to sleep to be together.

Before our baby came, my husband and I loved spending time together before falling asleep. This was often the only time all day that we were able to connect. Now that our baby is here, this time has only gotten more special. My husband often lies next to us while I nurse her to sleep and joins in the bonding by caressing my hair, praying, reading a book out loud, or singing a soothing song. Then when she is sleeping, we can cuddle by ourselves on the other side of the bed and fully focus on each other because we know by her breathing and little movements and sounds that she is okay.

intensifies the fear and the pain. Naturally, this child is going to wake up. Enter Dr. Mom and Dr. Dad, nighttime comforters and soothers of both physical and emotional pain. The child naturally feels safe and secure and less bothered by discomfort when snuggling next to his parents. Even after the source of pain is removed, the child still thinks, "Hey, this is pretty neat! I like this!" A smart child is

not going to willingly accept a downgrade in accommodations and go back to sleeping alone in the wooden cage in the dark room.

Now that you can understand the situation from your child's standpoint, use the co-sleeping-made-easier techniques on pages 122 to 127 or try the sensitive strategies for night weaning from the family bed on pages 149 to 155.

SEX AND THE FAMILY BED

How can we enjoy a normal sex life and continue to sleep with our baby?

Romance doesn't need to end when a baby enters your family — and your bed. In the early months, babies are not aware of lovemaking going on in "their" bed, so if you're comfortable, don't worry about baby. However, many couples feel inhibited by a third (little) person in the bed, even if he is sleeping. We have found that nighttime parenting actually encouraged us to be more creative in our sex life. Try these tricks:

Baby goes in the crib first. Put baby in his crib during the first part of the night, enjoy private time together, and then welcome baby into the family bed after his first night waking.

Play musical beds. The master bedroom is not the only place where lovemaking can occur. Every room in the house can be a potential love chamber: another bedroom, the living room couch, in front of the fireplace — wherever the mood strikes and the opportunity allows. (Our favorite love nest was our walk-in closet, complete with futon and soft music.) If you prefer your bed, carry your sleeping child into another bedroom while you enjoy your privacy. If baby is co-sleeping when the mood hits, either move baby or move yourselves.

Enjoy morning sex. Most new mothers are so tired after a day of baby tending that all

> ## FATHER TIP: ENJOY DAYTIME SEX
>
> Initiate sex during the day when baby is napping. Let your wife know that you are still interested in her and understand that she might be more available in the middle of the day than at bedtime. Also, there will be more time to get her interested if you do some of the chores to free up some couple time.

they want to do is sleep. As one mother so aptly put it, "My need for sleep is usually greater than his need for sex." If you can nurse baby back to sleep in the early morning, go for it when *both* of you are in the mood and better rested.

In deciding when to enjoy sex, take a tip from your basic biology. The body is actually programmed for sex in the morning, when more REM sleep occurs. REM sleep naturally stimulates erectile tissue in both men and women, setting the body up for more pleasurable sex in the morning.

Settle baby first. We figure that babies must have a built-in romance alarm. As soon as your intimacy starts to heat up, baby's radar goes off, she wakes up, and suddenly things aren't so hot anymore. Even if dad is in the mood to continue, mom's mind is with the baby.

Feed baby first. Trying to make love with full breasts is not only uncomfortable, it can be messy.

A NOTE TO DADS: BE SENSITIVE DURING SEX

Hearing your baby cry will instantly kick your wife out of lover mode and into mother mode. Don't try to compete with baby for her attention. You'll lose. Above all, don't get angry. Don't slam your fist down on the mattress and snarl, "Curses, foiled again! Darn that young 'un!" (Of course, if you can do this and get a laugh, that's another story.) Instead, be a loving, sensitive dad and bring baby to mom to nurse. Offer some reassurance: "Nurse the baby and we can make love later." The sensitive approach is a far more effective way to keep your wife in the mood.

One night during sex my milk went off like sprinklers.

Be prepared for inquisitive toddlers. When children get older, it's important that they get two messages concerning their parents' bedroom: the door is open to them if they have a strong need to be with their parents, but there are private times when mom and dad need to be alone. It's healthy for children to see affection between their parents, so don't hold back on hugs for your spouse when your kids are around. And, if the bedroom door suddenly swings open and your child catches you in the act, don't worry — though it's a good idea to keep the covers on just in case. It's better for a child to see his parents making love than fighting. If this happens, resort to the old standby "Go watch your video" unless your child is really frightened by what he has seen and needs your attention. And teach your toddler that when your door is closed, he needs to knock first.

Cover up if you co-sleep. Mothers will often ask, "My husband likes to sleep nude. Our baby sleeps in our bed. At what age could this be a problem?" To help your children develop healthy sexuality, you want them to learn that the body is good. That's why there is no need to panic and dive for cover when your toddler runs into the bathroom as you exit the shower in your birthday suit. Just casually reach for a towel. Yet, it can be overwhelming for a child to see a parent nude in other settings. To avoid this happening, it is prudent for dads to start wearing undershorts if they don't like pajamas, well before the time that an older baby would be observant — by around eighteen months, two years at the latest. Moms, too, may use this minimum of cover-up.

OVERCROWDED FAMILY BED

Our four-year-old and two-year-old love to sleep in our bed, with no signs of wanting to move out. How can we ease them into their own beds?

Too many people in one bed means that nobody gets enough room. The kids usually don't mind. This is what they're used to. But parents can take only so much. Here are your options:

Extend your bed. Put another bed, such as a twin or queen-size bed, next to your bed and have one big family bed. Tell the kids that the nighttime rule is "If you want to sleep in Mommy and Daddy's bedroom, you need to sleep in this bed."

Make special beds. You can get a lot of mileage out of the word "special." Put a futon or mattress on the floor at the foot of your bed. Encourage your four-year-old to sleep in his "special bed" and then gradually move the two-year-old into his own "special bed" next to his sibling. When they both become comfortable with this arrangement, move their "special beds" into their own room. Then make a fun trip to a children's furniture store and let them pick their own "big boy" or "big girl" beds. Children are more likely to use the bed they choose.

Consider weaning your kids to a double bed in their own room. Since they are accustomed to sleeping with other people, they may sleep better together than in separate twin beds. Plus, you can lie down with both of them at the same time to read stories or say prayers at bedtime.

MAKING ROOM IN BED FOR A NEW BABY

We're expecting a new baby soon. How can we ease our two-year-old out of our bed?

It usually does not work — nor is it safe — to have a young baby and an older child in the family bed at one time. If you do all sleep together, be sure that the new baby sleeps between mommy and the wall or rail and that the toddler sleeps next to daddy. Children should not sleep next to babies under nine months.

To ease your toddler out, try the "special bed" suggestion mentioned above. Or have dad sleep next to your toddler in the "special bed" or in another room while you sleep with your new baby. As the older child gets used to sleeping without being next to you, dad can rejoin mom and baby. Try these easing-out strategies well before the new baby enters your bed so your toddler doesn't feel displaced by the little "intruder." If you do wait, spin the move in a positive way and do what you can at other times of the day to reassure him that he hasn't lost his importance to you.

FEAR OF ROLLING OVER ON BABY

I want to sleep with our new baby, but I'm worried I'll roll over and smother her. Is this possible?

Each night all over the world millions of parents sleep with their babies, and their babies wake up just fine. The same subconscious awareness of boundaries that keeps you from rolling off the bed prevents you from rolling onto your baby. Mothers we have interviewed on the subject of co-sleeping report that they are so physically and mentally aware of their baby's presence, even while sleeping, that they know they would be extremely unlikely to roll over onto their babies. Even if they did, their babies would put up such a fuss that mother would awaken in an instant (unless, of course, she is under the influence of alcohol, drugs, or medication — in which case she should not be co-sleeping). Experiments have shown that even newborns vigorously fight to remove a cover placed over their heads during sleep.

Fathers, on the other hand, may not always have the same keen awareness of baby's presence while asleep. It's possible that dad might throw an arm out onto baby or roll over onto baby. Because of this possibility, it's safest not to position a tiny baby between mother and father. Baby should be next to mommy, and mommy should be next to daddy.

The controversy about the safety of co-sleeping goes back to studies done in New Zealand in the late 1980s. The data seemed to show that co-sleeping babies were in greater danger of dying during sleep than babies who slept solo, because of the risk of a parent "overlying" the infant. But when researchers went back and reexamined the data about overlying, it was found that in almost all of the cases where this happened, there were other factors involved, such as the co-sleeping parents being under the influence of drugs or alcohol. When the data were reexamined and families with these dangerous sleep-sharing practices were excluded, it was found that co-sleeping was actually safer for babies than solo sleeping.

Sleep researchers use the infant car seat analogy when evaluating co-sleeping studies. If we looked at all the traffic deaths and injuries to infants in car seats, the number would be alarmingly high. Yet, if we separate out from the statistics infants who were not properly and safely secured in their car seats or who were in unsafe car seats, the stats would be much, much lower. Rather than discouraging car travel with infants as unsafe, it's better to teach parents how to travel more safely with their babies. Ditto this approach to co-sleeping. Rather than discourage co-sleeping as unsafe, parents need to be taught how to do it safely. (See also Safe Co-sleeping, page 77, and Co-sleeping Is Safer, page 120.)

PETS IN THE FAMILY BED

We have a cat who likes to curl up with all of us at night. Is it dangerous for the cat to be in bed with our baby?

Yes. Pets and babies should not co-sleep. The pet needs to sleep on another bed, preferably in another room. If your pet nestles next to baby, its fur could interfere with baby's breathing enough to be concerning. Also, animal dander from all kinds of furry pets is a potential allergen that could irritate a baby's sensitive breathing passages, causing congestion and difficulty breathing.

Many toddlers, on the other hand, love to sleep curled up next to their pets. Providing the older child is not allergic to her pet, this is a safe arrangement. Sleeping next to a favorite pet as a "soothie" also helps some children enjoy a more restful night's sleep.

HUMOR IN THE FAMILY BED

My husband always slept with his shirt off, until our son started scooting around the bed in his sleep. One night, he woke up frantically to discover, much to my amusement, that our infant son was trying to latch onto his nipple and was getting very frustrated when it wasn't working! My husband has slept with his shirt on since then.

◆

I woke up and started shouting to my husband to find the baby. He pointed to our son and said, "He's right here," but I continued to shout about finding the "other baby." I was dreaming I had had twins and couldn't find the second twin! It took a few minutes for my husband to calm me down and convince me that we only had one baby and he was happily sleeping right there between us.

◆

"Fathers, please evolve and lactate," pleaded an exhausted mother of a frequent night nurser.

◆

A few nights after our baby was born, our dog was the one keeping us awake! Every time the baby whimpered or rustled the sheets, our dog would jump to attention and start barking at us while running from one side of the bed to the other. It seemed as if the dog was letting us know that the baby needed attending to. She was so excited about the baby and wanted to "help" us. At one point we locked her out of the bedroom, but that was worse because she sat on the other side of the door, whining and crying. She was very stubborn and knew she absolutely had to look out for the baby in case her masters were a couple of bozos. Luckily, by the third night, the dog settled down and realized that we did know how to take care of our baby. The dog now sleeps in her own room.

Night Feedings and Night Weaning — When and How?

W HY DOES MY BABY wake up so frequently to nurse?" This is the number-one nighttime parenting concern we hear about in our pediatric practice. Young babies need to nurse at night, and smart babies — especially high-need babies, or those with persistent personalities — are reluctant to give up night nursing as they get older. As babies become busy toddlers (especially if paired with a busy daytime mommy), they enjoy the private time of night feedings. In this chapter we'll discuss why babies nurse at night and how to make those night feedings easier. We'll also help you figure out what to do if baby's all-night nursing is keeping you from getting the sleep you need to be a happy mother during the day and help you decide if you are ready to have the night feedings come to an end.

AGES AND STAGES OF NURSING AT NIGHT

Breastfed babies need to be fed often, which keeps mother close by. Babies love to breast-feed, and the relaxing hormones released during feedings make it a pleasurable experience for mothers, too. Breastfeeding is an important part of how mothers get attached to their babies. Is it any wonder that you can't shut off this wonderful relationship just because it's time to go to bed? Since you're going to be spending time feeding your baby at night, you need to understand why your baby wakes up to be fed. The reasons change as your baby matures.

Birth to four months. Young babies breast-feed a lot. They are seeking both food and comfort at the breast. The sweet milk fills their tummies, and the sucking, combined with close contact with mother, calms their bodies and minds.

Tiny babies have tiny tummies, about the size of their fist, so they need to feed frequently around the clock. Breast milk is dubbed an "easy in, easy out" food because it leaves the stomach quickly and is digested easily and efficiently. Less wear and tear on the intestines is why breast milk leaves babies with a "good gut feeling." Formula and solid foods take longer to digest. A formula-fed baby may feel fuller longer but may have more pain in the gut from gas or allergies. In the first four months, expect babies to need at least two feedings during the night (from midnight to 6 a.m.).

Breastfeeding also helps young babies organize their behavior. Newborns are not very good at paying attention or staying calm, but breastfeeding helps them pull themselves together. It also eases the transition from being awake to being asleep. This tool that babies use to keep themselves happy has a human being attached to it, so when baby breastfeeds, he learns to associate mother with all kinds of good feelings.

Four to six months. By this time, baby has become conditioned to this pattern of association: wake up, need comfort, breastfeed, feel better, go back to sleep. It works! Babies depend on breastfeeding at night to cope with more than just hunger. When teething pains, stuffy noses, and other physical causes disturb baby's sleep, he looks for the breast to help him feel better and go back to sleep.

Naturally, babies come to regard nursing as the best source of comfort, so they think, why not use it? Here is where sleep trainers and others who believe that parents must be in control of their babies' behavior start to issue warnings: "If you nurse your baby for comfort, he is going to want to nurse all the time. He's got to learn to take care of himself." If babies could voice an opinion, they would say, "Nonsense! I'm not ready to handle life on my own." And they would be right. Eventually babies do

learn other ways of calming themselves and dealing with discomfort. But for now, they are learning about trust and security while nursing at the breast. These are important lessons that, later on, will help them be happier, confident, and yes, more independent.

Six to twelve months. Separation anxiety comes into play at night as well as during the day. As babies become able to hold an image of mother in their mind, they begin to worry and fret when this important person is not there. We believe that separation anxiety is a built-in survival mechanism. As babies develop the motor skills to move away from mother, their bodies say "let's go," yet their minds worry and say "not too far." Breastfeeding is an important way to reunite with mother, especially when babies feel anxious and alone in the dark of night. By this time, baby regards breastfeeding as a wonderful connecting tool, so that, naturally, when he feels separation anxiety, how does he spell relief? B-R-E-A-S-T!

Some babies are more separation-sensitive than others. High-need babies — those whose brains are wired in such a way that they need a lot of assistance from parents to stay calm and make transitions — may stick like glue to mom at night and nurse often, sometimes almost continuously. (Don't panic — we'll show you what you can do to help your baby not need to nurse *that* much.) When one of our high-need babies was going through one of those clingy stages, we dubbed her the "Velcro baby." Other babies may be more laid-back and will want to nurse at bedtime and once or twice before morning.

How breastfed babies sleep. How babies are fed affects how they sleep. If your formula-feeding neighbor is bragging that her four-month-old is sleeping through the night, while your breastfeeding six-month-old is still waking two or three times a night to nurse, you may be wondering what's going on here. If breastfeeding is so good for your baby, how come she's not a better sleeper? The fact is, breastfed babies tend to wake up more often than formula-fed babies, especially breastfed babies who sleep with their mothers. This isn't just an impression we have formed over the years. Researchers have documented this by comparing the sleep patterns of breastfed and formula-fed babies and those of babies who co-sleep and babies who don't.

Is this a hidden disadvantage of breastfeeding — something people kept from you when you signed on to feed and nurture your baby at the breast? Actually, not sleeping so soundly is a good thing for your baby. Remember what you learned about protective arousals? Babies need to be able to wake up easily. What if a baby were hungry in the middle of the night but didn't wake up? He would miss out on feedings he needed in order to grow. What if a baby who is left alone at night couldn't easily wake up and cry for someone to take care of him? A baby sometimes cries or wakes up to "check on" mother, to be sure she is close, which ups the odds that he's going to thrive.

The all-night nurser. If you suspect that breastfeeding and co-sleeping have something to do with how many times your baby wakes up at night, you are probably right. It takes

longer for breastfed babies to get to the point where they sleep a good four- to six-hour stretch at night. Hopefully, the inconvenience of waking up more often to feed your baby at the breast is offset by how easy it is to feed at night when she's right next to you. If you can get baby latched on and go right back to sleep as she breastfeeds, you may find that you are getting the sleep you need and that breastfeeding is actually helping you do this.

It was Snoozeville for me during night nursing.

Most babies' nighttime nursing starts to taper off in the second half of the first year, and they learn to sleep more soundly. As toddlers gradually wean from the breast, they also wean from night nursings and from co-sleeping. But what if you have a baby who is nine months old, twelve months old, even eighteen months old who still likes to nurse all night long? And what if this means that you feel sleep-deprived, depressed, and cranky during the day?

All-night nursing can take its toll on mom. At some point, mothers have to decide whether they're going to continue to nurse whenever baby wants to at night or find ways to encourage their child to nurse less or stop nursing at night. We often see mothers in consultation who have never been given tools to make night nursing easier on themselves. Baby is thriving, but mother is barely surviving. It is to these sleep-deprived moms that we devote this chapter.

This chapter is full of suggestions for how to make night nursing easier with both younger and older babies, and for how to get older babies who are very persistent about nursing at night to nurse less or not at all. It's up to you to figure out what combination of night nursing and co-sleeping allows everyone in your family to get the rest they need. And, as with so many other features of nighttime parenting, your approach to night nursing will probably change as your baby grows.

FIFTEEN WAYS TO MAKE NIGHT NURSING EASIER

In the early months, babies need to breastfeed at night in order to grow well. Throughout the first year and beyond, there may be medical conditions, family situations, growth spurts, or other reasons why a baby continues to nurse once or twice at night. High-need babies, who need more of everything, may breastfeed several times during the night, even in their second year of life.

Mothers who both survive and thrive with night nursing find efficient ways either to nurse without completely awakening or to go back to sleep easily after feedings. Here are ways to manage night nursing without setting yourself up for sleep deprivation:

1. Co-sleep. Most women who breastfeed for more than a few months sleep with their babies. Some of them make this decision before baby is born. Some experiment with different sleeping arrangements and gradually realize that co-sleeping is much easier on everyone in a breastfeeding family. Some night nursers learn to "self-serve." They find the nipple without waking mother. Co-sleeping mothers often lose track of how many times their baby nurses at night, since they are sleeping too

well to be certain or even to care. (See page 118 for more on the breastfeeding benefits of co-sleeping.)

I would be comatose during the day if I had to get up every couple hours at night, lift my baby out of the crib, rock and nurse her back to sleep, somehow get back to sleep myself, and then have the whole process start all over again all too soon.

2. Master the art of nursing while lying down. First, some pillow talk. Pillows are the key to comfortably nursing a new baby while lying in bed. Place two pillows under your head, a pillow behind your back, and one under your top leg, much like you did when you were trying to find a comfortable position to sleep in while pregnant. Does this seem like a lot of pillows? Maybe, but you're worth it! Night nursing should be relaxing for mom. Put your baby on her side facing you and nestled in your arm. Then latch her on, just as you do when you are sitting and holding her on your lap.

While you're still at the hospital, or in your first few days at home, have a lactation consultant or an experienced friend show you how to nurse lying down. Some mothers and babies get the hang of this side-lying position right away. Others take a little longer. Keep working at it until it's comfortable for you and your baby can latch on and nurse well enough to get a satisfying amount of milk and fall asleep.

Mastering side-lying nursing is the key to surviving night nursing. Side-lying nursing is much more restful than sitting up in bed and

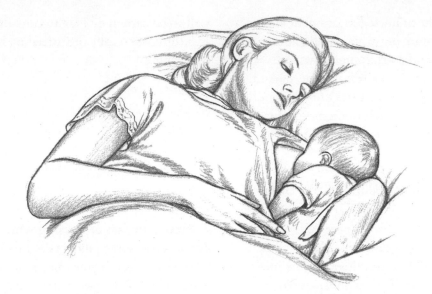

waiting forty-five minutes for your infant to finish nursing before you can go back to sleep. Nursing lying down lets you fall asleep while baby feeds. Getting out of bed and sitting up to nurse has many drawbacks for mommy and baby. You have to fully wake up to retrieve the baby and find the chair, and if baby falls asleep at the breast, you have to figure out how to get baby off the breast and into bed again without waking her up. When you nurse lying down, all you have to do is drift off.

Martha notes: *My sleep really improved when I finally figured out that I could nurse from either breast while lying on one side rather than flipping us both around every time she switched sides.*

3. Encourage a longer latch-on. When baby wakes up to nurse at night, encourage her to nurse long enough to fill her tummy. If she

keeps popping off the breast, you're likely to get sore nipples and she's likely to wake up hungry in a very short time. Try these suggestions for a longer latch-on:

- Be sure your baby is latched on well. She should get a good-size mouthful of breast. Once your milk lets down, you should see baby's jaw moving and notice her swallowing as she gulps down milk.
- Cuddle your baby in close to you as you nurse her in the side-lying position. If she has to reach and crane her neck to stay on the breast, she'll get less milk.
- Curve her body toward you by bringing her knees toward your abdomen. Bending baby discourages her back from arching, which leads to unlatching.
- When baby finishes the first breast, lean her against your chest and rub her back to gently bring up any air bubbles in her tummy. Then let baby nurse from the

other breast just by angling your torso toward baby to present the top breast. It can take a while to get the hang of nursing from either breast while lying on one side. At first, you may have to roll to your other side (reposition all those pillows!) to offer the second breast.

4. Make the breasts more easily available. Some mothers sleep better when they make their breasts easily available (baby sleeps near a topless mommy) to baby for self-serving. Even newborns can navigate themselves toward the nipple if they are close enough.

I slept with my breasts available to her. If she latched on, she could often do so without waking me when I was exhausted. I slept on my side, facing her, and her head was at nipple level, with my arm positioned above her head. I found she was happier with her head touching something.

5. Prehydrate yourself. Waking up to nurse is one thing. Having to get out of bed to go to the bathroom while baby fusses for a feeding is another. Yet you need lots of water to stay well hydrated while you're lactating. Here's one strategy: Drink a lot of water a few hours before bedtime. Then before you go to bed, be sure to empty your bladder well using the triple-voiding technique: after the urine flow stops, bear down with your pelvic muscles to squeeze out any urine that remains in your bladder. Do this three times.

6. Give a big bedtime feeding. Using a technique called "cluster feeding," try to feed baby every couple hours during the evening,

beginning after the late-afternoon nap. Then do the "tank-up feeding": Encourage your baby to nurse actively for a long time before he falls asleep. We call this the "dream feed." By nursing actively, we mean the kind of sucking where you can see a wiggle at baby's temple and baby is swallowing milk after every two or three sucks. Gentle comfort sucking puts babies to sleep, but it doesn't fill tummies. You might want to start this bedtime feeding before he gets too tired, so that he doesn't nod off after just five minutes of breastfeeding. If he does start to fall asleep at the breast too soon, take him off, burp him gently to wake him up a bit, and then latch him on again. Let him finish the first breast so that he gets lots of the high-fat milk, which will help him feel full longer. Then top him off by offering the other side.

Trying to load babies up with formula or solid food (or even too much breast milk) before bedtime may help them sleep longer, but it can also backfire. An overstuffed tummy may allow irritating stomach acids back into the esophagus, causing gastroesophageal reflux (see page 215). The pain that results will trigger night waking. Still, increasing the before-bed feeding is worth a try.

I tried to load and reload. I would feed him just before his usual bedtime and then wake him for another feeding before I went to bed. This combination helped both of us sleep for longer stretches.

7. Keep the bed dry. If you produce an overabundance of milk, put a few absorbent towels under yourself, since you're likely to soak through breast pads and nightshirts. A water-

MARTHA'S DE-LATCH

Some babies need to stay latched on at night to stay asleep. They startle awake when they lose the sensation of holding on to the nipple. If your baby falls asleep with the nipple clamped in his mouth, or if he continues to "flutter suck" as he would on a pacifier, this can be irritating. If you can't drift off to sleep that way, how do you get your breast back? Here's what Martha discovered and wrote about twenty years ago:

Wait until baby is barely sucking. Then use your finger to gently pry his jaws apart, ease your nipple out, and let him finish sucking for a while on your finger. It is easier to sneak your finger away than it is your nipple.

Babies older than around two months may not accept sucking on a finger. With an older baby, use a finger to release his jaws and slowly draw the nipple out of his mouth, keeping your finger there to protect your nipple in case he suddenly clamps down. If he gropes for the nipple, he is reacting to the change in pressure sensation in his mouth. Push firmly inward and upward under his lower lip or on his chin with the length of your index finger, keeping his mouth closed and applying enough pressure to keep him from awakening. Hold the pressure with your finger until he settles back into deep sleep. (Laying your other hand against his back may also help him settle.) If he does wake up, quickly give the nipple back to him, and try again after he is back to a deep sleep. You may have to do this three or four times before he stays still, but if the baby is in a deep sleep and you have been patient enough not to rush it, it usually works on the first try.

---

proof pad under baby will protect your mattress if his diapers leak.

8. Dress for the occasion. Wear whatever attire keeps you the most comfortable at night, with the least fumbling when it's time to nurse. Pajama pants and a loose top work well. Some mothers like nursing nightgowns, with special openings for breastfeeding.

I used a bed-rail cover that had pockets in it where I could put everything I would need during the night — a change of clothes, burp cloths, *diapers, ointment, and wipes. That way, I didn't have to get out of bed.*

9. Get comfortable. To get yourself back to sleep after nursing, lie in the position you find most sleep-inducing. Also, pull your baby toward you to nurse, rather than arching your back or contorting your body to get to baby. Falling asleep in a twisted position can cause you to wake up with a sore back.

10. Burp baby the easy way. Soon you'll find that traditional burping is no longer

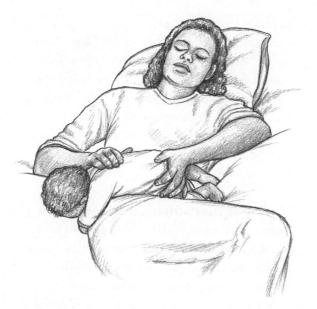

needed and you can do it in your sleep (so to speak). Simply prop baby up over your tummy or hip as you relax on your side and pat his back. After baby is a few months old, burping usually isn't necessary. Babies nurse in a more relaxed manner at night and so swallow less air.

After she's finished nursing, if she needs to be burped, I lay her on my chest while I lie propped up with a couple pillows. This enables me to stay in bed so that I don't fully awaken. If she wakes up, I give her a finger or pacifier, and that helps her go back to sleep without more nursing. Sometimes her dad does the burping duty.

11. Change nursing positions. Muscle pain and backaches are sometimes a side effect of night nursing and co-sleeping. It's possible to nurse from both breasts without turning over to lie on the other side, but if you find this leaves you feeling stiff and achy in the morn-ing, try to change positions during the night so that your baby sleeps on your right side part of the night and on your left side the rest of the night. Or switch off from one night to the next. Be aware of your body position as you lie there nursing your baby. Are your shoulders tight? Are your fingers tingling because of the position of your arm? Are you tensing the muscles in your neck, your back, or your legs? Relax into that pillow support-ing your lower back. (What? You're not using one? Trust us, it makes a difference.) Allow your body to sink into the bed and the pil-lows as you fall asleep. Ask your spouse for a back rub to help release any tension while baby nurses. Do some gentle stretches or some yoga during the day to counteract any tightness in your muscles from the way you sleep at night.

I used to nurse the baby on the first side, change his diaper, and then lie down on the other side and nurse him to sleep. This way, baby was already in position for the next feeding. This was a huge help.

12. Read baby's cues. Remember, your goal is to get yourself and your baby back to sleep as quickly as possible — no muss, no fuss. Reading baby's cues will tell you what to do to accomplish this. Most of the time, when babies wake up at night, they need to nurse — at least in the early months. If you can respond to baby's precry signals (squirm-ing, sputtering sounds, and so forth), you will get her back to sleep more quickly than if you wait for her fussing to escalate into a full-throated, angry cry. You can offer to nurse her right away or hold off for a minute or two and see if she goes back to sleep. She might settle with just your loving touch or a few soothing words. But if this doesn't do the trick quickly, offer the breast — or you may be awake for much longer than you'd like. When in doubt, err on the side of being more responsive rather than waiting to see if baby can soothe herself back to sleep without breastfeeding.

13. Offer an occasional sub. As baby gets older, you'll find that she is better able to settle without feeding. Try offering a substitute for breastfeeding when baby is less likely to be hungry at night. Dad can comfort baby, or you can pat baby's tummy or sing to her. This will help her learn that she can go back to sleep without always breastfeeding. Again, "nursing" implies comforting, not only breastfeeding. It helps to get baby used to other forms of night nursing. We call this approach "selective night nursing."

14. Seek out night-nursing friends. Don't complain about your baby's night nursing to friends and family members who find it hard to understand why you continue to breastfeed. They'll offer an easy solution — just stop nursing. Your "misery" needs the company of like-minded moms. Join your local La Leche League group and/or hang out with parents with a similar nighttime parenting mind-set. Veteran mothers who have "been there and done that" can probably offer you some helpful tips and you'll be able to gain some perspective on the challenges of nighttime nursing.

Each time my child woke at night to nurse, I would vow to wean him at night. Then, in the light of day, I would realize that I didn't feel that bad and that night weaning would be very difficult on both of us. Somehow when daylight hit, some kind of adrenaline kicked in and it didn't seem so bad. I also had some friends who were in the same boat, and it helped to know that I was not alone.

15. Adjust your attitude. Night nursing is a season of parenting. All babies need to feed at night, especially in the first six months. Since it's inevitable that your sleep will be disturbed, you might as well adjust your attitude and approach night nursing in a positive way. Let nursing relax you and help you get more sleep — rather than dreading each night feeding and filling your system with stress hormones that just keep you awake. (See more attitude-adjusting tips below and on page 68.)

Once I let myself enjoy the hours of rocking and nursing, the private time, and I regarded it as a passing privilege and not a chore, it became easier. I began to look at night nursing as an opportunity for relaxing and getting close to my baby. It's a time in your life when your baby will drift off to sleep easily in your arms. That time will pass too soon. Celebrate it while you can.

As we have previously said, night nursing is good for you and good for your baby. It may seem like a burden at times, but it also has benefits. During sleep, your levels of prolactin and growth hormone go up, and both of these increase your milk production. Babies get substantial amounts of the milk they need in order to grow from nursing at night. (We call the milk you produce at night "grow milk.") As an added hormonal perk, the higher level of prolactin has a relaxing, de-stressing effect. Also, researchers have discovered a sleep-inducing protein in mother's milk. So, night nursing helps both the baby and the mommy sleep.

Cherish this time. I remember that age like it was yesterday, yet my son is now two years old. It will be gone before you know it. Listen to the breathing of your little one, replay pleasant memories, talk to God, and so on. If you feel short on sleep, take a nap the next day when baby naps. Forget the household chores or other tasks calling you. Your baby will only be a baby for a short time.

Here are some other tips from seasoned night nursers on how to stay sane during the time your baby is waking to nurse at night:

- Don't look at the clock every time baby wakes up. Don't count the minutes (or hours) of sleep you're missing. An exact accounting won't make you feel any less tired. In fact, you'll feel worse.

- If you've been awake at night, be kind to yourself and make some adjustments in your plans for the next day. Grab a nap. Don't cook. Don't worry about the house-work when you're overtired.

- If you find yourself lying awake during or after a night feeding, don't fuss and fume and don't worry about how you'll feel to-morrow. Do something to take your mind

off the fact that you're not sleeping. Read a book that will amuse or relax you. Keep a pad and pen handy so you can do some journaling or meal planning. Listen to music softly (keep the stereo remote control next to your side of the bed). Enjoy watching your baby sleep. Turn this problem into an opportunity to enjoy some "me time."

- Pick a relaxing favorite movie and turn it on at night when you night-nurse. This makes the nursing time seem shorter and gives you something to look forward to.

- Place a sound machine on your nightstand (one that makes peaceful sounds, like waves, rain, or streams). Turn on a soothing sound before you settle in to go back to sleep.

Just as medications come with both benefits and side effects, night nursing has its good points and its drawbacks. Certainly the benefits outweigh the side effects: Baby is secure, thrives and grows well, and gets to enjoy all the health, nutritional, and developmental benefits of breastfeeding. Besides this, quite honestly, babies love to nurse at night. For mothers, night nursing helps them maintain an adequate milk supply, which is especially important for moms who work outside the home during the day. Night nursing also prolongs the period of time in which a lactating mother doesn't have menstrual periods and therefore has less chance of getting pregnant again (for more on this, see page 115). The major "side effect" of night nursing is

NIGHTTIME BOTTLEFEEDING MADE EASIER AND SAFER

I have fallen into the habit of giving our fifteen-month-old a bottle as a way of putting her to sleep at night. She also wakes up in the middle of the night asking for her "ba-ba." Should I break this routine? And, if so, how?

Formula-fed babies tend to wake up less often than breastfed babies. Formula is digested more slowly than breast milk, so tiny tummies stay full longer. Also, bottles and formula do not seem to be as strong a motivation for waking up as the breast and mother's milk are. But many infants, including bottlefeeders, need to suck to relax themselves into sleep. Here are some tips for making bottlefeeding easier and safer.

- Try to give baby an extra ounce of formula in her last nighttime bottle. For example, if she takes 5 ounces at most feedings, see if you can get her to take 6 ounces. Don't force it, though — if she gets too full, it could backfire by causing discomfort. Try giving your child nutrient-dense solid foods as a before-bed snack. Nutrient-dense foods are those that pack a lot of nutrition in a small volume and keep the tummy full longer. See page 45 for suggestions.

- Prepare the nighttime bottle early in the evening. Put it in the refrigerator so that it gets nice and cold. Place the cold bottle next to baby's bed just before you go to bed, along with an electric bottle warmer. When baby awakens for a feeding, you can warm and feed without making that long trip to the kitchen.

- Share night feedings with your spouse whenever possible.

I pumped once in the morning when I had extra milk, and my husband used this milk to feed her at 9 to 10 p.m. on those days when I went to bed earlier. She slept longer because she got some of my morning milk, which seemed to satisfy her more than the before-bed nursing, when my milk supply was lowest.

- Remember, there should always be a person at both ends of the bottle. Don't prop the bottle and let her suck herself to sleep unattended. Also, though it is

that baby learns to associate sleeping with feeding and may not want to go back to sleep any other way. This is okay with some families — they're happy to have a guaranteed way of getting baby to sleep — but may not be okay with others.

THINKING ABOUT CUTTING BACK ON NIGHT NURSING AN OLDER BABY?

Mothers who breastfeed all night (or what seems like all night) every night can get very tired and burned out. Even the most tempting to leave a bottle in the crib for a 3 a.m. self-serve, don't! Not only does this practice contribute to tooth decay, but baby can choke on the contents with no one there to help. Also, lying down during formula feeding allows formula to enter the middle ear through the eustachian tube and triggers ear infections.

- Try to gradually wean your baby from nighttime bottles between one and two years. The bottle itself is not harmful; it's what's in the bottle that matters. Bottles of formula or juice are not friendly to a sleeping baby's teeth. When baby falls asleep, saliva flow decreases, diminishing its natural rinsing action on the teeth. The sugary stuff bathes the teeth, resulting in severe tooth decay called "bottle mouth." To ease baby off the nighttime bottle, try the "watering down technique": gradually dilute the bottle contents with increasing amounts of water until baby figures out it's not worth waking up for the bottle.

- After giving her the bottle of milk or formula, brush her teeth gently, trying not to awaken her if she has drifted off to sleep. Toothpaste is not necessary. Use either a baby toothbrush or a piece of gauze wrapped around your finger, whichever method is easier. You may then need to walk her around to resettle her without the bottle. If your baby still needs a middle-of-the-night bottle, be sure to brush her teeth as soon as she wakes up in the morning.

- Don't give a juice bottle before nap time or bedtime. Reserve juice bottles for times when the child is wide awake (juice should always be served diluted to half strength with water). In fact, it's best to serve juice out of a cup, so baby doesn't get used to walking around with a juice bottle during the day and wanting it at night. Besides, juice is not as filling as milk or formula, so it serves little purpose for satisfying nighttime hunger.

- If baby is hooked on a nighttime bottle as a pacifier rather than a source of nutrition, try feeding her with a cup instead of a bottle before bedtime. Then offer a friendly pacifier, such as her thumb (see page 28) or a cuddly lovee. If she is old enough to understand, show her how her teddy bear goes to sleep without a bottle: "See, Bear-Bear doesn't need a bottle to go off to sleep."

on-fire mother needs sleep to keep going. If you are the burning-out mother of an all-night nurser, you may need to make a change. It may be time to figure out how to get baby to nurse less at night or how to wean baby from night feedings completely.

If you wean your baby partially or totally from night nursing (you can still nurse during the day), your baby will probably wake up a lot less, since there's no longer anything pleasurable to wake up for at night.

A baby's need for night feedings usually lessens with time and maturity. But some babies become toddlers who are very reluctant to give up night nursing. Because they have always been breastfed whenever they awoke at night, they've been conditioned to expect this, and they won't settle for anything less. They may be nursing more out of desire or habit than out of need.

What's the difference between a habit and a need? Habits can be changed. Needs don't go away so easily. If you give some night-weaning techniques a try and baby adapts fairly easily, you'll know that night nursing was a habit he was ready to lose. He may protest a bit. He may be unhappy for a couple of nights. But then he will settle into the new way of sleeping. If night nursing is meeting a genuine need, baby will protest strongly if you try to wean him. He may also become more clingy or anxious during the day. You'll know you are dealing with a need, because baby will become much more needy.

Martha notes: *Let baby be the barometer. When trying any behavior-changing technique on a child, don't persist with a bad experiment. Use your baby's daytime behavior as a barometer of whether your change in nighttime parenting style is working. If after several nights of working on night weaning, your baby is her same self during the day, persist with your gradual night weaning. If, however, she becomes more clingy, whiny, or distant, take this as a clue to slow down your rate of night weaning.*

If multiple nighttime feedings are leaving you burned out on breastfeeding and mothering, it's time to change something. Here is a sensitive approach to easing off nighttime nursing. We want to help you meet both your child's need for closeness and your own need for sleep.

How much of a problem is it? Be honest! Remember, babies need happy, rested mothers. If night nursing is disrupting your sleep to the extent that you can't function well the next day mentally or physically, your body and mind are telling you that you need to make a change. Listen to these signals! (And don't feel guilty about it.) If you've tried many strategies to help you sleep better and to catch up on your sleep during the day and you're still sleep-deprived, that's even more evidence that you need to make a change and try something else. If you dread going to sleep because it's work rather than rest, you know that something's got to give. If your health, your marriage, and your ability to care for your family during the daytime are being negatively affected by your efforts to meet your baby's needs at night, you need to get some balance back in your life. Many kids ago we learned a valuable survival principle:

> IF YOU RESENT IT, CHANGE IT!

I love her dearly, but I'm tripping over the bags under my eyes.

◆

When she reached fifteen months, I decided enough was enough! She was waking me up to nurse every two hours. So my husband took over the job of comforting her when she woke at night. It was very hard to listen to her cry on that first night, but I knew that she was just angry, not lonely, scared, or alone. She caught on very quickly and now sleeps consistently from about 8:30 p.m. to 6:30 a.m. Then I nurse her and have a morning cuddle until she falls back to sleep. She sleeps for another two hours. (Comment: Babies may give up the middle-of-the-night nursings more easily if they know they're going to get some nursing and snuggle time in the morning — sort of like skipping an evening snack when you know you're going to go out for breakfast the next morning.)

If, on the other hand, you are coping reasonably well with your baby's night nursing, then there is no reason to change. You may be tired occasionally because your baby has kept you awake more than usual the night before, but most of the time you manage to get enough sleep. While you may be wondering if your toddler will ever sleep through the night, you find that meeting his nighttime needs with nursing works pretty well in your family.

Once I got her used to other ways of going to sleep, I felt less pressure and actually enjoyed breastfeeding more. I knew I didn't HAVE to nurse her to sleep.

Also, don't feel pressured by neighborhood norms. When mothers talk among themselves, some tend to exaggerate how long and how well their babies sleep instead of being honest about their babies' sleep patterns. They want to make themselves look good — in their own eyes as well as in others' — and mothers often end up believing that everyone else's baby is sleeping through the night at age three or four months. (If they really are, there is probably a lot of night crying going on.) This is not the norm, even for formula-fed babies and those who do not co-sleep.

Anthropologists tell us that prolonged night nursing is actually the norm in most human societies outside of Western cultures. Babies seem to be "wired" for it, and these other cultures are more accepting of how dependent babies are on their mothers. In Western cultures, especially in America, we value independence and push children to be independent at an early age. But we fail to recognize that babies have to go through a prolonged period of being dependent on others to achieve the kind of emotional security that is the foundation of later independence. We think of weaning as a goal we must strive toward, whether it's weaning from the breast, from the parents' bed, or from childish behaviors. In ancient writings, the term "weaning" means "filled" or "completed." Children are not truly ready to move on to the next stage until the needs of this stage are filled.

Many mother-infant pairs continue to night-nurse throughout the first year or two without mom getting overtired and baby becoming overdemanding. Baby's needs for closeness, security, and nourishment are met, and mother gets enough sleep because she doesn't wake up completely while baby nurses, or she goes back to sleep easily afterward. In fact, some mothers feel night nursing helps them sleep better. Some of the physically and emotionally healthiest children we have met through the years are those who have been allowed to wean from their mother's breast and their parents' bed in their own good time.

I became a sleep nurser. Some people walk in their sleep and don't remember it. I was able to nurse in my sleep. I remember the first time I realized he had nursed during the night and I didn't remember it the next morning. I woke up and my PJ top was up and my bra flap was down.

Check on yourself frequently to be sure that you are mostly happy with your nighttime nursing situation. Also, think about how you can help your child accept other forms of comfort. If you meet all of your child's nighttime needs with the breast, you may not be giving him opportunities to learn other ways of falling asleep. This may be fine if your baby is only a few months old, but if your "baby" is a fifteen- or eighteen-month-old toddler, he may be able to wean a bit at night. Just as you encourage him to learn to eat solid foods, to walk around on his own two feet, or to solve problems as he plays, it's also your job to show him more grown-up ways of falling asleep and going back to sleep. Some of the tips listed below will help you do this, and you will be able to make a gradual transition to bedtimes and nighttimes without nursing. Knowing that you aren't going to be breastfeeding at night forever can make it easier to enjoy night nursing now.

Consider what you will lose by night weaning. (A word of caution: We're talking about older babies and toddlers here. Trying tricks to lessen night nursing in the early months can lessen your milk supply to the point where baby fails to thrive.) Besides losing the milk baby needs in order to grow, when you wean, you lose the relaxing and sleep-inducing perks of night nursing, which you may have gotten used to. Some mothers find that during the first three days of night weaning, they have more trouble falling asleep and staying asleep. Finally, you lose the ovulation-suppressing effects of those night-nursing hormones, so you can become pregnant again more easily.

I actually feel more tired now that my baby is weaned. Nursing had helped me drift quickly back to sleep. I can't imagine settling a baby in the middle of the night (or indeed at any time) without having recourse to nursing.

Balance your needs with baby's. Sometimes we see babies who are thriving with mothers who are just barely getting through the day. This is why a few years ago we added another B to the Baby B's of attachment parenting — BALANCE! If baby is doing great but mom is marginal, things are out of balance. Does this sound like your situation? Does the message playing inside your head say, "My baby needs me so much, I don't have time to take care of myself"? (Many mothers have this "baby-first, mom-whenever" mind-set, especially in the early weeks of parenting a newborn.) A healthier mind-set for mothers is "I need to take care of both of us." As we say throughout this book, a thriving baby and a barely surviving mommy is not a healthy combination. If achieving balance means that mom has to get more sleep, some nighttime changes may be necessary.

It helped to cut out the night feedings once we knew he was wanting them out of habit and not from hunger.

"But if I try to cut out night nursing, my baby will cry!" you may say. "And I can't just let my baby cry, can I?" One of the tenets of attachment parenting is that you should respond to baby's cries. Some take this to mean that parents must do whatever it takes to stop their babies from crying. But what we really mean is this: Don't let your baby cry alone.

To expect an avid night nurser with a persistent personality to give up without a protest is unrealistic. Yet, crying in itself isn't a bad thing. Babies often need to cry to release frustration and other negative emotions that are a part of everyday life, just as adults do sometimes (though, of course, a lot less).

It's the message that baby gets from his parents while he cries that matters. This is why we feel that the cry-it-out-alone sleep-training method is bad for babies. A baby who is left alone to cry feels abandoned, left by himself to solve big problems. But how about using techniques at night that might involve some crying, but not crying alone, and not at an inappropriate age? Even breast-feeding parents have nights when baby is fussy, won't nurse, and all they can do is carry baby around the house and hope that the motion will lull her to sleep while she cries. Baby is getting the message that her parents are there with her to help her through this fussy time. This stands in sharp contrast to the message that a baby gets when left to cry himself to sleep alone in a crib.

What we are saying is that *if* you are at the point where you need to wean baby from night nursing, and *if* your intuition tells you that it will be okay for your baby to go through some periods of fussing to sleep in mom or dad's arms, and *if* you feel this is the right thing for you and your baby right now, we believe that you can gently and humanely wean your baby from night nursing without endangering your baby's trust in you, because *you* are still going to be there. However, if you feel that it will harm this trust, then you shouldn't do it.

THIRTEEN TIPS FOR GETTING BABY TO NURSE LESS AT NIGHT

We love co-sleeping, but our nine-month-old uses me as a pacifier. She sucks while she sleeps. In the early months I didn't mind, but now I'm not sleeping well. I find her constant sucking irritating. How can I break this annoying habit?

For older baby night nursing, it's important that both mother and baby enjoy it. The key to enjoying it is to night-nurse your baby because you *want to,* not because you have to. Your lack of sleep and your annoyance at your daughter's all-night nursing are signs that you need to make a change. Your baby may be very comfortable nursing while she sleeps, but it is no longer working for you.

Night weaning is often difficult for mother and baby because both parties have become what we call "conditioned night nursers." Baby awakens, you are programmed to nurse, and it works — baby goes back to sleep. Because it works so well, it isn't an easy behavior to change. (One really conditioned mother shared with us, "I heard the cat me-owing and I tried to latch my infant on while she was sound asleep. Another time I tried to latch the cat on when she climbed into the crook of my arm during the night.") If you are a conditioned night nurser and it's work-ing for you, there's no need to change, as your baby will wean in due time. If you are an exhausted night nurser and baby is condi-tioned to night-nurse, expect the reprogram-ming process to take some time. Understand that night weaning will not occur overnight. It will be a gradual process over several weeks. Realize your baby will have to adjust and that he will resist a change to a new pattern, but he is not starving from giving up night nurs-ing. How strongly your baby protests depends on his personality and the length and frequency of his previous night nursing.

1. Tank your baby up during the day.

Many toddlers get so busy during the day that they forget to nurse. They make up for the food and closeness they miss during the day by nursing more at night. Or, mom may be too busy or unavailable during the day, and night nursing becomes a baby's way of reconnecting. Many babies nurse more at night after their mothers return to work. In-fants will "cluster-feed" (feed more often) at night because the breasts are more available at night. If possible, try to reverse this pattern and help baby cluster-feed during the day instead.

When we say "tank baby up," we don't mean stuff your baby with solid foods right before bedtime. This rarely helps babies sleep better and can even backfire, since a gassy baby with an uncomfortable tummy is more likely to wake up at night. Yet we suspect that some babies who nurse a lot at night aren't eating much during the day. Many parents have told us that their babies had little ap-petite for solid foods until they were weaned from night nursing. Snacking all night can depress baby's appetite during the day. If this sounds like your all-night nurser, try offering more food during the day. If baby is less than a year old, always offer solid foods in addition to, not instead of, the more valuable breast milk. Offer more nursings during the day as well. Try to work in one or two extra feedings during late afternoon and early evening. If baby breastfeeds while falling asleep, be sure he nurses for ten or fifteen minutes before he drifts off.

Cluster feedings before bed made a big improve-ment in how long he slept, once we both got the hang of it.

2. Increase daytime touch.

As babies get older and spend more time out of your arms, they get less touch time each day. All-night nursing can sometimes be a baby's way of getting more of the physical contact he is missing out on during the day, either because he's busy crawling around on the floor or because you are busy and not spending as much time with him. Night nursing reminds mothers not to rush their baby into independence. A child develops independ-ence at her own pace. Baby leaves and comes back, lets go and clings, takes two steps forward and one step back until he is away from you more than he is with you. Many mothers have noticed that their babies and toddlers show an increased need for nursing and holding as they enter a new stage of development or are coping with a change in lifestyle. Changes such as learning to crawl or walk or staying with a new sitter are stressful, and baby copes by nursing more.

To give your baby more "sling time" during the day, wear her in a sling when she's tired or needs a break from her active play. Use the sling rather than the stroller when you go out. Sit down and play with her. Cuddle together while you read stories. Give her a back rub at nap time and bedtime.

3. Introduce change during daytime naps. To help baby learn to accept alternative ways of comforting at night, introduce other ways of falling asleep at nap time, when it's not dark and you are not exhausted from a long day of mothering. When dad is home, encourage him to "father-nurse" baby down for naps. But be aware that some mothers find that if they nurse less at night, their babies need to nurse at nap time more. Nap nursing also helps to tank baby up so that he doesn't get hungry at night. Do whatever works best for you.

4. Awaken baby for a full feeding just before you go to bed. This may help your baby sleep for a longer stretch at night. If baby goes to bed at eight o'clock, you go to bed at eleven, and baby wakes up hungry at midnight, you get only one hour of sleep before he wakes. If you wake baby and feed him at eleven, the two of you can go to sleep then and probably get three or four hours of uninterrupted sleep. Nurse him in a rocking chair and then hand the almost-asleep baby to daddy to add the finishing touch.

Waking baby to feed will work only if baby is in the state of light sleep and about to wake up anyway. Awakening baby out of a deep sleep can throw off his natural rhythm and actually cause more night waking. It's probably better to "let sleeping babies sleep." Yet, it's worth a try — and it may work for you. An extra before-bed feeding is especially helpful during growth spurts, when baby really needs that extra feeding.

5. Get baby used to other "nursings." As we have frequently reminded you, "nursing" implies comforting as well as breastfeeding. Get your husband to "father-nurse." (To persuade him, tell your husband that when you are more rested, there'll be more of you to go around.) Wearing down is a good way for dad to take over part of the bedtime routine. After baby is fed but not yet asleep, have dad wear him in a baby sling while he walks around the house or around the block. When baby is in a deep sleep, he gently lays him on your bed and eases himself out of the sling. As your baby learns to associate father's arms with falling asleep, he may be more willing to accept comfort from dad in the middle of the night as an alternative to mom. Other ways to ease your baby into sleep without breastfeeding him include patting or rubbing his back while you walk with him, singing and rocking him, or even dancing in the dark to some tunes you like or lullabies you croon.

My wife had me "dad-nurse" the baby at night when he was a "little leech" and wouldn't let up.

6. Nurse to sleep — but not completely.
Help your baby learn that there are other ways to fall asleep besides breastfeeding. This works best if you start when baby is young. Toward the end of the feeding, ease her off the breast before she is completely asleep. Then you or dad can add the finishing touch with other sleep cues, such as "night-night" or finger sucking. She will associate these cues with the sleepy feeling she has and will eventually learn to accept them during the night hours. (For more on dad adding the finishing touch, see page 179.)

7. Offer a sub. While a baby with discerning tastes is unlikely to settle for anything less than the softness of your nipple and the sweetness of your milk, other things can fill in for mother when she is trying to sleep. Here are some time-honored subs for a baby who has just been fed:

- Dad's pinkie finger to suck on. (This works for young babies but not for older babies and toddlers.)
- Baby's own thumb or fingers.
- Water in a sippy cup (a possible compromise for a toddler who wants to nurse at night).
- Pacifier.

Let your child hold a favorite toy, such as a teddy bear, while nursing during the day and at night. Eventually he may go to sleep, or back to sleep, with the teddy bear only. It won't happen overnight, but at least he'll get the picture.

I let him gently play with my hair while nursing during the day, and at night he can touch my hair to get back to sleep without nursing.

8. Make the breast less accessible. Co-sleeping is a setup for night nursing. It's a nighttime parenting package babies love. If baby is sleeping in his favorite restaurant, inches away from his favorite food, he's going to want to eat. (Wouldn't you?) It's hard to tell a baby he can't eat when he smells the milk. That's one reason babies who co-sleep often nurse a lot at night. If you want to cut down on the frequency of night nursing but still enjoy co-sleeping, here are some suggestions for ways to keep the food in the cupboard (as it were).

- Put a barrier between breast and baby. A baby who doesn't sense the nipple readily may not be stimulated to think of it ("out of sight, out of mind"), though some babies with persistent personalities will keep searching and fussing until they find what they're looking for.

After I nursed him to sleep, I would "close up shop" (put the bra flaps up securely), pull my nightgown all the way on, and sleep covered up. This helped a bit.

- Have the older baby sleep on the other side of dad instead of next to you.

When our little boy wants me all night but I really need to sleep, we put him down next to my husband, and I sleep on the other side of the king-size bed. This way our son still has a warm body to snuggle up to, but he is less likely to wake up wanting to nurse. My husband loves this, and I get a good four hours or so of uninterrupted sleep. Then if he is really fussy, we switch back.

- Turn your back on baby. Sleep facing away from baby to make your breasts less available.

- Try a co-sleeper. To increase the sleeping distance between baby and breast, try putting your baby in a bedside co-sleeper (see page 127). Or, put your toddler on a mattress or futon at the foot of your bed and have dad lie down beside him to comfort him if he awakens.

- Try creative positioning. With an older baby or toddler, especially in the summer, when few or no covers are needed, sleep so that baby's head is not at breast level. Maybe turn baby upside down so her head is next to your thighs. Of course, her feet will then be at your breast level, so if she's a night kicker, this trick won't work.

- Find a behavior barrier. One mother told her two-year-old: "I have to brush your teeth every time you nurse at night." That slowed down the night nursing.

So my breasts aren't so close to his mouth, I sleep with my head close to his abdomen, or even sometimes with my feet at the head of the bed.

9. Move out! No, not out of the house. If your toddler still wants to nurse way too much, relocate "Mom's All-Night Diner" to another room and let baby sleep next to dad for a few nights. Baby may wake less often when the breast is not so available, and when he does wake, he may be willing to accept comfort from dad. Naturally, baby is going to fuss when his "breasts" are not within reach, and his protests may start to escalate. That's why mom is sleeping down the hall. You can reappear if necessary.

No, you are not going against what you said you'd never do — let him cry it out. As we've repeatedly discussed, we believe it's wrong to let baby cry unsupported and alone. But crying a bit in the arms of dad or another familiar and nurturing caregiver is different, especially when you consider how high the stakes are. A sleep-deprived and burning-out mom is not much good to anyone — dad or toddler. Although *you* may be crying it out alone in another room, try to give dad and baby some time and space to work this out. You'll be surprised by what creative strategies dad can come up with, if he's willing.

10. Just say no! One night when Martha was desperate for sleep, I woke up to hear this dialogue between her and two-year-old Matthew: "Nee" (his word for nurse) . . . "No!" . . . "Nee!" . . . "No!" . . . "Nee!" . . . "No, not now. In the morning. Mommy's sleeping now. You sleep, too." A firm but calm, peaceful voice almost always did the trick.

11. Just say yes! Dr. Bob's wife, Cheryl, found a creative way to help two-year-old Joshua resettle at night without nursing. If

Cheryl said, "No nursing," he would get more upset and awake. Instead, when he woke and asked for "nummies," Cheryl snuggled up to him and said, "OK, here's nummies." She slowly went through the motions of preparing to nurse him and he would quickly settle down and fall asleep while waiting.

12. "Nummies go night-night." By eighteen to twenty-four months, most children have the capacity to understand basic sentences and the idea that the breasts are sleeping. Use simple concepts to explain to your toddler when she can nurse and when she has to wait. Tell her, "We'll nurse again when Mr. Sun comes up." You can even show your child that it is dark outside. In the morning when she wakes up, show her that it is daylight outside and announce, "Mr. Sun is up. Time for nursing."

When he was able to understand what I was saying, I explained that he could have milk to get to sleep but not after that until the sun came up. Then he started to rise earlier (with the sun, of course). That's the price I paid for getting him to sleep through the night without feeding. I guess you can't have it both ways!

Or try this routine: As your child nurses off to sleep, tell her, "Mommy go night-night, Daddy go night-night, baby go night-night, and nummies [or milkies or whatever cute word you use] go night-night." When she wakes during the night, the first thing she should hear is the same gentle reminder: "Nummies are night-night. Baby go night-night, too." You may have to do this for a

week or two, but soon she will get the message that nighttime is for sleeping and she will stop waking up to nurse at night. If "nummies" stay night-night when it's dark, hopefully baby will, too. If sunrise comes too early for you, blackout shades, available at home-improvement stores, may buy you an extra hour of sleep.

Martha notes: *When weaning Erin, I showed her some pictures I'd gathered of babies sleeping without the breast nearby, and I talked to her about how the babies were sleeping without "nummies." Daily reminders helped.*

13. Share night duty. Honor your husband with his share of night nursing so your toddler does not always expect to be comforted by your breasts. This gives dad a chance to develop nighttime fathering skills and your child a chance to expand her acceptance of other nighttime comforters. High-need babies are not easily fooled; they don't readily accept substitutes. Still, it's worth a try. (See chapter 8 for nighttime fathering tips.)

Martha notes: *One of the ways we survived toddlers wanting to nurse frequently during the night was for me to temporarily go off "night call." Bill would wear the baby down in a baby sling so he'd get used to Bill's way of putting him to sleep. When the baby woke up, Bill would again provide the comfort he needed by rocking and holding him in a neck nestle position (see page 177) and singing a lullaby.*

Babies may initially protest when offered father instead of mother, but remember, crying and fussing in the arms of a loving parent is not the same thing as crying it out alone. Moms, realize it will be really hard for you to hear your baby crying. But, if you "rescue" him, it will be harder the next night because he'll expect you again. Dads, realize that you have to remain calm and patient during these nighttime fathering challenges. You owe it to both mother and baby not to become rattled or angry when your baby resists the comfort you offer.

Try this weaning-to-father arrangement on a weekend or at another time when your husband can look forward to two or three nights when he doesn't have to go to work the next day. You will probably have to sell him on this technique, but we have personally tried it, and it does work. Be sure to use these night-weaning tactics only when your baby is old enough and your gut feeling tells you that your baby is nursing at

night out of habit and not out of need. It's best to wait until your baby is around eighteen months. By then he'll be old enough to manage a certain amount of frustration.

A final note. When a toddler is night-weaned before he is willing, he *will* cry. If he is crying in dad's arms, mom will be tempted to rescue baby, and dad may become quickly frustrated and hand baby off after a few minutes. Deciding how long to let baby cry is a personal decision. We can't give you an exact number of minutes to endure. In chapter 8 we discuss in detail how to approach this situation.

In chapter 4, page 98, we share how one family successfully worked through this challenging night-weaning process.

Moving Out! Tips for Transitioning to a "Big Kid" Bed

YOUR TODDLER is beginning to wear out his welcome in your room. Your bed no longer seems big enough for three, especially when that third person seems to take up more than his fair share. It's time for him to move out (if not out of your room just yet, at least out of your bed). Or maybe your child has been sleeping well in his crib for a while, but this morning you found him standing on top of the railing, getting ready to dive off, in your room, where he sleeps.

Wherever you are right now with your kids, you will reach a point when it's time for a "big kid" bed. This age will be different for every family. Some parents enjoy sharing their room or bed with their kids for years, while others can't wait to reclaim their own private bedroom once again. There is no right age for this transition. Your own instincts will tell you when it's time.

In this chapter we discuss how to tell if your child is ready to move out, how to tell if you or your spouse is ready for your child to move out, how you can make the move happen in a stress-free, happy way for everyone involved (usually the happiest person is dad), and how to transition your child from crib to bed if applicable. We will also give you tools to use if your child begins resisting this change.

FIVE STEPS FOR EASING YOUR KIDS OUT OF YOUR BED, OUT OF YOUR ROOM, AND INTO THEIR OWN ROOM

Okay, so you've been co-sleeping for a year or more, maybe two years or more. It's beginning to look to you like all your kids will be in your bed forever, and you'll be sleeping as a family until they go off to college. You're not too crazy about this, but you don't want to just shove them out of bed and say, "See ya in the morning, buddy." Don't worry that you're turning them loose in the hard, cruel nighttime world at too early an age. This is going to be a very long process. If you work through the suggestions in this chapter, your kids will get out of your bed and room and go to sleep without you — and they will do so happily. Eventually.

AVOID LONG-TERM SLEEP STRESS

One of the best gifts you can give your child is the feeling that bedtime is a happy, peaceful, stress-free time to look forward to every night. You can achieve this goal by sensitively meeting your child's needs at bedtime and during the night. If a child is pushed into sleep independence before he is ready, he will grow up feeling anxious about sleep and may experience a variety of sleep problems.

Here is our five-step plan for moving your kids out of your bed and into the world.

Step 1. Decide When the Time Is Right

Is your child ready to sleep by himself? Are you ready to have him sleep elsewhere? You may not have firm answers to either of these questions. That's okay. Learning to sleep alone is a process. It's not something your child will achieve overnight. Here are some points to consider as you decide when you should try to move your child out of your bed or bedroom or out of his crib into a toddler bed.

Is your child ready? It can be very hard to persuade a co-sleeping, night-nursing toddler to sleep alone all night every night. If you have chosen to co-sleep and your child is still nursing frequently at night, you may find that trying to move her out of your bed now

will be near to impossible. What's more, it will create a great deal of nighttime stress for both you and your child. Since avoiding nighttime stress was one of your main reasons for co-sleeping, you may not find this acceptable, and you may want to concentrate more on decreasing baby's night nursing first (see chapter 6).

If your co-sleeping child is starting to sleep longer stretches without waking up, this may be a sign that she is ready to sleep by herself for part or all of the night.

Realistically, you are likely to be ready before your child is. It's not like she is going to tell you one day, "Mommy, I'm ready for my big-girl bed." You're going to have to sell the idea. Getting your child into her own bed all night will take some time. Just like weaning from the breast, weaning a child from her favorite place to sleep should be done gradually and with love.

Are you ready? Before you decide to ease baby out of your bed, be sure you're doing it for the right reasons. Do you want to move baby into his own bed because you are worried that he will never sleep on his own? Are you tired of criticism from friends, family, even your spouse, who complain that you're making him too dependent or spoiling him? The real question you should ask yourself is "Is our current sleeping arrangement working for us?" If it is, there's no rush to make a change. Your child will leave your bed when he's ready, or when you're ready to help him be more ready. Meanwhile, why mess with an arrangement that helps everyone sleep better at night? But if co-sleeping is no longer working for you, meaning one or more of you are not getting enough sleep, or you simply want the bed to yourselves, it's time to make a change.

Is baby becoming a bed hog? There comes a time when many co-sleeping toddlers become thrashers, and parents just can't take it anymore. You get poked and kicked throughout the night or you wake up with your toddler sleeping on top of you. Maybe you want to put some distance between yourself and a child who will nurse all night long if your breasts are readily available. Remember our motto: *If you resent it, change it!*

Time to put away the crib? Most kids will transition out of a crib between eighteen months and two and a half years. It's more a matter of the crib no longer being a safe place to leave a child unattended than it is a matter of a child wanting to move into a toddler bed. Watch for these ready-to-move-out signs:

- Rattling the cage. Baby stands up, holds on to the side rails, and starts shaking the crib.

- Trying to climb over the guardrail. If you have the mattress at the lowest height and baby is trying to climb out, take this as a sign that he's no longer safe in his crib and he's ready for a less confining space. Removing the padded bumpers will delay the escape artist, but your child will eventually monkey his way out of the crib.

- Baby wakes himself up when he scoots around his crib and bumps into the rails or end. He needs more room so that he can stretch out like a giant starfish.

Step 2. Decide on the Type of Bed and Where to Put It

When it's time to get baby out of your bed or room or his crib, where do you move him to? And what type of bed do you transition him into? It depends on where he is sleeping now and what his age is.

You'll need to decide if the new bed is going to be in your room at first or in a separate room for your child. The advantage of putting the bed in your room is that you are nearby when your child wakes during the night. The advantage of putting the bed in a different room is that you will have your child not only out of your bed but out of your room as well. You'll have attained both objectives as part of the same project. Most kids are comfortable changing to a new room as long as you come along at first.

Here are some factors to consider before you decide what kind of bed to get and where to put it.

If your baby is in your bed. The most logical next step is a small bed placed next to your bed. If your child is still a baby (under age eighteen months), you should move baby into something criblike for safety reasons. Here are the options:

A bedside crib or co-sleeper. We call this the "sidecar arrangement." A co-sleeper clamped to your bed frame or a crib alongside your bed allows you and baby to each have your own separate bed space, yet you're within arm's reach of each other for easier nursing and comforting during the night. This alternative works well for parents who want their babies to sleep close to them but not in their bed. (See the illustration on page 177.)

A crib in your room. This arrangement gets baby out of your bed so that you can enjoy some separate sleep — at least until baby wakes up. You can experiment with getting baby to fall asleep in the crib, or baby can go to sleep in your arms, and when he is sound asleep, you can place him in the crib. It will take some time for baby to adjust to sleeping solo. Be prepared and willing to take baby back into your bed for part of the night if he wakes and needs your presence. Cribs work well for babies and younger toddlers, who need the bars to keep them from falling out of bed at night and from getting into trouble when they awake.

If your toddler is in your bed. If your "baby" is no longer really a baby (over eighteen months), moving her to a crib isn't necessary. Here are your options for this age:

A futon or crib mattress on the floor next to your bed. This is the easiest transition to make. It's conveniently next to your bed for

---

SEARS SLEEP TIP:
GRADUALLY INCREASE THE DISTANCE

Once baby settles well in the bedside crib, gradually move it farther and farther away from your bed, but not yet outside your bedroom. If you find you are all waking up more often as baby sleeps farther away, decrease the distance again.

---

when your child awakens, and it's close to the floor, so there's no worry over injury from rolling out of bed.

An adult mattress on the floor next to your bed. You may find this easier if you need room to snuggle in this bed with your child during the night. But the space it takes up can be a drawback.

When she was seventeen months, I decided I would sleep in a twin bed beside her crib. The first few nights she woke up every hour and sat up and cried. I didn't get out of bed, but I would talk to her gently and say, "It's okay, I'm right here, lie down and go to sleep," and she would! After a week, she woke up only once or twice a night, and then by a month, she was sleeping through the night two to three nights a week.

Moving to a child's own room. When you feel your child is ready for her own actual room, here are some ideas for choosing a bed:

A crib mattress in a toddler bed frame very close to the floor. This is the standard choice, and it works well for most young kids.

A full-size mattress on the floor. We strongly caution against putting a young child up high on an adult bed with a box spring and bed frame. Your child is likely to fall off. Put the mattress right on the floor instead.

A futon on the floor. This is a relatively inexpensive and portable option.

Keep a home base. Realize that your child will wake up during the night and want to return to the old nest. Let him do this at first. Keep things positive and stress-free. You can expect children to take two steps forward and one step backward as they make progress toward a goal. If you want to discourage your child from joining you in your bed, try taking him back to his own bed and sleeping with him there (a good reason for skipping the toddler bed and going straight to a big one). Or keep a futon on the floor by your bed and lie down with your child there as he (and you) fall back to sleep. Another option is to keep a toddler bed set up in your room for a few months (or years) that your child can use when he comes into your room in the night.

Step 3. Sell Your Child on the Idea

Make a special family trip to the "big-girl bed" store. Just as when they pick out a potty for toilet training, kids are more likely to use the bed they choose. Pick out special bedding, too. Set the bed up at home, but don't push your child to start using it just yet. Let her play at putting her dolls or toys to sleep in this bed. Read stories there. Try napping in the new bed. Get to know the new bed as a comfy, safe place to be. If you sense that your

---

DISCOURAGING THE MIDNIGHT VISITOR

Even when kids begin sleeping in their own room, they will on occasion want to return to the old nest. Nighttime can be a scary time for little people, and a child's desire to be with you at night may be an actual need, not an annoying habit to be broken. This desire for nighttime contact may be particularly strong if your child has had little contact with you during the day and needs to reconnect with you at night. The need for nighttime contact also increases when a child is dealing with stress during the day, such as the birth of a sibling, a move, problems in her parents' marriage, or if she is starting preschool or day care. You need to handle these visits in a way that respects both your need for privacy and sleep and your child's need for nighttime security.

Above all, don't feel that you are spoiling your child or that she is psychologically disturbed because she can't yet sleep all night on her own. Many emotionally healthy children simply enjoy the nighttime security of sleeping close to their parents, especially when they are coping with challenges and upsets during the day. Remember, the goal of nighttime parenting is to nurture a healthy lifelong attitude about going to sleep and staying asleep. One thing that helped us cope with our many midnight visitors was realizing that this time of nighttime closeness was a passing stage and that losing sleep was an inevitable part of parenting. If you invest some nighttime energy now in helping your child feel secure and happy, you'll probably end up sleeping a whole lot better when your children are teenagers. (For more information on the midnight visitor, see page 49.)

child is resisting the idea of hanging out in this new bed, back off and try again in a week or two. Don't force the issue. Sit your child down by the bed some afternoon and explain what the bedtime plan is going to be. Be up-beat and positive. Focus on what your child is gaining — her own place to sleep! — not on where she isn't going to sleep anymore.

Step 4. Continue Your Usual Bedtime Routine for a While

Just because your child has a new place to sleep doesn't mean he is happily going to lie down and fall asleep there on his own. You are going to have to continue your previous bedtime routine, only now with a new end location. Only when your child is sleeping well in his new bed can you begin weaning yourself from the bedtime routine.

Step 5. Use the Fade-Away Strategy

Now the fun starts as you begin the long process of teaching your child to fall asleep without you. Once your child is used to going to sleep in her new bed with you there, you can work on helping her go to sleep without you. The fading-away process can be done as fast or as slowly as you feel is right for your child. As you will later read, Dr. Bob faded away over a five-year period. (That was one l-o-n-g fade away.) Try these fade-away strategies:

Snuggle to sleep. Lie in bed with your child while he falls asleep. If he's on a crib mattress, sit on the floor and lean over to snuggle with him. Wait until your child is completely asleep. If you try to sneak away early and

your child wakes up, he'll realize you aren't actually falling asleep with him, and he may become stressed about the new arrangement.

Dr. Bob notes: *One way I could tell that Andrew was completely asleep is that he would have muscle twitches. As soon as I felt those, I knew I could leave in another minute or two.*

Camp out next to the bed. As your child becomes comfortable in the new bed, begin sitting on the floor next to your child while she goes to sleep. You may need to lay your hands on your child during this time. This can be an opportunity to read to yourself, using a flashlight or small book lamp. When your child is comfortable with this setup, begin moving yourself away night by night until you are no longer in actual physical contact with your child or the bed.

Watching my daughter learn to fall asleep on her own has been so funny. At first, after her story and good-night prayers, I would lie beside her and use a book light to read my own book until she was sound asleep. She always knew what I was reading and would always ask if I had finished it yet. Then we went through a

---

SEARS SLEEP TIP

When your child isn't falling asleep "by the book," try not to become impatient. If you do, he will sense that you are wanting to hurry things along, and that will make the process even more drawn-out.

stage where she pretended to read her own chapter books, which she brought home from the library by the armful, while I read my book close by. After a few minutes, she'd turn out her reading light, turn her face to the wall, and go to sleep. Now, because my reading light is broken and I am borrowing hers, she goes to sleep with just a prayer and a hug. There was no master plan behind any of this. It's just how it happened.

Move in and out. Once your child is comfortable without being in physical contact with you while she falls asleep, begin leaving the room for brief intervals every five minutes or so. Tell her you have to check the laundry, go get your book, or anything else. Step out of the room for five seconds (longer if you know she can handle it), then come right back and sit down again for a while. Over a few weeks, gradually lengthen the time you step out of the room. Use a catchphrase each time you leave, such as "One minute" or "I'll be right back." If your child gets anxious during the seconds or minutes you are out of the room, sing a song while you are gone. Leave her door open so she can hear you singing.

Check on your child. You will eventually find that you are out of the room more than you are in it. After you tuck your child in, tell her you'll be back to check on her. Return every few minutes and peek your head in the door. You can even keep yourself busy in the hallway or next room, making quiet noises so your child knows you are near. Gradually lengthen the intervals at which you check on your child. Soon you will find yourself checking on your child every ten or fifteen minutes, and you'll find a peacefully sleeping child after only one or two checks.

This fading-away strategy is perhaps the gentlest way to move your child into falling asleep independently. It may seem too drawn-out for some parents. You can go through each step fairly quickly if your child is willing. Just remember the important goal of creating a stress-free bedtime routine.

Many parents have shared with us their own versions of fading away. Some find it helps to sit quietly in a chair and not move or make a sound, pretending to sleep until baby is asleep. If baby wakes up and seems not to be resettling, they issue a reminding sleep cue, such as "Sleepy-sleep," and then quickly pretend they're going back to sleep. Depending on baby's sleep temperament and the persistence of her personality, they may have to occasionally compromise a bit and help her resettle by taking her into the chair and rocking her and then putting her back into bed. If you try this, ideally, you'll gradually lessen the number of responses needed until your visual presence alone will be enough and you and the chair will gradually fade toward the door and eventually be gone from sight.

My husband was responsible for getting our two-and-a-half-year-old daughter into her own bed. I was pregnant with our son and needed the extra sleep. The process took several months. First, he read to her and slept with her all night in her bed. Then he slept on a futon next to her bed so he'd be close if she woke up and needed his reassurance. Gradually, he crept out of her room into ours — literally. At first he slept on the floor next to her bed. Each night he'd sleep a little farther from her bed, until just his toes were in her room. She'd sit up in bed and see him (even if just his toes) and be comforted by his presence. Then he was on the floor outside her room, inching closer to our room each night. Eventually she was used to sleeping by herself.

Here's another happy-ending sleep story parents in our practice shared with us:

We brought our nine-month-old infant, Tori, in for a sleep consultation because, although she was a happy, wonderful baby, we were wiped out. After hearing that she used to be a colicky, restless sleeper, Dr. Sears suggested that in the early months she probably had reflux and that she was conditioned to associate sleeping with pain rather than with pleasure. Now that the reflux was over, she needed to be retrained to associate sleep with pleasure. That made sense to us, since she had never liked to sleep horizontally and she had had so much pain in the first three months. Here's how we used the fade-away strategy:

◆

On days 1 to 3 we placed the rocker next to her crib. We consoled her through the bars and said, "Sleep-a, sleep-a, Tori." We never picked her up. She played and crawled around her crib, but she didn't fuss much. Many times we had to stand up to help her lie back down. On night 3, I put all six of her pacifiers in her crib because I noticed she would often drop the one I put in her mouth. It took her about an hour to fall asleep.

On days 4 to 6, we moved the rocker to the

middle of the room and verbally consoled her. By now it took her only about twenty to forty minutes to fall asleep. She again fussed a little, but she played mostly. Her biggest struggle was finding the pacifier when it dropped or she spat it out of her mouth.

On days 7 and 8, we stood or sat in the open doorway to her room. By now she knew the routine well enough that it took her only twenty minutes. If Tori stood up in the crib, we moved toward her bed, and she quickly fell into her sleeping position. At this time, we also moved her bedtime up to 8:30 from 9:00.

Day 9 was the night to do the short routine and then put her in the crib and slowly walk away. She slept from a little after 9 p.m. to 6:45 a.m. This was our first time to sleep through the night without interruption since she was born. She whimpered twice in the night but never really cried, and both times she fell right back to sleep.

As you can see, these fade-away strategies give baby two healthy messages: It's okay to go to sleep, and it's okay to use your own self-comforting tools to do it.

GETTING YOUR CHILD TO SLEEP INDEPENDENTLY — DR. BOB'S STORY

Dr. Bob has had experience weaning three kids from the family bed into their own. Here's his story:

My wife, Cheryl, nursed our three kids to sleep every night until they were weaned. At age two years, our first child, Andrew, had weaned from the breast, and getting him to sleep became my job. Andrew didn't care where he slept as long as Cheryl or I fell asleep with him. So getting him out of our bed was easy. I just had to go with him. We set up a twin bed in our bedroom next to our bed. (I was an intern at the time, living in a one-bedroom apartment, so nobody got their own room.) Every night, Andrew and I snuggled into bed together while he was falling asleep, which usually took about forty-five minutes. I often drifted off as well.

Sounds easy, right? Well, actually there were a couple of problems. Often I was so groggy from dozing off that I was useless to Cheryl for the rest of the night. Other nights, I would get very irritated when Andrew took longer than usual to fall asleep. Even more annoying was when I'd think Andrew was asleep and I would start to sneak out of the room only to hear "Dad!" Nuts. I was frustrated because I was losing anywhere from thirty to sixty minutes of my "finally the baby is asleep" part of the night. I had to change something. So I changed my attitude. I decided that by spending this time with Andrew, I was making a commitment to his long-term happiness and self-confidence.

When Andrew turned three and showed no signs of nearing bedtime independence, I decided I might as well make use of my time. I love to read, so every night, I brought a flashlight to bed, aimed it away from Andrew, and read. Andrew snuggled up to my leg or my back and went to sleep. I actually loved this. Free time to myself! When Andrew was four or five, I moved myself and my book to the floor next to his bed. At first I had to keep one arm touching him, but after a while I was able to wean him from that, too.

When Andrew was six (many books and many flashlight batteries later), our second child, Alex, was three years old and newly weaned, and he joined our bedtime routine. By now we were in a house, and the kids shared a bedroom. I found myself once again back in bed, because Alex needed snuggling. But this time the weaning went faster. Alex would fall asleep right away, and then I would move to the floor until Andrew fell asleep.

Soon I started to leave the room for brief periods after Alex was asleep, telling Andrew I would come right back. Andrew took this just fine. I then began to stay away for several minutes, telling Andrew I'd check on him every five minutes. I'd come back into the room, lean over and kiss his forehead, and say "I'll be back in five minutes" over and over again until I'd find him asleep. He wanted to be able to hear Cheryl and me during this time, so we would be sure to make some noise. This five-minute check time turned into ten minutes, then fifteen, and by the time Andrew was seven, I was able to simply tuck him in and leave the room. He'd fall asleep without any problem. I'd check on him twenty or thirty minutes later. Occasionally he'd still be awake and smile at me peacefully. I'm sure having Alex sleeping there in the room helped. The kids moved to their own beds, and Alex had no problem with my leaving before he was asleep.

Of course they still woke up from time to time. Between ages two and four, when Andrew woke up, he'd climb into our bed (often without our even knowing it — we'd wake up the next morning and there would be an extra body). Between ages four and six, Andrew would come to our bed and tap one of us on the shoulder, and I'd walk him back to his bed and tuck him in or let him fall asleep on the futon on the floor next to our bed. From age six to eight, Andrew would just climb onto the futon during the night without even waking us up. Alex almost never woke up during the night. But there was something about Andrew — he just needed to touch base with us, and then he'd go back to sleep. After age eight, Andrew stopped waking up at night.

Now, at nine and twelve, Alex gets tucked in at bedtime, prayed with, and kissed good night, and he falls asleep without a hitch. Andrew just tells us good night and heads to his room. They even have separate bedrooms. Unlike many kids, they aren't anxious sleepers. They never feel night stress, they never get up and ask for water, they almost never complain that it's bedtime, they never get up during the night, and they have never had a problem with sleep terrors or bed-wetting. Alex told me just the other day, "Dad, I haven't had a nightmare in years. I still have lots of dreams, though." Andrew added, "I had a nightmare that I forgot to turn in a homework page and got an F. I never have nightmares about monsters or anything scary."

Our third child, Joshua, is three, and we recently put a crib mattress on the floor next to our bed and dubbed it his "big boy" bed. Since he is at the age when everything is all about being a big boy, he loves this idea. He is weaned, so it's my job to snuggle him to sleep in our bed. When Cheryl and I go to bed, we move him into his little bed. He sleeps most of the night there, and we finally have our king-size bed to ourselves. Joshua wakes up and comes into our bed sometime during the night about twice a week.

Okay, you moms are probably thinking to yourselves, "Wow, that would be so awesome if my husband would take over the nighttime routine." You dads are probably thinking, "I can't spend an hour every night for five years putting my child to bed." We're not about to tell you that it will take five years to teach your child to sleep independently. Looking back, I realize I could have moved through this weaning process with Andrew a lot faster. I could easily have sped up the transitions we went through and had him falling asleep independently by age four, but it just never occurred to me. I really, truly loved the closeness that Andrew and I developed, and I was in no hurry to change it. Plus, I got to lie around and read lots of books, all in the name of sensitive nighttime parenting.

Here are some points to consider as you decide how to move your child to sleep independence:

- Be sensitive to what your child needs and find strategies that work for both of you.
- Go as fast or slow as you and your child are comfortable with.
- Share the bedtime routine with your spouse.
- Consider the long-term sleep goal we shared with you at the beginning of this chapter: to help your child learn to sleep stress-free. If you push too fast, your child won't develop the self-confidence and security needed to achieve happy sleep independence.

Twenty-three Nighttime Fathering Tips

DADS, NIGHTTIME IS WHEN you can really shine! How often have we heard tired moms lament, "I wish my husband would help more during the night." Yet dads often develop an acute case of nighttime hearing loss after a newborn joins the household, especially when mom seems to be so much better at getting baby to sleep. Big mistake! Skip the earplugs and get ready to take an active part in nighttime parenting. When we look through our "survivor" files — the stories of parents who have made it through those early months without succumbing to utter exhaustion — one feature stands out: the presence of a sensitive and involved dad. This chapter is all about how you can help your baby and your baby's mother get more sleep.

Moms, we want to say a quick word to you at the beginning of this chapter. We know that you are probably reading this chapter before your husband does. The second part of this chapter is all about how you can encourage your husband to get more involved with nighttime parenting if he hasn't

volunteered already. There we give you some helpful insights (from the male standpoint) into how to tell your husband about your needs and your baby's needs in a way that he'll understand. We also help you understand what your husband is feeling during this time, in case he isn't effectively communicating this to you. Even if he is reluctant to read this whole book, we hope that he will read this chapter to understand why a sleep-refreshed wife is more pleasant to live with.

Now, back to dad. Dads, if your wife is handing you this chapter to read, it's likely she is getting burned out. Take a hint!

PART ONE — FOR DADS

Here are twenty-three tips that will help you support your wife, be involved with your baby, and enable your family unit to function better at night.

Be a Supportive Father by Day

Nighttime fathering starts with things you do in the daytime. The relationship you have with your wife and baby during their waking hours will carry over into what happens in the wee hours of the night.

1. Understand the switch to mother mode. As soon as that umbilical cord is cut, your wife moves into mother mode: all baby all the time. All of her energy is focused on nurturing baby, and she may forget her own needs. Mother mode is nature's way of giving little human beings the right start in life. After all, for your baby to thrive, he needs almost constant care. Your wife's intuition is to put baby's needs above her own need for sleep — and certainly above your need for sex.

In those early months of marathon giving, many mothers are on the verge of burnout but won't admit it. What's the biggest contributor to mother burnout? Father walkout! By that, we mean fathers who are not involved in their babies' care and who fail to be sensitive to their wife's needs. If you want your wife to go through the mother-mode stage with romantic feelings about you, respect her need to nurture her baby and help her take better care of herself.

My husband does what he can to free me up to be a mother.

2. Keep the nest tidy. A neat, orderly home is more conducive to mothering than a home in which chores pile up, waiting for the woman of the house to do them. Because she already has so much to learn and worry about, you may find that your wife is easily upset by the slightest mess. During the postpartum period, Martha was upset by even one dirty dish, though ordinarily a sink full of dirty dishes wouldn't have fazed her. An upset mother often translates into an upset baby. Remember this acronym: TIDY — Take Inventory Daily Yourself. Don't wait for your wife to make a "honey-do" list. You need to make out the list yourself, and then do the things on it! Hire some help if you can; otherwise, take over the housekeeping yourself. Each day, walk around the house and look for things you can do so that your wife will have more energy for mothering. Sort through the junk mail. Wash the dishes. Clean the bathroom mirror. Put away the laundry.

If you are a night owl, use that time to make the house look more tidy for your wife the next day. If you have older children, enlist their help. Show them how to pick up after themselves and remind them to do so. (Preschoolers will need hands-on supervision.) Tell them that it's an important time for them to care for mom. Remember, you are bringing up someone's future mate, and someday that mate's spouse will hug you and thank you for training your child to do housework. One day a grandfather in my office told me, beaming, "My daughter-in-law gave me the supreme compliment: 'Thank you for bringing up such a sensitive man!'"

3. Be sensitive. Stan, a new father and professional tennis player, asked me how he could help with his newborn baby. I advised him, "Improve your serve!" Think about what you can do to help before your wife has to ask. Many new mothers are trying to do everything for the baby and everything in the household all by themselves. They are trying to be perfect mothers in their own eyes and in their husband's. This is completely unrealistic, yet their husbands seem clueless about their need for help. As one mother told me, "I'd have to hit my husband over the head before he'd realize I'm giving out." Try to figure out how you can help, and intervene before your wife is so drained that she begins to feel overwhelmed and depressed. For example, if you notice mother and baby are sleeping, turn off the ringer on the phone and hang a "Do Not Disturb" sign on the door. If baby wakes up before mom, quickly pick him up and take him outside for a walk, so that your wife can sleep a bit longer. That extra bit of sleep will get you a big hug. As one father summed it up: "I can't breastfeed, but I can create an environment that helps my wife breastfeed better."

Realize that some moms will not ask for help because they don't want to seem less than the Supermom they hope to be.

4. Be a "shareholder." Don't wait until the middle of the night to learn how to comfort your baby. If you are comfortable holding and comforting baby during the day, it will be easier for you to figure out what to do at night to ease baby into sleep. Baby will get to know your ways of holding and comforting and will learn to trust that dad can make everything all better. Experiment with various holding positions to get baby used to your unique way of comforting. Wear your baby in a carrier as much as possible throughout the day so that baby gets used to your unique motion, scent, and voice and you get used to various ways of daytime comforting. The more baby is accustomed to your special ways during the day, the more likely he will be to settle for you at night.

If you have a toddler and a new baby, spend time during the day to strengthen your bond with your older child. Some nights you and your wife will do tag-team nighttime parenting: daddy snuggles the older child while mommy nurses the baby. Or, baby is handed over to daddy while the older child is snuggled to sleep by mommy. If both of your children are comfortable with you, you will have more flexibility in solving nighttime problems.

5. Get involved early. During pregnancy and in the first weeks after birth, most mothers worry, "I wonder how my husband is going to handle all of these changes?" The sooner you can alleviate this worry, the better. Don't be a distant dad — day or night. Be part of the parenting team right from the start. When your baby is born, take as much time off from your job as is economically feasible. Also, when you do return to work, cut back on evening meetings and out-of-town travel.

Newborns become creatures of habit very early. The sooner you give your baby the message that both mom and dad are going to care for him, the easier it will be for your baby to adapt to your style of nighttime fathering. And the sooner you start, the sooner you will gain confidence in your abilities to care for your baby. Learning how to comfort your

MY HUSBAND . . .

"Nothing turns a woman on like seeing a man nurture her baby," a rested mother once told us. From our happy-family gallery, here are some inspirational quotes from mothers about sensitive fathers.

- . . . rubs my back or gives me a foot massage while I nurse if I'm having a middle-of-the-night meltdown.
- . . . tells me (over and over) that I am doing a great job and that everything will get better.
- . . . encourages me to go to bed when baby does, even if it's only 7 p.m.
- . . . brings me a midnight snack.
- . . . becomes a night-light. He holds a soft light for me to get our newborn latched on correctly for the night nursing in the first few weeks.
- . . . did the daddy dance. He would take our twins downstairs and dance to his favorite CD in the living room. Years later, these songs continue to calm them immediately. We call them "Daddy's songs."
- . . . lets me SLEEP IN on the weekends, which is like paradise.

- . . . and I put our baby to bed every night as a FAMILY.
- . . . lies next to us when baby nurses to sleep.
- . . . treats nighttime parenting as an EQUAL responsibility. None of that "I'm a hero for taking turns with a wakeful baby" stuff!
- . . . helps when our son is hyper and playful and doesn't look like he's going down anytime soon. He walks around the house and sings to him to wind him down.
- . . . got baby used to being comforted by him, which gave me a break now and then. At night we were a "nursing team." It was great!
- . . . takes over baby duty when he comes home from work so I can make dinner and do other things that need to be done.
- . . . gets up and uses his "magic shoulder" to burp the baby for me.
- . . . leaves the room with the baby when he's helping out. There is no point in both of us listening to the screaming.

baby at night builds daddy-baby trust. Early on, your child learns that mom is not the only one who can make boo-boos better.

Because our son was a marathon nurser and was attached to my breast much of the time, my husband was a little afraid in the beginning. He

didn't know how to get involved. By the time we decided to get him involved in nighttime shifts, our son did not want a change in routine. It wasn't until he weaned at seventeen months that he began to want his dad at night. With our next baby, we'll know better and start nighttime fathering earlier.

HOW DO YOU SPELL RELIEF?

F-A-T-H-E-R

6. Be a weekend warrior. On weekends, holidays, and other days when you don't have to work, care for your infant when he wakes up in the morning and allow mom to sleep in. After baby nurses in the morning and is wide awake and eager to play, whisk him away to another room, or even outside, so your wife can stay in bed and sleep. Take the phone off the hook as you go out the door. Put baby in a carrier and stroll around the block for a nice baby-daddy walk. If your walk puts baby back to sleep, keep him with you instead of laying him down next to mommy. Let her enjoy a morning of waking up baby-free. If your work schedule permits, try this arrangement on the occasional weekday, too — especially days when baby wakes up early. Keep baby with you in another part of the house and let your wife catch another hour of shut-eye.

Bill notes: *When Matthew was eleven months old, he and I both enjoyed going for a walk around the neighborhood right after his morning nursing. Eventually, Matthew got so used to this habit that after nursing he would give me the "go" cue. Then he would crawl toward the baby sling hanging near the door.*

◆

My favorite thing that my husband did was that every Sunday morning, he took the baby and went to get doughnuts and coffee and then *went to the grocery store, the hardware store, or anywhere he could go. He tried to stay out until noon most times, and that 6 a.m.-to-noon stretch was the longest sleep I would have all week. I LOVED that!*

You can also take over nap-time duties on the weekend. This is a good time to practice your getting-baby-off-to-sleep skills. Meanwhile, your wife gets a chance to enjoy some "just for me" time.

7. Support your wife's mothering style. Whatever nighttime parenting style your wife chooses, be supportive. Most new mothers are a bit shaky about trusting their own wisdom. But mom really does know best! Let her know that you support whatever she chooses to do. If your mother, her mother, or a friend criticizes the way she cares for your baby or starts pressuring her to do something differently (maybe they're telling her not to "spoil the baby by picking him up all the time"), do what you can to shield her from these bearers of bad baby advice. Don't bring home stories about friends' babies sleeping through the night after "only one night of crying it out." Your friends' babies are not your baby. Your baby has a unique temperament, and you and your wife have a unique parenting style. Besides, making comparisons like this gives your wife the message that you think your baby is waking up because of something she's doing or not doing. Don't pressure her to figure out how to get baby to sleep better at night. Read this book together and discuss sleep strategies as a team.

The best fathering my husband does — besides some one-on-one time with our son — is when he supports me and our choice to co-sleep and night-nurse in the face of a lot of criticism.

8. Actions speak louder than words. Don't just tell your wife to get more rest. Make it happen. Your reminder to "nap when baby does" sounds pretty lame if you are also complaining about the house being a mess or if you are expecting your wife to entertain your toddler while caring for the baby 24/7. Hire some help with the housecleaning. Pay a teen to come in and look after your toddler so that your wife can nap. When she starts to worry about "getting something done," remind her that she is doing the most important job in the world right now — raising a human being. It's okay to let other things go for a while. Lower your standards. Easy meals and quick cleanups are the norm when there are small children to care for.

If your wife is going through one of those "I don't have time for myself" phases, *make time* for her. Tell her, "I've scheduled an hour for you at the spa and have already paid for it, and I can't get our money back. I'll drive you there and look after baby while you enjoy yourself." One time when Matthew was going through a high-need stage, Martha said, "I don't even have time to take a shower, my baby needs me so much." I lovingly reminded her, "Martha, what our baby needs is a happy, rested mother."

My husband is what we call "daddy magic" with our son. If I hand our son to him so I can do something else, I often return to find that our son has simply fallen asleep. I think part of it has to do with my husband's voice and calm demeanor (and his lack of lactating breasts!). My husband always had greater success putting our son to sleep when he was a newborn. I think that it is simply a dad thing.

Support the Tired Mom at Night

If your baby falls asleep at the breast every night and goes back to sleep by breastfeeding in the middle of the night, you may be thinking, "Hey, this is great! I don't have to do anything." You may be right. This style of nighttime parenting works for some families. But it may not work for yours. Mothers who breastfeed a couple times every night can get very tired. They may also resent a dad who sleeps through it all. Here are some things you can do to make nighttime nursing easier on your wife:

9. Change your attitude. Instead of dreading nighttime and viewing it as an occupational hazard of having a baby, change your attitude. Try a principle that we teach our kids as one of the keys to happy living: *View a problem as an opportunity.* Becoming more involved with your baby's nighttime care will earn you double rewards: You will deepen your relationship with your baby, and you will enjoy the gratitude and admiration of your wife. It's going to be a while before your infant reaches the Promised Land of Nod, where she sleeps through the night. You might as well make nighttime fathering a positive experience.

It's normal to feel that you have the right to sleep at night. You work hard during the day to provide for your family. Maybe you are the sole breadwinner, and you need to be alert in the morning so that you can go to work and ensure your family's economic well-being. In some families mom shares the attitude that it's more important for dad to get a good night's sleep. But some burned-out and sleep-deprived moms don't agree:

Don't make any comments about having to go to work the next day. Moms work, too. Imagine working twenty-four hours a day at your main job and living at the office. That's what full-time mothering is like.

◆

I felt my husband worked all day to provide for me to stay home, so I was not about to wake him to feed the baby. I viewed this as my job. I did mine and he did his. I did, of course, encourage him to care for her in the evening, change diapers and so forth, so I could rest, and he delighted in it.

◆

I think a lot of stay-at-home moms try to do it all at night. They don't realize that their sleep is just as important as their husband's.

◆

Don't shush mom and baby when you're half-asleep. Get up and help. Otherwise, your attitude conveys that something is wrong with baby or something is wrong with mom's method of getting baby to sleep. Your wife may feel that it's

her fault that baby wakes up and that you think she's not a very good mother when she can't get baby back to sleep more easily.

10. Serve baby to mommy. If your baby awakens in the middle of the night in her crib, wanting a feeding, don't roll over, play dead, and incur your wife's wrath. Instead, get up, get baby, and deliver her to mommy. Murmur some sweet and encouraging words to your wife and enjoy this beautiful middle-of-the-night family moment. Baby, mom, and dad can all drift back to sleep while baby nurses. Many mothers prefer to let their babies sleep with them after the first night feeding. But if baby needs to be returned to the crib when the feeding is over, let sleeping mommy lie there (she's zonked out on relaxing breastfeeding hormones), and you be the one who shuttles the sleeping baby back to the crib. This is just one example of the importance of learning how to handle baby on your own.

Don't pretend to be sleeping when baby cries. We know you are awake! Don't fake snore and roll over like you are so wrapped up in sleep that you can't possibly wake up and help.

◆

We do tag-team nighttime parenting. Daddy gets baby, and mommy nurses baby. So, in a way, daddy nurses mommy.

11. Support the nursing pair. You may feel that since mom is nursing, there is nothing you can do at night, so you might as well sleep. There may be nights when, because of your work schedule, you need to sleep. Yet, as

POINTS — OR REWARDS?

A quick word about points. We use this word a lot in this chapter because we know that men think this way. The problem is, mothers don't. Or if they do, they see men's puny "point total" as laughable. What would happen if mothers kept score on how much they give to baby versus what baby gives back? In the first weeks of parenting, the score would be about a million to three. So if you think that eighty or ninety accumulated points are going to win you some rewards (i.e., sex), you'd better forget about it. Chances are, your wife will resent the fact that you are keeping score. Just keep on giving, and think of points as a way of accumulating long-term rewards, not gaining short-term victories. Your contribution to parenting your baby will give you a happy, well-rested wife and a close marriage. And yes, sex will be part of that.

often as possible, be available during nighttime feedings. Even though you can't breastfeed, do whatever you can to help your wife breastfeed more comfortably: fluff her pillows or massage her back. If she's lying on her side curled around the baby, wedge a pillow between the bed and her lower back for extra support. Keep her company. Just knowing you are there and that you care helps the nursing pair. If you tend to fall back to sleep quickly, as least give your wife an encouraging word of support as you drift off.

My husband would wake up when he heard the baby and me wake up. He didn't do anything, he just sat there in the dark with us. It was at those times that I loved him the most. He was providing nighttime fathering in the most unselfish way . . . by supporting his baby's mom!

12. Offer a nighttime relief bottle. If your baby is bottlefeeding or going through a stage of marathon night nursing and you sense your wife is giving out, once in a while in the middle of the night, give baby a bottle (of pumped breast milk if mom is breastfeeding) so that mom can get a few uninterrupted hours of sleep. Notice we advise only an occasional relief bottle when mom is on the edge of nighttime burnout. Don't try this until baby is at least six weeks old and mom's milk supply is well established. Substituting a bottle for the breast on a regular basis can interfere with the balance between baby's demand for milk and the breasts' ability to make milk. Also, mother may wake up feeling uncomfortably engorged.

Getting dad to give the 2 a.m. bottle of pumped breast milk sounds attractive, but since I have to get up and pump anyway to keep from getting engorged, what's the point?

Not all breastfed babies will accept a nighttime bottle. It might be easiest to get baby accustomed to the occasional bottle during the day first before you try to offer one at night. It's common for an avid breastfeeder to protest both the milk's container and the milkman who is delivering it. Try these tricks:

SHOULD YOU COMPLAIN TO YOUR WIFE THAT YOU NEED MORE SEX?

Okay, let's talk about sex. While the doctor may have okayed having sex six weeks after childbirth, the doctor is not the one recovering from childbirth. It may be many months before your wife has sexual feelings again. The reason for this is her body chemistry is telling her, so to speak, "Recover from childbirth, make milk, and don't even think about having another baby." So even if your wife actually begins having sex with you again six or eight weeks after the birth, the reality is, she may not really feel like it. When wives are not sexually attracted to their men, it is a blow to the male ego. But should you complain to your wife about this? You go right ahead, if you think it will do any good. At least she could reassure you that, of course, she still loves you and thinks you're hot. She's not too worried that you'll cool down before she starts warming up to the idea.

Men don't understand hormones, but at least it's something to blame the lack of sex on. Here's what happens to a woman's hormones after she becomes a mother: Before pregnancy and birth, a woman's hormones to mate are higher than her hormones to mother. After birth, a reverse occurs, and here's why. Not only do babies do what they do because they are designed that way, but mothers also act the way they do because they are designed that way. A shift from mating hormones to mothering hormones seems to ensure survival of the young of the species. Face it, guys, according to the rules of nature, babies can't thrive without their mothers, but dads can survive without sex for a while.

Another reason for your wife's apparent lack of interest in sex is just plain old fatigue. After being drained by a needy baby all day (and other demands in the

---

- Warm the bottle nipple under warm water to make it more supple.

- Hold your baby in a position similar to how he is used to being held during breast-feeding. If that doesn't work, hold him in a position that is completely different from breastfeeding.

- Walk around or rock your baby as you offer the bottle.

- Don't force the bottle nipple into your baby's mouth. Instead, encourage baby to

open wide and latch on as he does at the breast.

A policeman dad in our practice offered this tip: "I hold the bottle under my arm like I hold my flashlight and let baby nurse on the bottle that way. That's as close as I can come to doing it like she's used to at the breast."

13. Be the water boy! While your wife is nursing, bring her water, juice, a snack, or whatever she needs for comfort. Ask, "What household), all she wants to do is sleep. Mothers describe this end-of-the-day feeling as being "all touched out" or "all used up." So, as you can see, the best way for her to have any energy left over for you is for you to pitch in and share the baby care and household chores.

Want to make points the affectionate way? In the first few months after the birth, "sex" does not have to equal intercourse. Many times your wife simply wants holding, loving words, or even a soothing massage. After a bit of postpartum courtship all over again, you may be surprised that your wife is more ready and willing to go all the way. Also, acting like a sexually thwarted male who is ready to pounce is a guaranteed turn-off.

Be open about your wife's sexual feelings and your frustrations. Have sex, but don't expect it to be the "bouncing off the walls" kind of sex you may have enjoyed during your honeymoon. Tell your wife that you love her and understand the state of her body and mind right now. Tell her you simply want to have sex every so often and you understand that in time (in a very long time) your sex life will return to its B.K. (before kids) status. No pressure, no expectations, no problem, right? Well, not always. Some men get more frustrated about the temporary loss of great sex than others, just as some women get their desire for sex back sooner than others. If you feel she is neglecting you too much, tell her so in a very, very understanding and patient way, preferably when she is well rested and not nursing the baby. Do not blame her because her postpartum hormones are keeping her from feeling sexy (that's partly your fault, anyway — you helped make the baby). If you are open and understanding about this whole subject, who knows, maybe your wife will surprise you one night. (See also Sex and the Family Bed, page 129.)

do you need?" or "How can I help?" Be the "gofer," fetching diapers or a change of baby clothing. Do whatever you can so mother does not have to leave her nest. If she needs to get up to go to the bathroom, hold and comfort baby while she does and keep her side of the bed warm. Even though you're tired and would rather be sleeping, try to do night chores with a willing attitude. Resenting the loss of sleep won't help you feel any more rested, and it won't "make points" with your wife.

Breastfeeding and night nursing was my job. My husband would change baby's diaper before and after nursing and I would assume the job of burping the baby. Many times I would wake up starving in the middle of the night from all the nursing and he would go down to the kitchen and fix me some toast and juice.

14. Encourage earlier bedtimes and morning sleep-ins. Couples often want to stay up late to have some private time after baby is in bed. But this can backfire. Baby's longest stretch of sleep is likely to come during the first part of the night, say from 8 p.m. to midnight. If mom goes to bed at 11:30, she may have to wake up thirty minutes later and every two hours thereafter to feed the baby. She has missed out on her chance to get four solid hours of sleep. In the early months, encourage your wife to go to bed when baby does, at least a couple nights a week, so she can catch up on her sleep. Or, if mom is tired but baby isn't, encourage her to go to bed while you tend to baby for another hour or two. If some night you discover that mom has drifted off to sleep while nursing but baby is still awake, ease baby away from sleeping mommy and enjoy some baby-and-daddy time until baby is ready for sleep.

In addition to becoming a weekend warrior (see page 170), try to do daddy duty during an occasional weekday morning. Once a week try to schedule your work so that you can care for baby for a few hours when he first wakes up, which will allow your wife to sleep in.

The best thing my husband did was an early-morning thing. When our son was six months old and I was suffering from severe sleep deprivation, he started getting up with him for "guy time" in the early morning. This allowed me to catch an extra hour or so of "private" sleep. This truly made me love him in an all new way. He and our son now have an incredibly close bond, and when our son wakes in the morning, he automatically says "Dad!" and wants to go play with him.

15. Exude confidence. You and your wife both know that baby settles down easily when mom breastfeeds her, but mom, the starting pitcher, is wearing out. It's time for you to enter the game as a relief pitcher at nighttime or nap time. Your wife may be wondering, "Can he really handle this?" Put on your game face (even if you have to fake it) and give your wife (and baby) the message "Relax, I can do this!" (We call this the "Caribbean attitude" — "No problem, mon!") Try to be calm and confident. When you exude confidence as a nighttime father, mom and baby will both relax and you'll do a better job. Eventually, your wife will be more willing to go to the bullpen for relief because she'll know she can count on you to get the job done.

This man deserves a blue ribbon. He sees nighttime parenting as part of his "job," too. Our baby is adopted, and once a week he sleeps with the baby in our room while I sleep in another room. He takes over night feedings just to give me one full night's sleep a week.

◆

My husband would walk with baby in a football hold. She loved this and would fall asleep easily.

◆

Occasionally, dad needs to sleep in another room and "freshen up" for work. But we have settled into a sense of shared responsibility at night where we each respond to the fusses we hear. Often we are up together helping each other out. We are a family at night.

◆

Take baby out of earshot of the mother, so she can get some GOOD sleep and not just lie there awake listening to daddy try to calm the baby.

My husband, left to his own devices, has been great at finding innovative and successful ways to get our son to sleep.

Try Our Favorite Nighttime Fathering Strategies

We feel that fathers have a unique and different way of holding and comforting babies. It's not better or worse than mom's — it's just different. And babies enjoy that difference. While there is no way dads will ever beat the breast as baby's favorite nighttime pacifier, they can use the assets they do have — stronger arms and a deeper voice — to "nurse" the baby.

Okay, so your wife's breasts are like a magic button for putting baby to sleep or stopping baby's crying. This doesn't mean that you can't find your own way to comfort your child and get your child to sleep. Babies need to be able to count on both parents for comforting, even if, in the early months, they settle down most easily when put to the breast. There's no dishonor in coming in second to breastfeeding. You, your wife, and your baby will all know that baby can trust dad, too, to help him calm down and feel better.

So how do you comfort a breastfeeding baby when you don't have lactating breasts? Early on, help baby learn to associate other kinds of comforting with falling asleep. As you learned in chapter 1 (you did read this chapter, didn't you, Dad?), babies should have more than just one sleep association. Here are some of our favorite ways for dads to help babies fall asleep:

16. Use the "neck nestle" and "warm fuzzy" holds. The neck nestle and the warm fuzzy are two favorite holding positions for dads.

The neck nestle. Hold baby in your arms or in a baby sling against your chest with her head snuggled into the curve of your neck and your chin gently touching the top of her head. Baby's head will then rest against your voice box, and she will feel the comforting vibrations as you talk or sing in a low voice. Here's where dads shine, since the male voice is lower and the vibrations of the larynx are stronger. Just before nap time, bedtime, or even during the night, I would put Lauren in the neck nestle position and in a low, droning

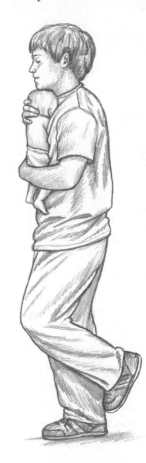

voice sing (to the *Lullaby and Good Night* tune):

> *Go to sleep, go to sleep,*
> *Go to sleep, my little baby.*
> *Go to sleep, go to sleep,*
> *Go to sleep my little girl.*

Oftentimes, my little girl and "big girl" would go to sleep to this tune. Double points!

My husband and I had a deal. If I could comfort baby without getting out of bed, I did it. Most of the time this was the case. If baby needed to be walked, then my husband would do it.

The warm fuzzy. While lying down on the bed or relaxing in your favorite recliner, drape your diaper-clad baby over your bare chest with his ear over your heart. The combination of your heartbeat, the rise and fall of your chest as you breathe, and the warm air from your nose flowing over baby's scalp will soothe and lull him into a sound sleep.

From the start, our baby loved to snuggle up against daddy's chest and feel him breathe. I think she immediately knew the difference between her small, soft mommy and her big, strong daddy. She seems to also need daddy. It's amazing what both parents, being so different, individually offer the baby they love.

17. Be a hands-on dad. Dads, the comfort of your loving hands on an awakening baby can often lull her back to sleep. We call this baby calmer the "laying on of hands." Use it to help baby stay asleep as you transfer her from your arms to the mattress. Use it again

> ## READ THE RULES!
>
> Dads, now that you are co-captain of the Nighttime Parenting team, you must read the sleep safety rules listed on pages 76 to 81.

during the night when baby fusses in her sleep and seems like she might be waking up. Put your hand gently on baby's chest for a minute or so. You can gently pat baby if that seems to be what she needs. Gradually ease your hand away, even letting it hover for another minute an inch or two over baby's chest. Baby will get used to that special touch to go to sleep, and it will also help her go back to sleep.

If she wakes up when we put her back down to sleep at night and I know she's not hungry, my husband ever so gently puts one hand over her chest and the other on her stomach and softly holds them there. She feels like she's being held, even though she's in her crib, and she nods off. She has moved from the bedside bassinet to the crib only recently and seems to need this extra reassurance. It is also great for my husband, because he's a loving, hands-on father, and this gives him the feeling of being able to really nurture and comfort her.

Adults lie still to fall asleep. Babies like to be in motion. Some babies need you to get up out of your chair to help them sleep. Snuggle your baby into a comfortable position in your arms or put her in the baby sling and then get moving. You can take a walk outside, stroll through the house, or do the "daddy dance" around the living room. Babies fall asleep most easily when you move in all directions — back and forth, up and down, and from side to side.

One night I woke up to find my husband sitting at his computer at 2 a.m. listening to rock and roll with the baby bouncing to the beat.

18. Try freeway fathering. If your baby is so wound up that he won't wind down with any of your usual techniques, secure him safely in the car seat and take a ride, preferably on a long, monotonous road that has few stop signs or curves. Babies are usually lulled to sleep by the motion and sound of the car. When you return home, carry the sleeping baby — car seat and all — into the house for nap time or nighttime. Years ago, when our son Dr. Jim was seventeen years of age, he was babysitting for two-year-old Erin, who was asleep when we left and asleep when we got back. In between, Jim told us, he had had to do some "freeway fathering" to get her back to sleep. Years later, when he became a dad himself, he remembered this technique.

19. Add the finishing touch. You and your wife may decide that you want your baby or toddler to learn to fall asleep without always breastfeeding. You can make the transition from breastfeeding at bedtime to going to sleep with dad easier on your child by doing it gradually, using the "finishing touch" technique. With this technique, baby continues to be breastfed at bedtime but does not nurse completely to sleep. When baby's tummy is

full and she is getting drowsy, your wife eases baby off her breast and into your arms.

Now what do you do? We hope you are prepared with some comforting tricks that have worked for you during the day. Try all of the strategies we listed above, or whatever else you think might work. Your goal is to soothe and comfort your baby until she is in the state of deep sleep, when you can put her down without her waking up.

If baby sleeps in a crib. After mother has rocked or nursed baby, use these finishing touches before putting baby into her own bed:

- Your voice. Say a sleep cue (such as "Sleepy-sleepy" or "Nighty-night") or sing a gentle, repetitive sleep song.

- Your body. Snuggle baby into the neck nestle or hold her against your chest in the "warm fuzzy" position.

- Motion. Rock baby in a rocking chair, or if baby begins to wake up, start walking around with baby in the "neck nestle" position while you continue your sleep cue or sleep song. If baby wakes up from the almost-asleep state, put her in a baby carrier and wear her around the house. (See Wearing Down in a Sling, pages 19 and 20.)

If baby sleeps with you. If baby is in your bed between you and your wife, mom simply eases baby off her nipple (see how-to suggestions, page 140) and rolls over, and you add the finishing touch by patting baby's tummy and softly repeating a sleep cue or sleep song. Baby should sleep on her back, or you can cuddle her in your arms and pat her back and bottom as she lies on her side. Continue humming and singing until baby is in the state of deep sleep (see chapter 3 to learn about the states of sleep). If baby is beginning to wake up instead of drifting off, give her more body contact. Lay her on your chest, tummy to tummy, and continue the patting and humming. If this doesn't do the trick, you may have to get up and add motion to the mix. When baby finally drifts off into a deep sleep, ease her onto the mattress to sleep on her back.

If baby is still young enough to need night feedings (most do under six months), add the finishing touch after each feeding instead of having mom nurse baby all the way to sleep.

On weekends my husband would put our baby on his side of the bed (between him and a guardrail). On those nights, I felt a bit of relief and could focus on sleeping. When she woke to feed, I would nurse her on my side, and after he burped her and changed her, she would go back to his side of the bed. Oh, how I looked forward to weekends.

◆

My husband always uses the same song to put our son to sleep, "Barbara Ann" by the Beach Boys. Our son even asks for it by name. It's very sweet!

20. If bottlefeeding, take turns doing bedtime. With bottlefeeding, you and your wife can take turns covering the nighttime shift. Work out a routine that fits your family's nighttime schedule and your individual sleep needs. Try this shared feeding arrangement so

---

> ## SWITCH PLACES!
>
> When baby becomes a toddler and your wife is working on cutting back on night feedings, after baby is sound asleep, do a quick switch in sleeping positions. If baby wakes up next to mom, he will gravitate toward mom's breast like a heat-seeking missile. Instead, if baby wakes up next to you, it's easier to get him back to sleep without waking mom to feed. Move baby over to your side of the bed, between you and the guardrail (or move baby into the co-sleeper, if that's what you're using), and then get yourself into position to sleep between baby and mom. If baby doesn't settle for dad, mom may have to wake up and move to your side of the bed, which you'll have pre-warmed for her. Make points! (And did you notice that your wife is now sleeping next to you, without baby in between? Clever, eh?)

that baby gets used to being bottlefed at nighttime by both mom and dad. If baby learns to go to sleep when father gives a bottle, he is more likely to go back to sleep for dad in the middle of the night. You may want to teach your baby other sleep associations besides bottlefeeding. Use the finishing-touch technique after feedings but before baby falls asleep.

My husband helps me by taking the baby just before bedtime. This allows me to be ready for my middle-of-the-night shift.

21. Enjoy fathering-to-bed rituals. There's more to getting baby off to sleep than adding the finishing touch. Older babies and toddlers depend on bedtime rituals to get them in the mood for sleeping. These bedtime rituals can be a wonderful way to enjoy special time with your child, especially if you are apart all day long. Bedtime is prime time for dads. Even if your baby usually breastfeeds to sleep, you can get him ready for that last feeding while mom rests or has some time to herself. A bedtime ritual might include a bath, saying "night-night" to everyone and everything, story time, prayers, or other quiet activities.

My husband is so good at it we call him "Daddy Night-Night."

Be prepared for your infants and children to string these rituals out for as long as they can. Take this as a compliment. It means that your child wants to spend more time with you, especially if he hasn't had you around during the day. Expect your toddler to prolong the bedtime ritual after a new baby comes into the home. It's as if he's thinking, "This is my special time with dad before bedtime and I'm going to make the most of it."

22. Help transition your child into a big bed. Dads have the starring nighttime role when it's time for a toddler to move from mommy and daddy's bed or a crib into a big bed of his own. Refer to the transitioning tips in chapter 7. Dad's involvement is especially important if this transition is part of preparing for a new baby. In that case, dads need to take over the nighttime parenting of the toddler so that mom can nurse the newborn at night.

23. Just be there! Stay cool. Some babies adapt more easily than others to alternatives to mom's breast. Those with persistent personalities may fight your clever tries at nighttime fathering. Other more easygoing infants may actually enjoy dad's novel approach. Try not to take baby's protests personally. If baby is looking at you with an expression on his face that says "There's something really wrong with this picture," stay calm and keep reassuring him that all is well. Realize, too, that there may be nights when you've tried all these strategies and nothing is working and baby needs mom. That's just the way it is, and mothers understand this.

Having my husband up with me in the middle of the night was unbelievably comforting. Even if he didn't physically do anything, just having him next to me was wonderful. Eventually, we settled into a nighttime routine of daddy = diapers, and mommy = milk. He's in charge of changing nighttime diapers and I'm in charge of nursing. It works for us.

PART TWO — FOR MOMS

Moms, you have, of course, read the first part of this chapter so that you'd know what we were telling your husband. We are not going to give you another twenty-three long points to read. We just want to tell you a few things that we, as dads and husbands, along with Martha as a wife and mother, think you should know as you work together with your husband in your shared (or not) nighttime parenting career.

1. Get dad involved early. For bottlefed babies, this is easy. Simply ask your husband to share in the bedtime and middle-of-the-night waking duties. Sure, you will probably end up doing most of it (unless you married Superdad), but it's helpful to get your baby used to being fed and bedded down by dad early on before baby gets completely hooked on you at night.

For breastfeeding moms, however, it is all too easy to take on all the nighttime duties yourself. You may feel that the only way baby will go to sleep is by breastfeeding. If this really is the only way baby is put to sleep in the early months, then you are right — you will be the only person who is able to put baby to bed at night. If, on the other hand, you do want your husband to help at night, let him get started early. Baby may not like it quite as much, but over time, you may find the occasional night off a blessing.

I didn't "sleep through the night" while our baby was learning his father's comforting style. I was so used to waking up at every little sound, plus I thought I'd better stay "on call" just in case I was needed. I usually wasn't.

2. Allow your husband to help. What? *Let* your husband help? You are probably saying, "Of course I'd let my husband help. It's he who doesn't want to do his share of night duty." Ask yourself this question: Are you allowing your husband to develop his own techniques, instincts, and ways of being with baby? Are you giving your husband some time and space in which to master nighttime fathering? Or are you hovering nearby to rescue baby at the first fuss? Are you getting exasperated when your husband can't calm baby after thirty seconds? There are times when you can't, either. If you constantly give your husband the message that he can't comfort baby as well as you can, then he will probably gladly let you have all the nighttime duty for years to come. Even if he can't comfort baby as well as you can in the beginning (and believe us, he knows this), if you are patient, supportive, and encouraging, he will get better at it. You will come to appreciate his baby-comforting skills, and you will both sleep more.

3. Don't be too quick to rescue baby. When you hear your baby crying in dad's arms, of course you want to come to the rescue, for your husband's sake as well as for baby's. But before you rush in to help, use your knowledge of your baby to decide if you are really needed. A baby who is screaming hysterically does need you. Rather than persist with a bad experiment, this would be the night to intervene and nurse baby and encourage dad to try again the next night. (You don't want either one of the pair to start associating this hysterical screaming with bedtime.) You and your husband can even agree beforehand about how he will decide when enough is enough. That way, he can develop the instincts he needs for deciding when it's time to bring baby to you. But if baby is simply fussing and taking a while to settle down and not growing more and more upset, let your husband be a dad and do the job.

4. Don't be a martyr. Tell your partner what you need. It's very easy to start feeling like a

WHEN TO RESCUE DAD

There will be times when baby just won't settle for anyone but mom. Here are some clues that you need to intervene:

- Baby's protests are escalating instead of winding down.
- You sense dad is becoming frustrated and angry.
- Your gut instinct says you need to help (unless you're just being a control freak!).

During times when we were sure he was not hungry, my husband would take him and rock him to sleep. If he didn't go to sleep, he was probably hungry, and then I would nurse him.

◆

My twenty-one-month-old son woke up one night, and my husband went in to try to soothe him and give me a little break. Our son continued to wail, so I finally went in. He stopped crying immediately, smiled, and said, "Mommy!" throwing his arms around my neck. Then he said, "Daddy, out! Mommy, in! Bye, Daddy!" It's pretty clear that even when the vocabulary isn't all there, kids still know how to communicate their needs.

There may be times when it's actually easier and more restful for mom to get up with baby than to have dad do it. Some parents take one week on and one week off night duty.

My husband is an extremely heavy sleeper, and early on, it became very frustrating to try to rouse him to help me out. And, truthfully, since my sleep is in sync with the baby's, it's a lot easier for me to wake up.

◆

My son never did anything as quaint as fussing. He screamed. It's all well and good to say dad needs to learn to comfort baby, but when the baby turns purple from crying, it's time for the mom to intervene.

martyr when your baby is waking you every two hours and your husband just rolls over in bed or, worse, doesn't wake up at all. But if you don't tell your husband about your feelings and your needs, he may just assume that you're doing okay and that you don't need his help at night.

5. Talk openly about sex. Sex (or lack of it) is a common frustration dads reveal to us during sleep counseling. We have been through this with our wives (and one of us has been the wife) many times, and we've found that the best way to approach the topic of sex after giving birth is to be very open and talk about it now and then. We told your husband that you may not feel like having intimate sex for a while and that he should be sensitive to this. We want to say a few words now to you moms so you can understand how your husband might be feeling about sex during the months after a new baby comes along. Remember, your husband's hormones don't change after childbirth like yours do.

We know that you know that your husband is probably feeling neglected. He is trying to be patient and deal with it. What can really help your husband is for you to acknowledge that he feels neglected. Men get frustrated when they think that their wives don't even know or care about their sexual needs. A new dad is likely to feel, "All she thinks about is the baby. Doesn't she know that I have needs, too?" Try telling your husband every few days, "Honey, I know you really miss sex, and I know you wish that I would feel sexual toward you. I will again soon, I promise." It will mean the world to him. Your husband can then grumble about not getting enough sex instead of grumbling to himself that you are oblivious to his needs. At least he'll know that you understand.

Can you actually give your husband enough sex to keep him happy during the first year after you have a baby? Maybe, maybe not. So what can you do besides talk about it? Let your husband know that you are aware of and sensitive to his needs by actually having sex with him — maybe not as often as he'd like, but at a frequency that you are comfortable with. Sometimes you may find that once you get started, sex is actually pretty nice. Other times, you may feel like you just aren't into it and that you're having sex just for your husband's sake. If he's being too demanding, let him know.

One sure way to get him to back off a bit is for you to occasionally initiate sex yourself. Nothing will make him feel more appreciated. Such an experience will probably last him (and his sexual ego) a good week or two.

When our baby was going through a frequent night-waking stage, my husband suggested that we bring her into our bed. I slept better, but he didn't. So he began sleeping in another room. Sometimes, after quickly nursing baby back to sleep, I would sneak into the other bedroom and surprise my husband.

Nap-Time Strategies That Work

I'T'S HARD TO SAY who needs naps more: children or the grown-ups who take care of them. Tired parents need babies and small children to take naps during the day so they can tend to needs of their own and, sometimes, so they can nap, too!

Napping habits vary tremendously from one child to the next. How well babies and children nap depends a lot on their temperament. An easygoing baby will tend to nap longer. High-need babies will take short naps (unless you hold them and carry them around while they're sleeping — then they'll sleep for hours!).

In this chapter, we share practical tips for getting the most out of nap time. We will help you work with your child's individual nap needs. We want nap time to be a pleasant oasis in the middle of a busy day — not a time when you have to struggle to get your child to fall asleep.

CREATING HEALTHY NAP HABITS

Don't you wish that babies came equipped with a sleep switch that you could use to put them in sleep mode at nap time and bedtime? You could put your baby to sleep the same way you turn off your computer, with just a click of the mouse. Too good to be true? Yes. You can't force a baby to nap, just as you can't force a baby to sleep at night. You can, however, create conditions that allow sleep to overtake your baby when it's time for a nap. Babies are creatures of habit. Develop regular sleep conditions around baby's nap time and you will have the next best thing to a nap switch. Here's how:

Observe baby's need-to-nap signs. Babies who are not tired will not nap, no matter how hard you try to help them fall asleep. If you want your baby to nap at more predictable times, you need to know when he will be sleepy. Watch for clues that your baby needs to nap. Just as you learned to read your infant's need-to-sleep signals at bedtime, learn to recognize the signs that your baby or toddler is ready for a nap. As you notice that certain behaviors lead to napping, record them in the nap log on page 189 to help yourself remember and identify the signs in the future. Also note the time of the day and anything else that might shed light on baby's need for sleep (such as a busy morning, outdoor play, or not enough sleep the previous night).

Pre-nap signals might include:

- a change in behavior, such as a wiggly baby slowing down or a toddler stopping his active play and wanting to cuddle
- a change in mood from happy to cranky
- nodding head, drooping eyelids, yawning
- baby wanting to nurse, but more for comfort than for food

Seize the opportunity. As soon as baby gives you clues that she is tired, get her down for a nap without delay. If you wait even a few minutes (say, because you want to finish what you are doing), you may miss your window of opportunity. Baby will rev herself up again, and it will be much harder to wind her down into sleep. If you help your baby fall asleep as soon as you notice that she is tired, you will set up patterns of association in her brain between feeling cranky or drowsy and drifting off to sleep. The more you strengthen these associations, the easier it will be to get your baby to nap. It's even better to begin getting her down before she shows tired signs.

Set the scene. Retreat into the bedroom. Dim the lights, pull the shades (or put blackout shades on the windows), turn on soothing music, and set the tape or CD player for continuous play. Use background white noise from a fan or air conditioner. Cut out distractions. Turn off the phone ringer, put tape over the doorbell, and set your other kids up with a quiet activity. Read, rock, or nurse your baby to sleep. This nap-enticing scenario is called a "setting event." Baby learns to recognize these changes in his environment as the prelude to sleep. Circuits in his brain learn to connect the dim lights and the quiet music with rest and sleep. The more often you follow a pattern, the easier baby will go down for a nap.

Try to create a nap routine that you enjoy. You are more likely to use the routine if it is something you look forward to each day. Play music that you enjoy, or use this time to relax and read a book.

Don't sneak away until baby is fully asleep. If baby falls asleep in your arms or cuddled up next to you on the bed, be sure he is in the state of deep sleep (with hands unclenched, arms dangling loose, and facial muscles still) before you put him down or try to leave. If baby is still sleeping lightly when you try to exit (as indicated by closed fists, flexed limbs, facial and limb movements, or squirming), he may wake up a few minutes later. You can forget about doing whatever it was you were sneaking away to do. (When you do leave, place an item of your clothing with your body scent next to your sleeping baby.)

Co-nap. If your infant or toddler fights naps or won't stay asleep for very long, pick one or two times during the day when you are the most tired and snuggle up in bed with your child. Use this special time to enjoy napping together.

Most mothers discover that their infants sleep longer when they co-nap. Get behind the eyes of your tired baby. Wouldn't you sleep more peacefully if you were nestled next to your favorite person? Wouldn't you be content to stay there and sleep longer? Even toddlers sleep better knowing that mother will be there at the nap's end, just as she was at the nap's beginning.

Okay, so you won't be able to "finally get something done." But you will get the rest you need, and you'll get to enjoy a special time of touching and quietly being close to the baby or toddler who keeps you hopping the rest of the day. Trust us, this stage passes all too soon. You won't get to enjoy high-quality naps like these in the years to come, when you are busy driving your child to soccer games, gymnastics, and piano lessons. Enjoy co-napping while you can.

If baby sleeps better with you nearby but you really want to get something done, stay in the room and do something for yourself, like read, write letters (remember them?), catch up on e-mail, make shopping or to-do lists, sew, or knit — or whatever you can do quietly while she sleeps. She may sense your presence and sleep better when you are in the room.

When he sleeps by himself, he naps only twenty to thirty minutes. When we co-nap, he sleeps one to two hours.

Use a motion simulator. What is the number-one thing that keeps a baby asleep? Motion. That's why your baby will nap for hours in a baby sling or swing, in a moving vehicle or stroller, or in your arms. Most of these motions involve you. Some days you won't mind being the motor that drives your baby's nap, even for the whole nap, but when you need a break, call on a nonhuman motion source for help. Try settling baby into a baby swing. Wind it up and let it rock baby back to sleep each time baby stirs. Some babies, however, don't sleep well in swings. They need more than a back-and-forth motion to keep them asleep. When you walk around, you naturally move in three directions: back and forth, up and down, and from side to side. That's the style of motion baby was used to in the womb.

A hands-free alternative that best simulates being carried is the Amby Baby Motion Bed. This little hammock hangs from a spring, so each time baby stirs, the bed gently moves in all directions — from side to side, up and down, and back and forth. Baby may nap longer in it. See the picture on page 25.

Enjoy nap nursing. If you are breastfeeding, you will discover that your baby likes to nap and nurse. He will feed a little, sleep a while, wake up and nurse some more, and then drift off to sleep again. This is a great way to get more milk into your baby, especially if baby is easily distracted during daytime feedings. Nap nursing is good for moms, too. When baby nurses, your body responds by producing hormones that relax you and help you drift off to sleep.

"Wear down" to nap. When you know your child is ready for a nap (or you need him to nap), snuggle your baby into a baby sling and wear him around the house while you do simple jobs. Or just stroll around your home, your backyard, or your neighborhood until baby is lulled to sleep. Keep baby in the sling until he drifts off into a deep sleep, then walk slowly to his bed, bend over, and ease the sling over your head while you put baby down on the mattress. This "wearing down" technique has been very useful in our families. We find it's especially helpful when the toddler is hyperstimulated and so wound up that he can't relax and nap. Nestling baby in the sling contains his energy. The rhythmic motion of your walk while he is snuggled against your chest and you are gently patting his back helps him relax. Wearing down will help you relax, too, since you know it almost always works! A great tool for dads as well.

Enlist dad as nap coach. If your baby gets used to daddy putting her down to nap when he's available, she may more willingly accept dad putting her down to sleep at night.

Having daddy put the baby down to sleep at nap time helped a lot when we were transitioning our son to going to sleep without nursing. He was usually more calm falling asleep during the day and more willing to fall asleep with dad. Once he got used to the idea that dad could comfort him to nap, dad was able to help more with nighttime duty.

GETTING BABY TO NAP AT PREDICTABLE TIMES

While we don't often advocate strict scheduling, the truth is that if you want easy consistent nap times, you are going to have to create some routine. Many parents have baby nap whenever she seems tired, but if this isn't working for you, we suggest you try nap

---

NAP NEEDS

Here are some general age-and-stage guidelines for naps. Keep in mind that children vary greatly in their nap patterns. Some are born nappers who take long, regular naps. Others are catnappers.

newborn	three naps a day, 1 to 2 hours each, or frequent, irregular, short catnaps
1–3 months	two to three naps a day, 1 to 1½ hours each, with some predictability
3–6 months	two naps a day, 1 to 1½ hours each
6–12 months	1-hour morning nap and 1- to 2-hour afternoon nap
12–24 months	no morning nap; 1- to 2-hour afternoon nap
2–4 years	1-hour afternoon nap

scheduling. There's something to be said for consistency. If baby's lunchtime is always followed by twenty minutes of quiet play and then an opportunity to lie down and go to sleep, you may soon be able to count on a predictable nap time every afternoon. If more consistent nap times sound like a good thing to you, here's how to plan them:

Get to know your napper. Don't just jump right into nap scheduling. You first have to get to know your baby's natural nap pattern, since this will be the starting point for the nap schedule you create for your baby. Keep a nap log for a week or so. Don't try to force baby to take naps at certain times during this week. Just chart how your baby naps on her own. Fill in the log below:

Day	Time of first nap	Duration (hours or minutes)
1	_____	_____
2	_____	_____
3	_____	_____
4	_____	_____
5	_____	_____
6	_____	_____
7	_____	_____

Day	Time of second nap	Duration (hours or minutes)
1	_____	_____
2	_____	_____
3	_____	_____
4	_____	_____
5	_____	_____
6	_____	_____
7	_____	_____

Do you see any pattern? Is your baby naturally getting sleepy at a certain time each day? Are your baby's nap needs similar to those in the box on page 62? Or are they different? Don't worry if your baby isn't napping as long or as often as the numbers in the chart. These are just averages. What counts is your baby's nap pattern.

Your nap log will show you one of two things: Either your baby is already napping at a fairly predictable time each day and you just never noticed it before, or your baby's naps are truly unpredictable. In the first case, voilà! there's your nap schedule. Just keep putting baby down for a nap at those times. (If you want to modify this schedule, see page 190.) If your nap log doesn't show much consistency, you need to figure out why. Here are some things to consider:

- *Are you interfering with your baby's naps?* Perhaps baby would take predictable naps, but you are busy about town and baby can't get some shut-eye. If this is true, try to take a week off from your busy life and concentrate on baby's naps for a bit. (You realize, don't you, that if you want your baby to take naps on schedule, you are going to have to shape your day around baby's naps, instead of letting baby catch a nap around your busy day.)

- *Are you trying to put baby down for naps independently before she is ready?* Often parents try to teach baby to fall asleep on her own for naps, but baby just doesn't take well to that idea. Baby falls asleep stressed and then has a short, restless nap.

If you first teach baby to fall asleep (and stay asleep) in a way that is more comforting to baby, she will learn to crave these long, comfortable naps. This may involve a few weeks of feeding baby to sleep and then holding baby while she sleeps. Don't worry. Once baby learns to nap well, you can then teach baby more independent ways of napping.

- *Are you overlooking baby's tired signs?* Perhaps your baby is showing some signs of needing a nap at predictable times each day but you are missing them or can't stop what you are doing at that time to get baby down for a nap. By the time you get around to nap time, baby has gained a second wind.

- *Is baby sick or teething?* Don't try to meddle with your baby's nap pattern in the middle of a stressful time like this. Wait until this complicating factor is out of the picture, then try again. What? Your baby is always teething? Well, then, do the best you can. It may take every nap tip in this chapter to get a stressed-out baby to nap when you want him to.

- *Is your household simply too busy?* If you have older kids, this can be a problem. One way around this is to create a daily pattern for your older kids where they are engaged in quiet play at baby's nap time every day. They don't necessarily have to be quiet for baby's whole nap, just while you get baby to sleep. See what you can do to eliminate the factors that are getting in the way of your baby's naps. Then try another week of keeping a nap log.

Establish a set nap schedule. Once you have discovered baby's predictable sleepy times, you can create a nap schedule by first doing whatever it takes to get baby to nap at those times every day. Breast- or bottlefeed baby down for naps if this is a sure-sleep method for your baby. Once you have the sleepy times established and in keeping with baby's natural sleep rhythm, baby will more easily fall asleep at nap times using whatever method of falling asleep you choose.

In order for a nap schedule to sink in, you will need to not only program the nap times but also get baby to take long naps. During the learning stage, this means doing whatever it takes to get baby to nap longer. For some babies this will involve holding baby, wearing baby in a sling, or lying down with baby for the entire nap time. If your baby starts to wake up prematurely, try to soothe him back to sleep before he has a chance to become fully awake. Pat him, talk soothingly to him, offer the breast — do whatever you did to get him down for a nap in the first place. We know this may not be how you want to spend baby's nap time. But don't worry, this is just temporary. The idea is to program a nap rou-

> ### SEARS SLEEP TIP
>
> Sleep research has shown that babies usually enjoy longer naps and deeper sleep in the afternoon than in the morning. Consider napping with baby in the morning, and plan some time for yourself during baby's afternoon nap.

tine into baby's mind first. Once this routine is set, you can start working on less hands-on ways to keep baby asleep longer.

My baby napped longer if I held her. I made sure I had books, drinks, the TV remote control, a phone, and occasionally my laptop within reach. Sometimes she'd stay asleep if I moved her from my arms into her car seat, even though we weren't going anywhere. The car seat didn't upset her like the crib did.

Schedule the afternoon nap — the key to a consistent bedtime. Some babies go to sleep every night at a predictable time, no matter when their afternoon nap takes place. For most babies, however, bedtime depends on what time that afternoon nap happens and how long it lasts. Find your baby's tired time. In order to create a consistent and predictable tired time each evening, you need to have baby nap at a predictable time each afternoon.

So how do you achieve this? For a few weeks, do whatever it takes to get baby to nap at a certain time. What afternoon nap time is right for your baby? Here are some ideas:

- *If you want baby to have an early bedtime.* If your desire is for baby to go to bed around 8 p.m., the afternoon nap should be from around 2 to 4 p.m. (for a baby who is taking two naps). This gives baby enough energy to get through dinner in a good mood, leaving her tired by 7:30 or 8 p.m. Of course, with baby going to bed so early, she'll probably be up at sunrise, and she'll

probably take a late-morning nap around 10 a.m. As baby gets older and starts taking only one nap, you will find this one nap will fit best right in the middle of the day, around noon or one o'clock. These times are guidelines only. Try to work the

SLEEP SCIENCE SAYS NAPS ARE HEALTHFUL

Like nighttime sleep, naps are restorative. When babies and children awaken from naps, they are happier, calmer, and ready for another go at life. What makes just an hour or two of sleep (twenty minutes for power nappers) so healthful? Babies enjoy a lot of REM sleep during naps. While non-REM sleep mainly benefits physical well-being, REM sleep improves emotional well-being and improves brain maturation.

Napping also reduces levels of the stress hormone cortisol. This is why naps cure crankiness and why children who skip their naps are irritable and unhappy until bedtime. When it is finally time for bed, the child who has not napped may have trouble falling asleep. That unrelieved buildup of stress hormones makes it harder to relax. This explains why keeping your child from napping during the day is not a helpful strategy for getting your child to sleep longer at night. Children who have not had a chance to relax and unwind during the day bring all that fitful energy to bed with them. They have trouble falling asleep and don't sleep peacefully.

naps in as close to baby's natural tired time as possible. (For more on rescheduling a late bedtime, see page 194.)

- *If you want baby to stay up late.* If you enjoy late evenings with baby, time the afternoon nap to occur right before dinner, from around 4 to 6 p.m. Baby will likely sleep late each morning and then have a late-morning nap around eleven o'clock or noon. When baby switches to one nap, it will probably be around 2 or 3 p.m.

WINDING DOWN THE RELUCTANT NAPPER

What do you do if you have followed the suggestions above for cultivating good nap-time habits but nap time is becoming a struggle? Most babies and children go through stages when it is hard to get them to nap. Yet they still need to sleep, whether they want to admit it or not. Most babies need a morning and an afternoon nap. Most toddlers need at least one nap a day, usually about two hours long. What's more, caregivers need a break. But it's not always easy to get a busy baby or an active toddler to slow down for a nap. They get so involved in fun activities that they don't want to trade playtime for nap time. Yet, without an afternoon nap, they will be cranky and not much fun to be with in the evening. This can be especially upsetting to parents who work outside the home during the day and look forward to spending quality time with their child in the evening. It takes some effort to market the napping concept to a busy toddler, but it's worth it. Here are some tips:

Don't force the naps. If your toddler doesn't seem tired or consistently fights sleep at what used to be his usual nap time, take this as a clue that he is ready to drop that particular nap. If you drop the morning nap because your toddler just isn't settling into it anymore, the afternoon nap will come more easily.

She knows it's nap time but doesn't want to miss anything. She just loves hanging out with us and realizes she's missing something during naps, so she fights her naps. I try not to put her down for a nap unless the tired signals are clearly there.

Nap on the move. Try "moving naps." Put your baby in a baby sling and take a walk. Baby may think he is setting off on a fun adventure with you, but soon the walking motion will lull him into dreamland. This becomes a predictable nap-time pattern. When you begin the ritual of putting your baby in the baby sling and starting to walk, baby clicks into the preset pattern of association — first the sling, then the nap. Babies will often stay asleep longer while on the move nestled in a sling.

Or try buckling your toddler into his car seat and taking a ride around the neighborhood until he is fully asleep. Then return home and ease him from the car seat into his bed to complete his nap. If you have a busy day with lots of errands to run, let your child nap in the car seat while you drive home.

Martha would often try to time our infants' and toddlers' naps with the afternoon school pickup time. This became a predictable nap-time pattern.

The jogging stroller is great because I get to stay outside the entire time she sleeps, so I can get a good sixty minutes of exercise in. Ditto this for shopping. After two stores she is often ready for a long afternoon snooze in the stroller.

◆

Sometimes if she falls asleep in the car seat, I will just park the car in the driveway and lean my seat back and take a nap or relax with a book. Even if I don't sleep, I still get some rest.

Have an active morning. Fresh air, outdoor play, and socializing with other children will prepare a child for an afternoon nap. Adults also sleep better at night when they exercise during the day. Older babies and toddlers are more willing to take an afternoon nap when they have had a busy morning.

Make a nap nook. Some children fall asleep best if they fall asleep in the same place every time. Others can be enticed into napping in a new, special setting. Some children feel lonely in a big bed in a big room. A nap "nest" is cozier and more contained. If you are struggling to get your toddler to nap, you're probably willing to let him nap anywhere, just so long as he sleeps. He may find it easier to let go of fun activities if he gets to nap in the corner behind the family room couch. We would make a nap nook for our reluctant nappers by putting a futon or "special bed"

wherever the child wanted. The locations they chose included under the piano, in a little tent made of blankets, and in a large cardboard box with a cutout like a cat flap that the child crawled into when she was tired. In a tent or a large box a child can pretend to camp or to be sleeping with a favorite character from a story. Making these little hideaways capitalizes on children's natural desire to construct their own retreats in nooks and crannies throughout the house.

Naps are never in the place where we sleep at night. I think children regard naps as being different from sleeping at night. Sleeping at night is a "sleep till it gets light" thing. Nap time is a "wake up whenever" thing.

Nap with a "friend." Let your child snuggle up with a toy friend. Tell him, "It's time to put Teddy Bear down to nap." Your child will likely fall asleep, too.

Announce "special time." Nap time does not always mean sleep time for the older toddler or preschooler. Some children can get the rest they need with a quiet time in the afternoon when they lie down and listen to a tape or story. (Watching videos is too stimulating for a quiet time.) Market this as "special time," when mommy, daddy, or another caregiver and the child rest and nest together in a quiet room. Some days this will result in a nap. Other days it will just be a time to rest and relax while she looks at her books.

Sometimes I shut my daughter's bedroom door and lie on her bed and rest while she plays on the floor. Her mattress is on the floor, so she can crawl onto it with me if she needs a quick hug or wants to nap.

FREQUENTLY ASKED QUESTIONS ABOUT NAPS

Naps that are too short, naps that come too late in the afternoon, naps that don't happen at all — there are lots of reasons parents are unhappy with their children's napping habits. Here are some real nap-life questions and some helpful solutions:

NAPS TOO SHORT

Our nine-month-old sleeps great at night, but when I put him down for a nap during the day, he wakes up after only twenty minutes. Has he really slept enough? How can I get him to nap longer?

As a general rule, if your child sleeps well at night and is mostly happy during the day, don't change anything, especially his nap pattern. Be grateful for what you have. If you try to lengthen baby's naps, you could end up with a baby who sleeps less at night.

Is your baby happy and rested after a short nap? That may be all the sleep he needs. Some babies are what we call "power nappers." They can take a few fifteen- or twenty-minute naps and be refreshed and happy. But if baby wakes up cranky and stays that way, he may not have slept long enough and deeply enough to feel rested. If that's the case, follow the strategies for better, longer napping that we've laid out in this chapter. Re-

member to minimize distracting noises. Turn off the phone ringer, put tape over the doorbell, and close the curtains and the windows. And, if your baby starts to wake up prematurely, try to soothe him back to sleep before he has a chance to become fully awake. Pat him, talk soothingly to him, offer the breast — do whatever you did to get him down for a nap in the first place. If you can anticipate when baby is likely to wake up (check your nap log), you can be right there, on the spot and ready to help him go back to sleep. You may end up lying down with your baby to get him to sleep longer — but, hey, you had the first half of baby's nap to do what you wanted to do.

LATE NAP, LATER TO BED

Our nine-month-old likes to take a late-afternoon nap around 4 p.m., but then he's awake until 10:00. By then, we're exhausted. We'd really like to have some time in the evening to ourselves. How can we change this pattern?

Ah, the dreaded late-afternoon nap. Babies who fall asleep at 4 p.m. or later can keep going and going, on into the nighttime. They bask in their parents' attention, and they love staying up late with the grown-ups.

Believe it or not, this works well for some families. When dad, mom, or both are gone all day, they may enjoy having baby's company in the evening, and it's a lot more fun to play with a baby who is well rested. With today's busy lifestyles, the custom of early naps and early bedtimes may be a modern mismatch. A child who takes an early-afternoon nap will be tired and cranky by "happy hour," that predinner hour when adults are likely to be pretty crabby themselves. Before you try to change things, you might want to make sure that you really do want your child to go to bed earlier. There's no rule that says babies have to be in bed by seven or eight, or even nine o'clock.

If the late-afternoon nap is truly not working for you, you'll need to turn back your baby's internal napping clock. Here are some suggestions:

- Try putting your baby down for a nap fifteen minutes earlier each day. You can gradually work your way back to a regular nap time earlier in the afternoon.

- Consider eliminating your baby's morning nap. This will help him fall asleep earlier in the afternoon. Or try shortening his morning nap.

- Start watching for those need-a-nap signals in the early afternoon, and try all the nap-inducing tips discussed in this chapter as soon as you see them. If your baby takes short naps in the late morning or early afternoon, try the tips for lengthening his nap time.

- If baby does decide to take a nap at 4 p.m. or later, wake him after twenty minutes or so. A catnap may give him enough sleep to make him pleasant to be around but not so much that he's then awake until ten o'clock.

SOMETIMES SKIPS NAPS

Our two-year-old is usually a predictable napper, but sometimes he skips naps. How can we keep him on a regular nap schedule?

If there's one thing you can count on with babies, it's change. Just when you manage to get baby on a consistent nap schedule, his sleep needs change and you must make adjustments. How do you do this without throwing baby's bedtime routine out of whack? Here are some suggestions:

- **When baby misses a nap.** This will happen from time to time. Simply watch for baby's next tired time and put baby down for a nap then. But what if this catch-up nap comes too late in the day? Should you skip the nap and try keeping baby awake until bedtime? It's your call. Maybe you can compromise and let baby take a catnap. Wake him after twenty minutes or so, and he may be rested enough but not too much to go to bed at his regular time.

- **Giving up a nap.** You will see baby's nap routines change as baby gets older. Sometime between his first and second birthday, your baby will probably make the transition from two naps a day to just one. By the age of five, most children give up napping altogether. (There goes your free time!) Some children give up naps as early as age three, long before their caregivers are prepared to enjoy their company all afternoon. These changing nap patterns can wreak havoc on regular bedtimes, especially if your child manages to stay active and awake for much of the day, only to crash in the late afternoon and then wake up with enough energy to last until midnight. So what can you do when your child is in this no-man's land? Experiment. Try new nap times, quiet times, catnaps, earlier times for rising, earlier bedtimes, or even (shudder) later bedtimes to see what works best for you and your child. You may have to help your child through some cranky evenings and even a few late nights before the new nap — or no-nap — pattern settles in.

LAP NAPPER

Our two-month-old has no problem sleeping alone in her bassinet at night, but the only way she'll nap during the day is in my arms or on my lap. I don't mind holding her for now, but I worry that I am creating a bad habit. Will she outgrow the need to sleep in my arms?

No, you are not creating a bad habit, and yes, she will outgrow the need to nap in your lap. After all, your baby is only two months of age, and many babies this age still need the security of a womblike environment to sleep well. Celebrate and enjoy this special closeness, since it will pass all too soon. Like many "problems" in parenting, your situation can also be seen as an opportunity. Take it as a compliment that your baby loves to nestle in your arms. A perk for you from having your baby sleep in your arms is that you are forced to take time to relax. You certainly need this rest, but unless baby "demands" it, most mothers don't allow themselves the luxury of frequent rest stops during the day.

As your baby gets older, you can experiment with alternatives that will gradually teach her to sleep more independently. Most nappers who need to snuggle up to mom enjoy co-napping. You might be more comfortable lying down on your bed with your baby and actually falling asleep rather than sitting up in a chair. Lying down next to your baby also allows you the option of getting up to do your own thing after baby has fallen into a deep sleep. As babies grow, they learn to sleep more soundly, and they enjoy having more space in which to stretch out and sleep. Your little lap napper will eventually sleep in her own space. (For nap props instead of your lap, see the suggestions on page 187.)

SIBLING NAPS OUT OF SYNC

How can I get our six-month-old and our two-year-old to nap at the same time?

It's easy to tell the mother of just one child to "nap when your baby naps." But you can't do this with a two-year-old on the loose. Infants and toddlers have different nap needs, as do siblings with different schedules and different temperaments. But if they never nap at the same time, when does mom get to rest? With two children, you are likely to be doubly tired.

Ideally, you want both children to nap at the same time at least once a day. Here are some strategies that have worked for us:

Try a nap nook. It's probably easier to get your six-month-old down for a nap than it is your two-year-old, so work on the two-year-old's nap first. Try the nap nook idea (see page 193) to sell your older child on the idea of taking time out from her day to sleep. Put the nap nook in your bedroom so that once your toddler is asleep, you can lie down and nap with your baby.

Co-nap. Try co-napping with both children. Pick a time of the day when all three of you are ready for a rest and snuggle between your baby and your toddler. You can nurse and cuddle your baby to sleep in one arm while holding your two-year-old with the other. Sing something soft and monotonous so both children can nod off together.

Wear your baby down. Still another alternative is to wear your baby down to sleep in a sling (see page 187) and then settle down with your toddler for a quiet story, a song, or a back rub. Even if your toddler doesn't want to take a nap at that time, you can at least get into the habit of daily "quiet time." When there's a younger baby to compete with, the older sibling welcomes this special cuddle time with mom when baby is asleep and not bothering "me and my mommy." You may not get a nap, but at least you can put your feet up for a while and relax.

Play nap. When you really need to get some rest, try making a child-proofed play area in your bedroom for your toddler. You can lie down and nurse the baby while your toddler plays quietly on the floor. You may not be

able to sleep, but you can doze and rest, keeping one car open for whatever your two-year-old is doing.

Hire nap help. If simultaneous naps aren't working, call in some help. Get someone to play with your two-year-old while you nap with your baby. On weekends, have your husband take your older child outside or to the park. Hire a teen or a junior high school kid to come in after school and play with your toddler while you rest with your baby. Toddlers like young teens, and they're relatively inexpensive to hire.

TIME FOR SELF DURING BABY'S NAPS

I enjoy napping with my baby, but sometimes I'd like to be free to do things just for myself while she naps. But she doesn't sleep very long when I'm not with her. Help!

Just as many babies sleep better at night when a loving parent is close by, they also nap better when they know mother is near. Resting while baby naps is an important thing you can do for yourself, but there may be times when you need to do something other than sleep. Use the sleep science you've already applied to baby's nighttime needs to your advantage at nap time. Wait until your baby is in the deepest state of sleep before you try to put her down and sneak away. Sleep research has shown that babies usually enjoy longer naps and deeper sleep in the afternoon than in the morning. So plan your activities during baby's afternoon nap (or whenever your baby seems to sleep the deepest and the longest). Above all, don't try to sneak away when baby is in the REM, or lighter, state of sleep (recognized by baby's tight fists, flexed limbs, facial and limb movements, and squirming). Baby will know that you are gone and will wake up, and you won't get to do what you want to do. Before you leave her sleeping on her own, wait until baby is obviously in a deeper state of sleep, with a quiet face and relaxed fists and limbs.

If she wakes when you leave the room, another approach is to see if she'll stay asleep longer if you stay in the room, near her. You can still do something for yourself then, like read, write letters, catch up on e-mail, make shopping and to-do lists, pay bills, and so forth. She may sense your presence and sleep better if you are in the room.

NAPPING AT DAY CARE

Our eight-month-old will soon be going to day care part-time. At home she nurses to sleep, and we also co-nap. What can we do to get her to nap well at day care?

Since your baby loves to nap-nurse, you're going to need some creative strategies to get your baby to accept someone else putting her to sleep. First, try to get baby used to nap-time alternatives at home. Next, be sure your substitute caregiver has a parenting mind-set like yours. Watch out for red flags, such as, "I see she's spoiled and can't go to sleep on her own." As a clue, ask a prospective sub how she feels about the "let baby cry it out" advice. You certainly don't want your baby to be put in a crib and left to cry herself to sleep.

Ask your day-care provider to try to match the nap-time routine at day care to the one you use at home. Tell her when and how your baby is used to going to sleep. Explain that you want your baby to enjoy going to sleep without you. Ask her to "nurse" your baby to sleep by rocking, singing a lullaby, wearing her down in a carrier, or even lying next to her while she drifts off to sleep. At the very least, expect your sub to stay by baby's crib and sing or pat her off to napland.

Wearing a baby down to sleep in a baby sling may be a new concept for your day-care provider, so you may have to show and tell her how to do it. Show your caregiver how to use the sling and explain its advantages. (Carrying your baby in a sling makes it easier for her to walk around and tend to other babies.) Tell her how to recognize when baby is sleeping deeply enough to be put down, and then show her how to ease herself out of the sling and lay baby down in her crib. Most experienced day-care providers realize that babies are happier and easier to manage throughout the day if they are well rested.

On the other hand, it may be helpful for baby to get used to novel sleep associations. If you have a sensitive and nurturing caregiver, you may wish to let her devise her own sleep plan. If it's working, stick with it.

NAP SAFETY IN A BIG BED

I lie down with my baby in my bed to help her fall asleep at nap time. Once she's asleep, I like to get up to do other things. But I'm afraid she's going to roll or crawl off the bed when I'm not there with her. How can I keep her safe?

This situation is faced by many co-sleeping parents. Besides following the safe-sleep guidelines in chapter 5, here are some ways you can keep your mobile infant safe in your bed during naps.

- Use a baby monitor so you can hear when baby starts to awaken when you are in another room. Check on your infant anytime you hear rustling.

- Put guardrails up on both sides of the bed.

- Take your mattress off the bed frame and box spring and put it on the floor. If baby does scoot across the bed or crawl off, she won't have far to fall. Place cushions on the floor around the bed, so if she falls, her landing will be soft.

- Let her nap on a futon rather than in a big bed.

- During playtime, teach baby how to crawl backward off the bed so she can do it safely by herself when she wakes from a nap.

Should Baby Cry It Out?

THE DICTUM "LET YOUR BABY CRY it out" has been standard advice in childcare books for more than a century. We can trace it back as far as a baby-training book written by Dr. Emmett Holt in 1894. And you'll find that same tired cry-it-out advice in books published in the twenty-first century. Same advice — just a new package.

Sound familiar? You can't get through those first months of life with a new baby without having someone tell you that this is what you must do if your baby is ever going to learn to sleep well. Letting baby cry it out is regarded as a rite of passage for parents. After a month or two, they must harden their hearts and get tough about crying for baby's own good, or so the sleep trainers pontificate.

If babies could vote, they would all put their little thumbs down on the CIO advice: "I'm just a baby," they would plead. "Please don't *force* me to sleep. Instead, *teach* me to sleep." In this book we've given you the tools to do that.

Why does crying it out persist as part of the nighttime parenting advice package? One reason is that it appears to work, at least for some babies. If no one comes to comfort them, some babies do eventually stop crying. But the fact that this method works some of the time for some babies doesn't make it right for every baby.

In this chapter we are going to share with you our honest opinion of this method, based on our experience with our own kids, our combined forty years of pediatric practice, and scientific research on sleep and child development. We are also going to give you some ideas and alternatives to consider if you feel desperate enough to want to try this method with your baby.

WHAT "CRYING IT OUT" REALLY MEANS

"Let your baby cry it out" sounds easy enough. You simply allow your baby to cry until he's all done crying. But what really happens when you follow the cry-it-out ad-

WHAT SLEEP SAGES SHOULDN'T SAY

We have read a lot of books about how to get babies to sleep. Frankly, we think that some of them ought to be titled *How to Train Your Pet to Sleep Through the Night* because the advice they contain would be better applied to a dog than to a human infant. Dogs can — and should — be trained to do what their masters expect. Human children are more complicated. Yet sleep advisers offer the kind of inflexible rules one wouldn't even use to train a puppy. Here are some sad solutions from popular books on how to train your baby to sleep through the night:

- "If your baby cries, don't back down. Let him cry for up to an hour at nap time and for as long as it takes at nighttime."

- "Once your child is in bed, he is there to stay, no matter how long he cries."

- "Don't sing, rock, or nurse your baby to sleep. He may get used to it."

- "At nine months of age, there is no need to be fed." (Try telling that to a baby who *knows* when he is hungry and when he is not!)

- "Detach yourself from your baby's protests."

- "Harden your heart."

- "There is no evidence that babies are harmed when they are allowed to cry."

- "It's okay if he cries so hard he vomits."

This tough-love approach assumes that when babies cry, they are being disrespectful, defiant, and disobedient, like an undisciplined puppy. If your dog defies you, you scold him, exclaiming "Bad dog!" in your most authoritative voice. But a baby is just a baby. Is baby's crying really about defiance? Or do baby's cries express real human needs?

---

vice? There's more to this simple phrase than meets the eye — or the ear. Let's analyze the phrase "let your baby cry it out" in order to understand why this phrase has no place in parenting.

"Let . . ." CIO advocates often talk about night crying as if it's a control issue. According to some CIO advocates, if mother responds to baby's cries, she will give the baby the idea that he is in control — and parents should never ever let their children control them. Instead, parents should abandon their crying baby bit by bit, until she gives up. "Let the baby cry" equals "Let the baby alone." At least, that's how it feels to baby.

". . . your . . ." It's presumptuous for someone who isn't there at 3 a.m., who doesn't know your baby and who has no biological connection to your baby, to tell a tired and vulnerable mother to let her baby cry it out. We believe that the only person who knows if, when, and how long a baby should be left to cry is the person most involved in that baby's care. Usually this is the person who shared an umbilical cord with the crier: the mother — the person most dedicated to reading and responding to baby's smiles, cues, and complaints.

I was so tired that I tried the cry-it-out approach, since my friends recommended it. Big mistake! It tore me up inside to hear her cry. The next morning, my baby was hoarse and I had a hurting heart. She clung to me like a koala for the next couple of days. I will never do that again!

". . . baby . . ." Babies are different from adults. Adults do not need to eat in the middle of the night, but to grow adequately, almost all babies need one or two nighttime feedings in the first six months. They also have a need for close human contact and for comfort when they are in distress — a need that is almost as great as their need for food. Babies who do not get enough touching do not grow well. Babies who are not comforted become anxious and cry more.

When I try to put our usually co-sleeping baby to sleep in a crib, he cries. I believe he's trying to tell me, "Get me out of here!"

The CIO club insists that babies cry at night because they *want* mother's attention, not because they need it. In order for the CIO scheme to pass muster with caring par-

ents, it has to downgrade real needs into mere wants. Thus, the CIO philosophy tells parents that a baby cries at night because he wants to be held but that he doesn't necessarily need to be held, and parents shouldn't always respond to wants; they should respond only to biological needs. Babies' needs do change as they get older, and eventually, nighttime crying may have more to do with baby wanting company than needing food or comfort; but once again, we believe that only someone who knows a baby very well — a parent — can tell the difference between a need and a want. In young babies (those under four to six months of age), needs and wants are pretty much the same thing. And in older babies, wanting to be held can still be viewed as a need — an emotional need for comfort. Think of it this way. Perhaps your child is crying for help, and if your child could talk, he would say, "Mama, *help me learn* how to get back to sleep."

Listen to them when they are young, and they will listen to you when they are older.

". . . cry . . ." A baby's cry is a baby's language. It's an attachment behavior, designed to ensure the survival of the baby by provoking a response from the parents, especially the mother. A baby's cry is a baby's way of saying, "Something is not right. Please make it right!" As mothers know instinctively, *babies cry to communicate, not to manipulate.* If your natural maternal response to your baby's cry were measured in a laboratory, here's what would happen. The various wires and monitors used would detect an increase in blood flow to your breasts. Blood samples would show a sharp increase in the level of oxytocin in your blood, which makes you want to pick up your baby and nurse her. Your body might also respond to your baby's cries by producing stress hormones, which rev your body up to pick up your baby and comfort her. Mothers are hormonally wired to respond to, not ignore, their baby's cries. (Fathers, take note: You can't argue with biology!)

I am a speech pathologist who works in early-childhood programs. A cry is a form of communication. Children begin to communicate as soon as they are born, using cries and then differentiated cries. If a parent does not respond to their child's cries, I feel that it lets the child know that their communication is not important to the parent."

". . . it . . ." What really is the "it" in "cry it out"? CIO advisers regard the cry as a bothersome behavior that needs to be "extinguished." ("Extinction" is a term behavioral psychologists use to describe the process in which a

---

JUST NOISE?

With a little imagination, one could hear a baby's cry as actual words instead of just noise. "Mommy, Daddy, I need you. Please pick me up!" Do we as parents ignore an older child when he or she speaks to us? Do we ignore our friends or our spouse when they say "I need you"? Why should we ignore a baby's language?

---

behavior decreases or stops because it is not being rewarded.) Is crying a habit that must be broken? Mothers know differently. Their body's response is a clue that baby's crying indicates a need that must be met. Anthropologists who study the behavior of human mothers and infants believe that crying is a survival tool. Babies are programmed to cry when they are separated too long from their mother or trusted caregiver. The cry is designed to get baby the help he needs in order to survive in the world. Make that cry go away by letting baby cry it out, and baby loses a valuable tool for getting the attention he needs to stay safe, grow, and develop into a mature human being. For more on what "it" is, read on.

". . . out." What goes out of a baby who is left alone to cry? A baby has two choices when no one listens. Either she can cry louder and harder, hoping desperately that someone will finally listen, or she can clam up, stop bothering everyone, and become a "good baby" (meaning a quiet, undemanding, convenient baby). Either way, what goes out of baby is trust in her ability to communicate with her caregivers and her belief that they will respond to her needs. Parents beware. If you let your baby cry it out, you may get rid of much more than a simple night-waking problem. What goes out of your baby may be trust, security, and the desire to communicate. There's a lot more at stake here than a few hours of sleep.

Get behind the eyes of your baby. Imagine how you would feel if, in the middle of the night, you needed something and you tried

EXPERIENCE IS THE BEST TEACHER

A young pediatrician friend of ours told us that after she had her first child, she spent a whole year apologizing to her patients' parents for all the "packaged book" advice that she had dispensed during the first few years of her practice — especially the cry-it-out approach to getting babies to sleep through the night.

your best to communicate that need, but no one listened. No doubt you would feel powerless, unimportant, and angry that no one cared enough to listen and respond to you. Some babies in this situation give up on trying to communicate. They give up on trust and security at the same time. Other babies cry persistently for hours, night after night. They don't follow the CIO book, which says that crying at night is just a habit that is easy to break. Common sense tells us that a *habit that is not easy to break is really a need.* When babies are left to cry it out, their need for closeness may be extinguished. As a result, they may lose something valuable — the desire and ability to achieve *intimacy.* That is the "it" that gets cried out.

Something important also goes out of parents, especially mothers, when baby is left to cry it out. Parents lose their sensitivity. When you "harden your heart," as cry-it-out advisers insist you must do, you ignore your basic biology. You work hard to desensitize yourself to your baby's signals and to your intuitive responses. Many mothers whom we have

interviewed who have bought into this method have confided to us, "My baby's cry no longer bothers me." When I hear this, I think, "That's a problem. Your baby's cries *should* bother you. You're made that way. Why do you want to be less sensitive to your baby?" A mother once told me, "I can't let my baby cry." I replied, "If you can't, you shouldn't."

Dr. Bob relates: Friends of ours made the decision to let their baby cry it out, starting around one month of age. The mom honestly felt that this was right for her and her baby, and she was thrilled to report that this system "worked" immediately. When we asked about it, however, the mom would state that the baby cried every night for thirty to sixty minutes before falling asleep. Figuring this would diminish over time, the mom decided to continue with this method. At six months of age, the baby still cried for thirty minutes every night, and at one year it was still the same. The mother thought the method "worked" simply because the child did eventually go to sleep each night. At some point he did stop crying himself to sleep (we don't know when — we stopped asking about it). But, wow! At least a whole year of this! That child's cries either didn't bother the mom, or she refused to let it get to her.

Her child is now older and has been diagnosed with ADHD, learning disabilities, and other psychological and behavioral problems. We're not saying that crying it out is the only cause of this child's problems. Problems of attachment are not that simple. But clearly, this baby was trying to tell his mother that he needed help in settling down to sleep. Ignoring his signals did not make the problem go away. Instead, mother missed out on valuable opportunities for teaching her baby how to calm down without crying. Mother and father also missed an opportunity to sharpen their sensitivity skills, which they would later need for dealing with his learning and behavioral problems.

HOW CRYING IT OUT SABOTAGES THE PARENT-CHILD RELATIONSHIP

What's wrong with this picture? Baby is put down in her crib to sleep. Her parents leave the room. She cries, and the crying continues for ten minutes (or whatever time the book or doctor said). Her parents return. Father puts a hand on baby's tummy and says, "It's okay," but does not pick her up. Baby cries even harder as her parents again leave the room.

CIO weakens communication between parents and baby. In this scenario, mom and dad are following the instructions in the sleep-training book, which says that their baby has to learn to go to sleep in her crib, not in her parent's arms. CIO advisers tell parents to "reassure" their baby that all is okay, but "don't pick him up." Imagine how this looks from your baby's point of view down there on the crib mattress. There's mom, standing over you, mumbling some words that you don't understand. Then mom walks away. She may be in the next room, but you don't know that. (Babies don't under-

stand that people continue to exist when they can't see them.) You don't know if this important person will return. When mother finally does come back, she just stands next to your crib, with her arms folded. She says something, but the one kind of communication you understand — the comfort of being in mom's open arms — is withheld.

You can see how this would be confusing (and probably enraging) to a baby. Mother has to fight her feelings, too. She wants to open her arms and reach out to her baby, but the book warns her not to. The cry-it-out advice has somehow gotten in between mother and baby and is sabotaging their natural communication-response network. A distance begins to develop between them.

Here is how the cry-response system is designed to work: Baby senses something is wrong; for example, his tummy hurts because he's hungry, or he is growing anxious and worried because he is alone. He becomes restless, frets, complains, and finally cries. Mother comes to his rescue, picks him up, and tries various ways of comforting him until something finally works.

With practice, both mother and baby become more skilled at the cue-response pattern. Mother learns to recognize the early signals and respond to baby's restlessness or complaining even before he cries. Baby learns that he can depend on his mother to respond, so he works hard at communicating in more subtle ways. Baby learns to "talk" better, and mother becomes able to read her infant's signals more precisely. Eventually she knows when to come running and when she can hold off a bit before she picks baby up.

Because baby trusts that mother will come, he doesn't always even have to cry to communicate his needs. Mother and baby gradually become more independent of one another, but the close understanding between them remains.

I think rigid sleep-training methods make baby angry with mother.

Let's take a deeper look at how the CIO advice affects parents and babies. While cry-it-out advisers promise parents that they will have more independent children and more freedom for themselves, the CIO advice actually fails to deliver on these points, because it goes against much of what we know about the attachment between mothers and babies. More important, CIO fails to recognize the dangers to the healthy emotional (and even physical, in some cases) development of babies, who need solid attachment to thrive and grow into emotionally healthy adults.

CIO is biologically incorrect. As described above, a mother's body is programmed to respond to her baby's cries. Responding to the cry not only rescues baby from his misery, it also relaxes mommy. When you follow your biological signals and pick up and nurse your crying baby, you enjoy the relaxing effects of the calming hormones released by breastfeeding. Not only does nursing calm baby, it also helps you become less anxious about baby's cries. Enjoy the benefits of allowing your biology to work for you!

CIO leads to poor-quality sleep. Which baby do you think will sleep more peacefully?

---

95 PERCENT OF MOTHERS CAN'T BE WRONG

We use the families in our pediatric practice as a kind of focus group when we are working on a book. To gather information about nighttime crying and parents' responses, we gave questionnaires to several hundred families. One of the questions was "What advice do you most commonly get about what to do when your baby wakes up during the night?" The advice most commonly offered to parents was "let the baby cry it out." We also asked parents to tell us how they felt about this advice. Ninety-five percent of mothers who responded to our survey told us that the cry-it-out advice did not feel right to them. We concluded: 95 PERCENT OF MOTHERS CAN'T BE WRONG!

A baby who goes to sleep held in a parent's loving arms or a baby put down to sleep alone, left to face the innate fear that babies have when no one is with them?

To sleep peacefully you have to relax and wind down. A baby who cries furiously before falling asleep will sleep in a state of hormonal havoc. Crying releases stress hormones into baby's circulation. Going to sleep should be a relaxing process, a time when stress hormones go down, not up. Frantic, unattended-to crying that escalates in intensity can keep a baby from going to sleep, and when eventually he does drop off to sleep, he may have trouble staying asleep. Then the crying starts all over again. Listening to baby cry also releases stress hormones in the mother that will prevent her from sleeping. As a result, you have two or more anxious sleepers in the house.

You cannot force someone to fall asleep. It's better to try to create calming conditions that allow sleep to overtake the baby. The baby who falls asleep at mother's breast or in father's arms, rocked and soothed into a peaceful state, will sleep more restfully. What type of sleep memories do you want your child to have? The memory of warmth and comfort before falling asleep or of stress from being left alone to fall asleep from exhaustion.

CIO sabotages parents' sensitivity. When you choose not to respond to your baby's cues, you run the risk that you and your baby will drift apart. Letting baby cry it out can be a lose-lose situation. Both parent and baby are affected. When you go against your biological programming, you lose confidence in your own ability to understand your baby. Your baby loses trust in his ability to make himself understood. Because the two of you do not communicate as well, you drift apart.

I went to visit my friend and her newborn in their home. While we were talking, her baby started crying in the nursery. Her baby kept crying, harder and louder. Her baby's cries didn't bother my friend, but they bothered me. My breasts almost started to leak milk! Yet my friend seemed oblivious to her baby's signals. Finally, I couldn't stand it anymore, and I said, "It's okay, nurse your baby. We can talk later." Matter-of-factly, she replied, "No, it's not time for his feeding." Incredulous, I asked, "Where on earth did

you get that advice?" "From a baby-training class," she proudly stated. "I want my baby to learn that I am in control, not him."

This novice mother, wanting to do the best for her baby, had fallen into the wrong crowd of advisers. She was unknowingly starting her parenting career with distance developing between herself and her baby. This insensitivity to each other spells trouble for the relationship, now and in the years to come.

CIO can interfere with healthy growth. Above all, ignore anyone who tells you not to feed your baby once you've put him down to sleep. If you feel he's hungry, feed him. If he is telling you that he is hungry, feed him. Studies have shown that babies have a remarkable ability to know how much food they need and when. Trust your baby to know when he is hungry. Trust yourself to know when your baby is hungry. Don't trust a book or a class.

CIO is medically incorrect. Health care providers, please take note! In our pediatric practice we often see babies whose medical problems have been missed because of the cry-it-out advice. Someone makes the erroneous assumption that baby is crying at night out of habit and believes that ignoring the crying will make it go away. As a result, a medical problem is ignored, despite the baby's clear signals that something is wrong. See chapter 11 for possible medical problems.

CIO doesn't work in the long run. Studies have shown that most babies who are left to cry it out in the name of sleep training may

CRY IT OUT ON TV

Sitcom fans may remember the episode of *Mad About You* when Jamie and Paul put their little one through the cry-it-out experience. The program showed every excruciating detail of the new parents' anguish as they sat outside baby's door and resisted the urge to go in and pick baby up. Predictably, just as mom was about to rush in, baby stopped crying and fell asleep. It worked! There was a big sigh of relief across the nation, but not for the TV mom. Jamie looked stricken as she said, "I'm afraid we've broken her little heart."

not become such "good babies" after all. When their cries go unheeded, they learn to "cry it *in*" in ways that are disturbing. They often cling to their parents more and actually take longer to become independent, or they withdraw, shut down, and become "independent" way too soon. Many parents who have tried this method have told us that it doesn't work, or if it does "work," they feel really bad about it. Sometimes they tell us that it worked for a while and then the child went back to crying and cried louder and harder because he never really learned how to fall asleep. (See the description of "shutdown syndrome" on page 88.)

SENSITIVE SLEEP TRAINING THAT DOES WORK

We are going to be honest with you. The cry-it-out method appears to work — at least some of the time in some families. Many parents have tried it, and some babies have learned to go to sleep on their own fairly quickly, without too many nights of crying. Parents get some much-needed rest, and everyone seems happy.

But it does not work with every baby. It's the easygoing babies who learn to go to sleep on their own with minimal fuss who have made this approach so popular (or it's the parents who do it but don't tell you how awful it was). Because the cry-it-out approach worked on a neighbor's easy baby, parents naturally want it to work on their own baby, even if their baby has a different temperament. High-need babies with very persistent personalities have a very rough time if they are left to cry it out. They may eventually learn to fall asleep independently but at a high cost.

Also, whether crying it out works or not depends upon how you define "works." If you stop responding to a child's nighttime needs, of course she will eventually give up on asking for your attention and go to sleep. But she has not learned that it's nice to go to sleep by herself. She has learned that she has no other choice. For some parents and infants, this is the beginning of a distant, less sensitive relationship. Crying it out proves to be a bad investment — one with short-term gain but a long-term loss.

Parenting isn't about plans and programs. It's about relationships. Remember, you are nurturing a little human being, not training a pet. One-size-fits-all methods may work for puppies (or they may not). One-size-fits-all methods definitely don't work for babies and children.

But you wouldn't be reading this book if you didn't want to change something about how your baby sleeps — or doesn't sleep. In this chapter we have spoken out fairly strongly against the cry-it-out method. But we have also stressed that individual parents know what is best for their baby. So who are we to say that the cry-it-out method is wrong for your baby? We have never used it on any of our own babies, and we have never told a patient to give it a try. But we know that some of you reading this chapter will try this method. So we want to offer you some guidance on how to individualize a sleep-training approach for your baby (which, as you'll see, is really not CIO) — guidance that you may not receive from the people or books that advocate this approach.

A sensitive approach to sleep-training means that you adapt the cry-it-out program to fit your baby. You don't just follow the recipe in the cry-it-out cookbook. Instead, you learn to read the signs that indicate that your baby is sleepy. You think about your baby's unique sleep difficulties and find ways to parent him through the process of falling asleep. Remember, sleep trainers can offer only general advice — what works for some babies. But every baby comes with his own unique personality. No matter how hard or how long you work at it, you may not be able to get your baby to act like the baby in the book. Persisting with a bad experiment will get parents into trouble. Both you and your baby will end up frightened and frustrated.

Sensitive sleep training does not mean forcing your infant to sleep. Rather, it should mean creating conditions that make sleep more attractive to baby and teaching baby tools to help himself go to sleep and back to sleep. In toilet training (better called "toilet learning"), you wouldn't lock your child in a bathroom and let him cry until he removed his own diaper and used the toilet. Instead, you gradually teach him how to listen to his need-to-go signals and what to do. Before you embark on any sleep-training method, make sure you do the following:

Get connected. It's very important not to begin using any sleep-training method until you feel you are connected to your baby — you know her well, understand her cries, and can usually soothe them. Sleep training is only a small part of how you parent your infant. Parents who start off using as many of the attachment tools (the Baby B's listed on page 70) as they can will naturally be more sensitive about sleep training. Of course, because they are sensitive to their infant's needs, they usually decide that crying it out is simply not an option for them, and they are motivated to experiment with more sensitive alternatives.

Consider your baby's personality. An easygoing, mellow baby may learn to fall asleep independently without a great deal of fussing. However, if you have a high-need baby, one with a persistent personality who does not give up easily, please don't try the cry-it-out-alone method. It will be too tough on your baby and on you. Babies with persistent personalities will cry for a long time, and if you don't respond, you risk destroying the trusting connection between the two of you. To help your high-need baby sleep more independently, try the sleep tips offered in chapters 1 and 2, as well as the additional suggestions for night weaning in chapter 6 and the fathering tips in chapter 8 and at the end of this chapter.

Realize the difference between CIO and CIOA (cry it out alone). When it comes to crying it out, it's the alone part that we have the real problem with. All babies cry, some a lot more than others, and oftentimes (such as when they're teething) there's not much you can do about it but hold your baby and wait it out. And there are times when you feel it's okay to let your baby cry — but always in the arms of a caring person, such as dad when mom is desperate for sleep or when baby is old enough to handle the frustration of not getting what he wants at night.

Consider baby's age. As baby gets older, your response time can lengthen. You don't always need to respond to a nine-month-old as quickly as you would a nine-day-old. But no form of CIOA is appropriate for a baby at any age. A nine-month-old, or even a twenty-month-old, needs to know a person is going to show up fairly promptly. It's what you do after you show up that requires some planning.

Consider medical causes of night waking. Before you try sleep training, go through the checklist on page 214 to make sure that baby's night waking isn't due to a medical problem.

Observe the warning signs. Study the warning signs on page 211 so that you will know whether or not you and your baby are okay with this experiment.

SCIENCE SAYS: CRYING IT OUT MAY BE HARMFUL TO A CHILD'S HEALTH

Science tells us that when babies cry alone and unattended, they experience panic and anxiety. Their bodies and brains are flooded with adrenaline and cortisol stress hormones. Science has also found that when developing brain tissue is exposed to these hormones for prolonged periods, these nerves won't form connections to other nerves and will degenerate. Is it therefore possible that infants who endure many nights or weeks of crying it out alone are actually suffering harmful neurological effects that may have permanent implications on the development of sections of their brain? Here is how science answers this alarming question:

Chemical and Hormonal Imbalances in the Brain

Research has shown that infants who are routinely separated from parents in a stressful way have abnormally high levels of the stress hormone cortisol, as well as lower growth hormone levels. These imbalances inhibit the development of nerve tissue in the brain, suppress growth, and depress the immune system.[1, 4, 6, 22]*

Researchers at Yale University and Harvard Medical School found that intense stress early in life can alter the brain's neurotransmitter systems and cause structural and functional

---

* References can be found in Appendix C.

WARNING SIGNS!

No one method of helping a baby learn to sleep better works for all babies. If letting your baby cry isn't working, don't persist with a bad experiment. As we have said before, parenting is about building a relationship with your child, not about getting your child to conform to a program or a plan. Here are some clues that you need a change of direction:

- Your "parent gut" says what you're doing isn't right for your baby.

- Baby seems distant and withdrawn during the day.

- Baby seems anxious and clingy during the day.

- A distance is developing between you and your baby.

- Stress signs appear while baby is crying (for example, you or your baby is hyperventilating). Harmful physiological changes are often a clue to underlying stress that needs to be resolved.

EXTREME WARNING SIGNS!

If you are doing CIO and you observe these extreme warning signs, stop:

- Baby vomits while being left alone to cry it out.

- Your milk supply is dwindling. In this case, baby is way too young for you to even begin sleep training.

- Baby is not gaining enough weight.

- Baby is not making progress toward developmental milestones.

For a sensitive alternative to the cry-it-out method, see page 98 for a story of how two of our patients got through a difficult situation of night waking and mother burnout.

---

changes in regions of the brain similar to those seen in adults with depression.[20]

One study showed that infants who experienced persistent crying episodes were ten times more likely to have Attention Deficit Hyperactivity Disorder as a child, along with poor school performance and antisocial behavior. The researchers concluded that these findings may be due to the lack of responsive attitude of the parents toward their babies.[43]

Dr. Bruce Perry's research at Baylor University may explain this. He found that when chronic stress overstimulates an infant's brain stem (the part of the brain that controls adrenaline release), and the portions of the brain that thrive on physical and emotional input are neglected (such as when a baby is repeatedly left to cry alone), the child will grow up with an overactive adrenaline system. Such a child will display increased aggression, impulsivity, and violence later in life because the brain stem floods the body with adrenaline and other stress hormones at frequent and inappropriate times.[32]

Dr. Allan Schore of the UCLA School of Medicine has demonstrated that the stress hormone cortisol (which floods the brain during intense crying and other stressful events) actually destroys nerve connections in critical portions of an infant's developing brain. In addition, when the portions of the brain responsible for attachment and emotional control are not stimulated during infancy (as may occur when a baby is repeatedly neglected), these sections of the brain will not develop. The result: a violent, impulsive, emotionally unattached child. He concludes that the sensitivity and responsiveness of a parent stimulates and shapes the nerve connections in key sections of the brain responsible for attachment and emotional well-being.[19, 37]

Decreased Intellectual, Emotional, and Social Development

When infant developmental specialist Dr. Michael Lewis presented research findings at an American Academy of Pediatrics meeting, he concluded that "the single most important influence on a child's intellectual development is the responsiveness of the mother to the cues of her baby."

Researchers have found that babies whose cries are usually ignored will not develop healthy intellectual and social skills.[24]

Dr. M. R. Rao and her colleagues at the National Institutes of Health showed that infants with prolonged unattended-to crying in the first three months of life had an average IQ of 9 points lower than average at five years of age. They also showed poor fine-motor development.[34]

Researchers at Pennsylvania State and Arizona State universities found that infants with excessive crying during the early months showed more difficulty controlling their emotions and became even fussier when their parents tried to console them at ten months.[41]

Other research has shown that babies who cry it out alone have a more annoying quality to their cry, are more clingy during the day, and take longer to become independent as children.[14]

Harmful Physiological Changes

Animal and human research has shown that when separated from parents, infants and toddlers exhibit unstable temperatures, heart arrhythmias, and decreased REM sleep (the state of sleep that promotes brain development).[15, 17, 18]

Dr. J. E. Brazy at Duke University and Dr. Susan Ludington-Hoe and her colleagues at Case Western University showed in two separate studies how prolonged crying in infants causes increased blood pressure in the brain, elevates stress hormones, obstructs blood from draining out of the brain, and decreases oxygenation to the brain. They concluded that caregivers should answer cries swiftly, consistently, and comprehensively.[3, 26]

What can parents conclude from this research? All babies cry, and most babies grow up to be emotionally and neurologically healthy. Clearly, crying in and of itself does not harm the brain. Additionally, some research shows that crying while being consoled and cared for by a parent does not harm the brain. However, the research is clear on one point: Intense, extended periods of crying *alone* over and over again can permanently harm a baby's developing brain. Brain researchers have long known that chronically elevated stress hormones can damage neurological development, a condition called *glucocorticoid neurotoxicity.*

What does this mean for the CIO method? If a baby cries only for brief periods and learns to self-soothe himself to sleep easily within a few nights, there probably is no harm done. If a baby cries for many minutes, night after night for many nights, this may be harmful. Notice we don't say how many minutes and how many nights are safe, because no one has ever researched this. No scientific study has ever been done to determine what degree of the CIO method is safe.

Using CIO is analogous to giving a child a medication that appears to work well but has not undergone extensive safety testing, and preliminary testing shows some severe side effects. No doctor would ever dream of prescribing such a medication, and no parent would ever think of using one. Whenever any medication is found to have harmful side effects that outweigh its usefulness, it is immediately taken off the market. Why shouldn't parenting practices hold to the same standard? We look forward to the day when medical experts and parents alike will recognize the scientific basis for the harmful effects of CIO, and this alarming practice will become a thing of the past.

Hidden Medical and Physical Causes of Night Waking

WHEN PARENTS TELL US THAT their frequently waking baby seems to be in pain, we take this observation seriously. These parents have often "tried everything" to get their baby to sleep longer and more comfortably at night, but with no success. Some sleep advisers might dismiss their concerns and suggest to these "overly anxious parents" that a few nights of crying it out will teach their baby not to wake up. But in our practice, we take parents at their word. When babies who wake up seem to be hurting, there is usually a medical or physical cause for their night waking.

WHEN TO SUSPECT A MEDICAL CAUSE FOR NIGHT WAKING

As we said in previous chapters, babies wake up at night for lots of good reasons: they get hungry, they need closeness, their brains are not mature enough to sleep soundly. How do you tell the difference between normal, baby-will-grow-out-of-it night waking, and night waking caused by a medical problem? Here are some clues that indicate that baby's frequent waking may have a physical cause:

- Baby has not slept well since birth.
- Baby awakens suddenly with colicky-type abdominal pain.
- Baby is restless all through the night.
- Baby seems to gag or choke frequently at night.
- Baby spits up frequently day or night.
- A previously "good sleeper" suddenly becomes a restless sleeper.
- Baby has been labeled "colicky."
- Night waking is occurring more rather than less often.
- Baby cries a lot for no apparent reason (not tired, hungry, bored, and so on).
- The usual sleep-inducing strategies aren't working.
- Baby seems very cranky or excessively irritable.
- Your "parent gut" tells you your baby hurts somewhere.

Does this sound like your baby? If so, there may be a hidden medical cause behind baby's frequent night waking. This chapter describes common medical causes of night waking in babies and toddlers and what parents can do about them.

GASTROESOPHAGEAL REFLUX (GER)

Is your baby "colicky"? Suspect gastroesophageal reflux, or GER. GER, also called "acid reflux," "acid indigestion," and "gastroesophageal reflux disease" (GERD), is a painful medical condition caused by the regurgitation of acid-containing stomach contents into the esophagus. Adults call it "heartburn."

When you swallow, the food travels down the esophagus into the stomach. A circular band of muscle called the lower esophageal sphincter (LES) opens to let the food into the stomach and then contracts again to keep stomach contents in the stomach. If the LES relaxes and remains open, stomach acids can escape back into the esophagus and irritate the sensitive lining, causing a painful burning sensation. This backflow from stomach to esophagus is called "reflux."

Reflux can cause babies to spit up — a little or a lot. In some cases, the stomach contents stay in the esophagus, so there's no spitting up, just pain. Sometimes the stomach acids settle in the back of the throat, causing a sore throat ("throat burn"), choking, gagging, coughing, or, in older babies and adults, erosion of dental enamel. Sometimes the stomach contents can be aspirated into the lungs, causing wheezing and asthmalike problems. Most babies have some degree of reflux during the early months, and most gradually outgrow it during the second half of the first year as the LES matures. Mild reflux may not bother some babies. We call them "happy spitters." In this situation, what you have is a laundry problem, not a medical concern. Other babies are bothered a great deal by reflux, and the pain is worse at night, so that they cannot enjoy restful, peaceful sleep.

Susan, a wise and intuitive first-time mother, brought her six-month-old baby, Nathan, to our office for consultation about his "colic." We listened as this exhausted and angry mother related her baby's story:

"Nathan has never slept well since birth. I'm up with him three or four times a night, and the only thing that seems to settle him is nursing. An hour after I put him down, he wakes up screaming. The same thing for naps. The only way I can get him to nap longer than forty-five minutes is to nurse him as he sleeps. He seems fine during the day as long as I keep holding him and nursing him, but as soon as I put him down, he screams again. I'm so tired of people telling me I'm spoiling him by holding him so much. I've been to six doctors, and twice we've taken Nathan to the emergency room at night because he seemed to be hurting so much. All these doctors have told me that he's waking up out of habit, and if I would just let him cry and not nurse him so much, he'd quit waking up. But I know there's a reason that he keeps waking up. I'm not just an anxious, overprotective mother, as they keep telling me. I know something is wrong with him."

Susan's intuition was right. After delving into Nathan's history, I suspected he was waking because of severe pain from reflux. An esophagoscopy, a procedure that uses a flexible tube with a miniature camera on the end to examine the inside of the esophagus, revealed severe GERD (gastroesophogeal reflux disease), to the extent that Nathan had multiple ulcers, open sores, in the lining of his esophagus. Obviously, this baby truly did hurt.

When I saw the pictures of his esophageal erosions, I was angry at the "cry-it-out" crowd who had failed to take this baby's crying seriously, and who had also failed to listen to the person who knew the baby best, his mother. If this problem had been detected and treated earlier, this baby could have been spared six months of pain, and his parents would not have had to suffer through six months of sleep deprivation. Instead, because the reflux had damaged Nathan's esophagus, he required surgical treatment, following which he grew better, ate better, and eventually slept better. Because Nathan in those early months had been conditioned to associate sleep with pain, he had to be reconditioned into sleeping more normally. This took nearly six months.

How to Recognize Reflux

Signs and symptoms of GER vary according to the severity of the problem. Babies may have most of the following signs or just a few. Here are clues that your baby may be waking up from reflux:

- *An early start.* GER starts in the first few *weeks* of life. If your previously sound sleeper starts waking up in pain at four months of age, it is unlikely to be due to GER.

- *Frequent, painful night waking.* Baby wakes up suddenly, sometimes screeching, triggering your gut feeling, "He's hurting somewhere! It's that cry again!"

- *Sleeping position.* Baby sleeps soundly when held upright or semi-upright but poorly when lying flat. Or baby may sleep better on his stomach than on his back. (Note: Unless your doctor advises you otherwise, always put your baby down to sleep on his back, since back sleeping is associated with a reduced risk of SIDS.)

- *Poor-quality sleep.* Baby is restless, squirms, arches back, and has frequent jerky movements.

- *Spitting up.* Baby spits up frequently and forcefully, especially when lying down. Sometimes she spits up "like a volcano." (Note: Some babies with GER do not spit up.)

- *Daytime colic.* Baby experiences frequent bouts of inconsolable crying during the day — and not only in late afternoon and early evening, which is typical of "colic."

- *Irregular breathing during sleep.* All young babies show some irregular breathing during sleep, but GER is associated with prolonged stop-breathing episodes during sleep.

- *Throaty noises, as if baby is clearing his throat.* Baby swallows noisily and makes choking and gagging sounds.

- *Excessive drooling.* Baby has an incessant drool rash around her mouth, cheeks, and in the skin folds of her neck.

- *Wet burps.* Milk comes up with the air bubble most of the time.

- *Sour breath.* You smell a sour odor, especially after baby eats.

- *General fussiness.* Baby's fussiness diminishes when she is held upright or nursed.

Severe reflux can take its toll on the entire family. One sleep-deprived mother of a frequent night waker once told us, "I'm camping out in your office until you find out what's wrong with my baby." A father in our practice was so disturbed by his baby's incessant crying and night waking that he had a vasectomy, explaining, "I'll never go through that again!"

Why GER is worse during sleep. Normal physiological changes that occur during sleep can aggravate reflux. Saliva production and swallowing frequency diminish during sleep. We often refer to saliva as the body's natural "health juice" because it not only helps digestion, it also acts like a natural antacid and lubricant to soothe the inflamed esophagus. In addition, saliva contains a healing substance called "epidermal growth factor," which helps repair the damaged lining of the esophagus. But at night there is less saliva.

GER may also be worse during sleep because it takes longer for acid to pass out of the stomach when the body is sleeping. To add insult to injury, the LES, like most muscles, may relax more during sleep, which makes reflux more likely. And lying flat during nap time or nighttime makes it easier for the stomach contents to regurgitate back up into the esophagus. When baby is upright, gravity helps keep the stomach contents down. (However, in some infants and children with reflux, position changes seem to make no difference.)

GER may also affect baby's breathing at night. When a baby falls asleep, the muscles surrounding the airway relax, and the airway gets narrower. In babies with normal airway structures and no reflux, this does not compromise breathing. But this can be a problem in babies whose airways are already irritated by acid-containing throat contents. The inflammation can obstruct breathing, causing baby to wake up frequently, or it can cause wheezing and restless sleep.

How to Help a Baby with Reflux Sleep Better

As you can see, there are plenty of reasons for a baby with reflux, like Nathan, to cry out for help at night. You can also see that mom's "medicine" was instinctively right. Frequent holding kept Nathan upright, so that gravity helped keep down the stomach contents. And frequent doses of mom's milk acted like an antacid to soothe the burning esophagus. Over our many years in pediatric practice, we have been amazed at how often mothers

"COLIC" = REFLUX?

In our experience, "colicky" babies who wake up frequently and painfully at night often have gastroesophageal reflux. Babies who are labeled "colicky" during the day but who sleep reasonably well at night probably don't have GER. They want to be held and nursed frequently during the day because of their temperament and need level, not because they are in pain.

instinctively do what's medically right for their infants and children, even if it means going against professional advice. Because we see many infants like Nathan with medical causes of night waking, we are passionate about teaching parents to respond to their babies' cries and to avoid using cry-it-out-alone methods of sleep training.

If you suspect that your baby is waking up frequently at night because of GER, start keeping a journal about baby's symptoms and take it with you when you visit your doctor. Include in your journal your baby's responses to the following ten tips on how to lessen the pain of GER:

1. Feed smaller amounts more frequently. Here's our rule for reflux feeding:

> Feed half as much twice as often

Frequent feedings stimulate saliva production, which neutralizes stomach acid and lessens the irritating effects of the acid on the lining of the esophagus. Smaller amounts of milk and food empty out of the stomach into the intestines more quickly, so there's less opportunity for the stomach contents to flow back into the esophagus. Babies, just like adults, are more likely to have heartburn after a big meal than after a small one.

2. Breastfeed as often and as long as possible. Studies show that GER is less severe in breastfed babies. Mom's milk is a magic medicine for babies with reflux. Here's why: Breastfed babies naturally feed more frequently, so they get more frequent doses of this natural antacid. Breast milk empties from the stomach much faster than food or formula. Breast milk makes the stools softer and easier to pass, thus lessening the reflux-aggravating effects of constipation. Finally, breastfeeding mothers enjoy the effects of the relaxing hormones during breastfeeding, which helps them cope with the extra doses of mothering a baby with reflux requires. Here's a testimonial from a mother in our pediatric practice:

At age five months and after I had consulted four different pediatricians, Jacob was diagnosed with gastroesophageal reflux. I am forever grateful I did not give up! The goal of one of Jacob's reflux meds was to help digestion so he would not reflux. I figured, what could be better for him than the most easily digested food for babies . . . mom's milk! When the specialist first met Jacob, he was shocked to see him looking so happy. He told me that most babies with his degree of reflux fail to thrive and are very sickly. I am convinced that Jacob did not fail to thrive because he was breastfed.

3. Eliminate possible food sensitivities. If you are breastfeeding, it is possible that foods you are eating are getting into your milk and bothering your baby. Follow the steps on page 222 to eliminate possible culprits.

4. Use a predigested, hypoallergenic infant formula. If you are not breastfeeding, remember this reflux feeding rule: Get the stuff out of the stomach fast. In hypoallergenic infant formulas, the proteins have been predigested through processing, which helps the formula move through the stomach faster than standard formulas. Many infants with reflux also seem to be allergic to milk-based infant formulas. The special formula, though more expensive and less palatable, often helps. Ask your health care provider to recommend a hypoallergenic formula. Then feed half as much twice as often. Since an infant's tummy is about the size of her fist, place baby's fist next to the bottle and feed her an average of one fistful per feeding. For most infants during the first six months, this will amount to 2 to 3 ounces every couple hours.

5. Burp better. A tummy full of air aggravates reflux. Burp baby well when switching breasts during breastfeeding. If bottlefeeding, burp baby after every few ounces and use a

feeding system that prevents air bubbles from collecting in the bottle.

6. Keep baby upright and quiet after feedings. Shake up that tiny, full tummy and you're likely to get a splat of spit-up on your shirt. Instead, hold, cuddle, or wear your baby upright in a sling for at least thirty minutes after a feeding. Move gently with your baby. Bouncing him around may jostle the stomach contents and trigger reflux.

7. Pacify baby. Mothers of infants with reflux often report that their babies want to nurse constantly. This is because frequent sucking calms babies and increases saliva production. Expect baby to nurse for long periods to soothe her sore esophagus. The "half as much twice as often" idea does not mean that you should shorten your breastfed baby's time at the breast. If you're comfortable with long nursing sessions and they seem to help your baby, then relax and enjoy this soothing time together. If you find that the human nipple or the person attached to it is wearing out, try offering your baby a pacifier or a finger to suck on after feedings. But be aware that some infants will suck so vigorously on pacifiers that they swallow air, which can aggravate reflux. You may have to experiment with the pacifier to see what keeps your baby most comfortable.

8. Dress for sleep. Let baby "sleep loose." Avoid clothing that binds baby around the waist, such as tight diapers and sleepers with tight waistbands. Any increased pressure on the abdomen can aggravate reflux.

9. Position baby for sleep. Even though sleeping on the tummy may lessen reflux, during the first year, it's safest to position your baby to sleep on her back, since back sleeping reduces the risk of SIDS. For toddlers one year and older, sleeping on the left side may reduce reflux, since this position locates the gastric inlet higher than the outlet and helps gravity keep the food down. Elevate the head of baby's crib at least thirty degrees. If baby sleeps in your bed, try positioning baby on a reflux wedge (available at infant product stores).

10. No smoking, please. Nicotine has a double fault: It stimulates the production of stomach acids and relaxes the LES, two factors that aggravate reflux. Don't smoke around baby. And don't smoke at all if you breastfeed, since nicotine passes through your milk into baby.

Talk with your doctor about reflux. Try as many of these home remedies as you can and enter what works and what doesn't in your journal. This information will help your child's doctor determine whether or not your

FEEDING CHILDREN WITH REFLUX

Babies often outgrow problems with reflux, but for some it remains a problem — and a cause of night waking — into the preschool years. Here are some tips on feeding toddlers and children who have reflux.

• Avoid heavy meals just before bedtime. Serve dinner earlier in the evening and make bedtime snacks low-fat, low-fiber foods that empty from the stomach faster.

• Avoid giving your child foods that aggravate reflux, such as spicy foods, acidic foods (citrus fruits and juices), caffeine-containing beverages, chocolate, fried foods, peppermint and spearmint, and carbonated beverages.

• Raise a grazer. Continue the small, frequent feeding pattern you began in infancy. Offer small, frequent minimeals rather than three big meals. Try the "sipping solution." Encourage your toddler to sip on a fruit-and-yogurt smoothie throughout the day. Blended foods empty from the stomach faster.

• Raise a lean child. Obesity tends to aggravate reflux, perhaps due to the increased intra-abdominal pressure from excess abdominal fat.

• Play chew-chew. His mouth is your child's own blender. Encourage him to take small bites and chew his food well. Food chewed into smaller portions empties from the stomach faster, and children who eat more slowly tend to swallow less air.

infant has reflux, how severe it might be, and what type of treatment is needed. Oftentimes, working out an individual reflux plan using the above remedies is all that is necessary. If your doctor and you are fairly sure your baby has reflux and the usual home remedies aren't working, your doctor will likely prescribe an antacid medication as a trial to see if it helps. If reflux is still suspected, your doctor may choose to have a pediatric gastroenterologist do some special tests to determine if your baby has reflux and how severe it is.

Get support. Night waking from reflux ranks at the top of the list of causes of family sleep deprivation. As you probably gathered from the treatment tips above, medical treatment usually plays a minor role in helping reflux, and parental remedies play a major role. Support from other parents will help you figure out how to help your baby and how to cope yourself. We highly recommend that you contact PAGER (Pediatric/Adolescent Gastroesophageal Reflux Association) at www.reflux.org.

FOOD ALLERGIES AND SENSITIVITIES

Rumblings in the gut can keep tiny tummies awake. Because the intestines are richly supplied with nerves, what bothers the abdomen also bothers the brain. Ever try to go to sleep with a gas-bloated abdomen after indulging in an elaborate late-night meal? The same gut feeling happens in babies who are sensitive to certain foods. Here are some clues that food sensitivities may be keeping your baby awake:

- Baby generally seems gassy or bloated after feeding.

- You feel and hear baby's intestines churning, and he seems generally irritable after a feeding.

- Baby shows a change in bowel habits, either diarrhea or constipation, after you introduce new foods.

- Baby shows a "target sign" — a red, circular rash around the anus — which is caused by the skin reacting to overly acidic stools.

- Baby shows colicky, abdominal pain, irritability, or diarrhea following breastfeeding (suggesting baby may be intolerant to something in the breastfeeding mother's diet).

- Baby has a rough, raised, red, sandpaper-like rash mainly on the cheeks but also possibly on the elbows and knees. Also, typical "baby acne" progresses onto the scalp and down onto the shoulders.

- Baby has respiratory symptoms: sneezing, runny nose, wheezing, and a persistent cough.

- Baby experiences recurring ear infections.

- Baby has puffy eyelids or dark circles under her eyes.

- Baby suffers from persistent night waking, and his sleep is restless and fitful.

Food allergies generally affect four areas: skin, respiratory passages, intestines, and behavior (such as night waking). While it's easy to pin night waking on food sensitivities when you're desperate to find a cause, in our opinion, if a food sensitivity is severe enough to cause night waking, you'll also notice some of the above clues in baby's skin, respiratory passages, or intestines. If baby has reasonably clear skin, a happy, nonallergic-looking face, no congestion of the nasal and respiratory passages, and no digestive problems, it is unlikely (but not impossible) that baby is waking up because he is hurting from food sensitivities.

About 90 percent of food allergies in infants are caused by these nine foods (known as the "nasty nine"):

- dairy products
- wheat
- shellfish
- soy
- egg whites
- tree nuts
- peanuts
- corn
- tomatoes

Other suspects are strawberries, chocolate, and citrus fruits. The only food sensitivities that have been scientifically correlated with night waking in a breastfeeding mother's diet are to dairy and wheat, yet many mothers have reported their babies getting colicky, with facial and respiratory symptoms and night waking, when they eat lots of corn-containing foods. Caffeine-containing foods, such as coffee, tea, chocolate, and soft drinks, bother some babies. Also, beware of the caffeine in some over-the-counter cough remedies. Usually, but not always, a breastfeeding mother must consume a lot of caffeine to keep her baby awake. Very spicy foods usually do not bother breastfeeding babies, but these foods should still be on your elimination list if you're trying to track down the culprits (see below). Some mothers report that gassy foods such as broccoli, onions, brussels sprouts, cabbage, and cauliflower (usually only in the raw state) make their baby gassy and cause night waking. It's hard to scientifically explain how gassy vegetables eaten by a breastfeeding mother can cause gas in her baby, yet this does occur.

In many breastfeeding mothers and their infants, the food sensitivities are dose-related: Your baby may wake up a lot if you drink two glasses of milk one evening but not if you have a small dish of yogurt.

Tracking Down Foods That Can Cause Night Waking

Blood tests to detect food allergies are inaccurate in infants, especially in the first year. It's better to rely on your own observations. Here are four steps to help you become your baby's fuss-food detective:

Step 1: Make a fuss-food chart. From the list above, select the foods that are the most likely culprits. Next, list the signs and symptoms that you relate to food sensitivities and then note your baby's change after you eliminate the foods. It can take up to two weeks or more to see a change, especially if your baby is older when you are doing this. As we discussed, true food sensitivities usually show up not only as night waking but also in other ways, such as in baby's skin, breathing, and gastrointestinal tract.

SAMPLE FUSS-FOOD CHART		
Suspected Food	**Signs and Symptoms**	**Change After Food is Eliminated**
milk	facial rash, diarrhea, and night waking with gas	facial rash much less, stools firmer, and sleep less restless

Step 2. Eliminate suspect foods. Choose the most likely suspects and eliminate from your diet as many of these foods as you can for two weeks. Using the chart above, record changes, if any.

Step 3. Gradually reintroduce the suspect foods one at a time. If you've eliminated all of the most common allergenic foods, as listed on the previous page, and your baby gets better but you're not sure which foods were causing your baby's night waking, reintroduce one food at a time back into your diet in gradually increasing doses. If the symptoms reappear, put that one on your forbidden food list.

Avoid all the suspect foods for a few months and then, unless your baby has severe food allergies, reintroduce them one at a time in gradually increasing doses. Most food sensitivities completely or partially subside by two to three years of age.

Step 4. Try the desperation diet. If you've tried eliminating the most common foods but baby still isn't doing well, you can eliminate "everything" all at once from your diet and spend two weeks eating just six foods that are virtually guaranteed not to bother baby. These are turkey, lamb, potatoes (white or sweet), squash, rice (or millet, another grain), and pears (or pear juice). Use rice milk (which isn't milk at all — it should really be called "rice water") as needed. Rice comes in many forms — flour, cakes, cereal, and bread (available at health food stores). Do not use soy. And drink lots of water. Eat, drink, and take absolutely nothing else (including vitamins and any other natural supplements). If you are on any medications, ask your doctor if you can safely go off them for a brief time.

Sounds fun, huh? Fill your fridge and cupboard with these delights and enjoy them for two weeks. You may feel quite hungry at first, but you'll learn to eat more of these foods and be creative with them. The deprivation is worth it if you see that your baby hurts a lot less. If baby gets much better, then you can slowly add in your favorite foods (one food every four days), keeping a list of anything that bothers baby (and, obviously, don't eat that food for a few months). Martha's foods to avoid were dairy products, wheat, and corn. Our daughter-in-law could eventually eat anything but bananas.

FORMULA INTOLERANCE

If your formula-fed baby is waking up frequently and is showing some of the signs of food sensitivity listed above, suspect that your baby's formula is the culprit. Here are the formula changes you can try, in order, to solve the problem. Allow each formula about a one- to two-week trial to see if it works. If baby significantly worsens sooner, then move on to the next step right away. While you can try these changes without consulting your doctor, we suggest you do let your doctor know if you end up making a formula change for the long term.

Change the form of formula. If you are using powdered formula, change to the same brand in liquid form. If using liquid, try the powder.

Change the brand but not the type. Whatever type (milk- or soy-based, or other) of formula you are using, try a different brand of the same type. If you're using a milk-based formula, try a different brand that is still milk-based, since the protein formulation in a different brand may be more comfortable on baby's tummy.

Change the type of formula. If baby is on a milk-based formula, try changing to soy. If on soy, try milk. If neither works, try a hypoallergenic formula.

Consult your doctor. If changing brands and types doesn't work, consult your doctor. If you do find a "happy" formula, let your doctor know at your next visit.

STUFFY NOSES

Tiny babies prefer (even need) to breathe through their noses rather than their mouths, so even a slight bit of stuffiness in already narrow infant nasal passages can lead to difficulty breathing and consequent night waking. Even previously long sleepers often wake up more during a cold. The more severe the cold and the congestion of the respiratory passages, the more frequent the night waking.

It's common for children who once slept for long stretches to revert back to frequent night waking following an illness. An illness throws off a child's sleep rhythms, and once they start waking up, they seem to temporarily forget how to get themselves back to sleep. Also, when a child is sick, parents are naturally sympathetic and nurturing, especially at night, so waking up has its rewards. Your child got used to, and enjoyed, the extra tender loving care at night, and now it's hard to go back to the other way of sleeping. It's sort of like going back to real food after enjoying lots of popsicles and ice cream while you had a sore throat. Expect at least another month of retraining your child to sleep through the night. In addition to the sleep-inducing strategies we've mentioned throughout this book (patting, rocking, swinging, and so forth), try what worked for you to help him sleep longer stretches before he got sick. (See our two home remedies for unstuffing little noses in the Environmental Allergies section below.)

EAR INFECTIONS

Ear infections are one of the most painful causes of night waking. The fluid draining from baby's snotty nose collects in the middle ear and causes pressure on the eardrum (especially if baby lies with the affected ear down). Clues that an ear infection could be causing your baby's night waking are:

- Baby's cold worsens and the discharge from her nose becomes thick and snotty. There is yellow drainage from both eyes.

- Baby's sleeping patterns suddenly change and she wakes up with painful cries.

Ear infections bother infants and toddlers more at night for two reasons: The middle-ear fluid presses on the eardrum when baby is lying with the affected ear down, and at night there are no distractions from the sensations of a painful ear. Babies vary tremendously in their sensitivity to ear pain. Some are bothered by a slight bit of fluid in the middle ear, others are not. Usually, but not always, if an ear infection is severe enough to

cause night waking, baby will have other signs of a cold. To relieve ear pain, hold baby upright for a while. In a toddler, encourage him to sleep with the affected ear up.

Fevers that accompany colds and infections can also trigger night waking, mainly because of the overall bodily discomfort caused by the fever and the infection. Rarely is it necessary to awaken a sleeping child to take her temperature or administer fever-lowering medicines. Simply kiss her forehead to check the temperature.

ENVIRONMENTAL ALLERGIES

Allergens in the bedroom (animal dander, dust, and mold) can congest baby's breathing passages and cause night waking. Remove possible allergens from baby's bedroom. Use a HEPA-type air filter and put the dogs and cats out of the room. Perfumes and hair sprays may give off fumes that act like nasal irritants, causing a stuffy nose in a co-sleeping baby. Above all, no smoking where baby sleeps. (For detailed instructions on how to allergy-proof your baby's bedroom, see www.AskDrSears.com.)

Dry air, especially during the winter months of central heating, can cause the normal secretions in baby's respiratory passages to thicken and impair breathing. Try to keep the humidity in baby's bedroom around 50 percent by using a cool-mist humidifier. If baby's nose is stuffy, try a warm-mist vaporizer. Since hot vaporizers pose a burn hazard, be sure to place it safely beyond baby's reach. As an extra perk, the steam from vaporizers can act as an extra heat source, allowing you to turn down the temperature in baby's bedroom.

Try to put your baby to bed with a clear nose and clear breathing passages. To do this, try our two home remedies: a "nose hose" and a "steam clean." For the "nose hose," spritz a few drops of saltwater nose drops into the nostrils to loosen secretions. These nose drops are available at your pharmacy as "saline nasal spray," or you can make your own by adding 1/4 teaspoon of salt to 8 ounces of water. Using a nasal aspirator (veteran parents call this handy gadget a "snot snatcher"), gently remove the loosened secretions from baby's nose. For the "steam clean," steam up the bathroom with a hot shower. Then sit in the bathroom and read to your baby before bedtime. Steam loosens the thickened secretions in baby's airways.

ANEMIA

We see many babies who have a low hemoglobin level (detected by one drop of blood from a quick finger prick during baby's checkup) and restless sleep. After a month or two of increasing the iron content of their baby's diet, mothers report that their baby sleeps better. A low iron level not only bothers the blood, it bothers the brain, leading to poor-quality sleep. Iron-deficiency anemia is most common between six and twenty-four months of age. Your baby's health care provider will check baby's hemoglobin during his regularly scheduled exams. You might want to mention anemia as a possible cause of night waking to your baby's doctor.

PINWORMS

Occasionally, night waking can be caused by itching associated with pinworms. At night the pregnant pinworm crawls out of the rectum to lay her eggs around the anus. All this wormy activity around the anus can itch. The child scratches the itchy area and picks up eggs under his fingernails, and then when he sucks his fingers, the eggs travel from his mouth through the intestines, where they hatch and repeat the cycle.

Here's how to be a home pinworm detective. Suspect pinworms if your child has scratch marks on his bottom or complains of an itchy bottom. Sometimes you can shine a flashlight around your child's anus at night and see the pinworms. They look like tiny pieces of white thread about a third of an inch long. If you can't see the worms but still suspect your child has them, place a piece of tape (sticky side out) on a tongue depressor or popsicle stick and capture the eggs by pressing the sticky tape on the skin around the anus. The best time for the tape test is in the morning just before your child awakens. Take the tape to your doctor's office or a laboratory, where it can be examined under a microscope to look for eggs. If eggs are present, your doctor will prescribe treatment.

SLEEP APNEA

Children who snore loudly, sleep restlessly, and seem overly tired during the day may suffer from sleep apnea. Loud and persistent snoring is a clue to a structural problem in the nose or throat that partially obstructs the breathing at night. During sleep, the muscles that keep the airway open during the day relax, allowing the airway to become more narrow. The air passing through narrowed airways causes vibration of the tissues around the airway, producing snoring. Sometimes snoring is a clue to a condition called sleep apnea, in which the compromised breathing also compromises your child's sleep. Here's how you can tell if your child has sleep apnea. Make a video of your child's sleep during the first couple hours, especially when he is snoring the loudest. In the case of sleep apnea, the child will breathe very noisily with periods of noiseless stretches of ten to fifteen seconds when he doesn't breathe, followed by a loud catch-up breath. This sleep apnea pattern usually results in a restless, tired, and cranky child the next day and, if present in an older child, usually affects behavior and school performance.

The most common cause of sleep apnea is large tonsils. During the day, the tonsils do not compromise the airway, but at night the airway passages relax, become more narrow, and require more effort to move enough air through them, causing the noisy breathing associated with sleep apnea.

Have your child's nasal passages and throat examined by your pediatrician. If your doctor says the nasal passages are clear and the tonsils are not obstructively large, show your doctor the video. If the above pattern is not present on your recording, you can rest assured that snoring is not a sign of sleep apnea and no surgical treatment is needed.

To lessen snoring, have your child experiment with various sleeping positions, such as tummy or side sleeping. Be sure your child's sleeping environment is free of allergens, including dust collectors and animal dander, which can cause nighttime stuffiness and result in abnormal breathing. Put a HEPA-type air purifier in your child's bedroom to remove nasal irritants from the air.

If your child's doctor suspects sleep apnea, you will be referred to an ear, nose, and throat (ENT) specialist.

Take sleep apnea seriously. It interferes with a child's overall health and well-being. When airways are partially obstructed during sleep, a child often semiawakens with a startle from lack of air. This causes an adrenaline rush and revs up the child's nervous system at night, interfering with sleep. Incidentally, sleep apnea is a common hidden cause of bed-wetting because this adrenaline rush causes the bladder to empty. So, as an added perk, your previously bed-wetting child may enjoy nighttime dryness once those tonsils and adenoids are in a hospital pickle jar.

IRRITATING SLEEPWEAR

Several mothers in our practice went through the checklist of causes of night waking on page 230 and discovered their babies were sensitive to polyester sleepers. Once they changed to 100 percent cotton clothing, their babies slept more comfortably. (Flame-retardant cotton sleepwear is available.) Other babies don't like the sensation of fabric on their feet. A clue to this irritation is when baby starts pulling off his socks or pulling at the feet of his sleeper. (For more on dressing your baby safely and comfortably for sleep, see page 76.)

TEETHING PAIN

As those pearly whites push their way through sensitive gums, teething pain can cause frequent night waking, especially in babies between four and seven months. Even though you may not see or feel the teeth until six or eight months, teething discomfort may start as early as three or four months, as witnessed by the telltale signs of increased drooling, a drool rash on the face, constant finger chewing, and wet bed sheets. Also, the increased saliva production can collect at the back of the throat, causing normal gurgly breathing sounds and coughs that may sometimes awaken a sleeping baby. Beginning at six months of age, expect a tooth to erupt around once a month until your child is two to two and a half years of age. Theoretically, teething pain could cause night waking throughout this teething time. Tiny teethers often enjoy a few restful weeks between dental eruptions.

It would be nice if a tiny tooth fairy comfortably ushering those teeth in were not a fairy tale. If you suspect your baby is waking because of teething pain, in consultation with your baby's doctor, give an appropriate dose of acetaminophen (or ibuprofen, which may last longer) just before bedtime for a few nights, and repeat every four hours if baby wakes up. Also, let your tooth-sore baby gnaw on your knuckle when she wakes up. This readily available hard pacifier may help her go

---

IS IT TEETHING OR AN EAR INFECTION?

In our pediatric practice we have an inside joke we call "the five-month ear check." Here's the usual scenario: Baby starts teething and waking up at night and is pulling on her ears during the day. Parents rush baby in to check the ears. The night waking is almost never caused by an ear infection. How can you tell at home without seeing your doctor? If baby has no cold symptoms and no fever, then simple teething is probably the culprit. If baby does have cold symptoms and a fever, it could be an ear infection.

---

back to sleep. While during the day cold pacifiers, such as an ice cube in a small sock, may soothe baby's sensitive, swollen gums, they are likely to awaken baby even more at night.

Babies often intensify their nursing — day and night — when they are teething. At this time many babies become all-night suckers; this will temporarily interrupt your sleep plan. On the other hand, sometimes teething triggers the opposite of increased nursing — a nursing strike.

GROWING PAINS

While we think of growing pains as a cause of night waking in older children, parents often report that their babies seem to wake up more when going through growth spurts. Since growth occurs mostly during sleep (that's when the growth hormone is secreted), it's theoretically possible that the changing biochemistry and physical growth could cause enough discomfort to awaken baby. Some babies will go on five-times-a-night feeding marathons to get the extra nutrition they need to fuel their growth spurts. That's one time it's best to nurse often to supply the growing body's increased demand.

We have noticed that babies often wake up when going through major motor milestones, such as from sitting to crawling, and from crawling to walking. A half-asleep baby may sit up or crawl into the wooden rail of the crib to "practice" his newly found motor skill. Or, he may become a crib sleepwalker who stumbles and wakes himself up. Perhaps baby is dreaming about crawling or walking, and he tries to practice his skills while partially asleep. He falls, startles, awakens, and quickly summons his favorite comforter — mom or dad.

DIAPER IRRITATION

Since babies are used to the feeling of wet or soiled diapers, this is an unlikely cause of night waking. If your baby sleeps through wet or soiled diapers, there is no need to wake him up for a change. Yet, if baby has one of those "power poops," he will need a diaper change. If baby is suffering from diaper rash, the protective skin barrier breaks down when wet or soiled, allowing the diaper contents to more easily irritate baby's sensitive skin. In this case, slather a generous amount of a zinc oxide—containing barrier cream over the rash for protection against the irritating diaper contents.

This may help baby sleep through a wet or soiled diaper without a change. If she wakes up, try to change the diaper as quickly as possible.

BABY IS TOO HOT OR TOO COLD

Create a consistent room environment. A stable bedroom temperature and relative humidity help babies sleep. See page 12 for how to maintain a consistent and sleep-conducive temperature and relative humidity in baby's bedroom.

BEDROOM NOISE

Most tiny babies are used to sleeping amid the ambient sounds of a busy family, and older children seldom need to be advised to tip-toe around a sleeping baby. Yet, some babies are more noise-sensitive than others, especially if they are already going through a night-waking stage. Tighten and oil loose joints on a squeaky crib, especially if your toddler moves around a lot at night. Oil the hinges on the bedroom door. Close the window if there is a lot of outside noise, such as middle-of-the-night sirens or early-morning garbage pickup. If baby does seem to be noise-sensitive, try the white noise sounds listed on page 24.

SEPARATION ANXIETY

How can anxiety be a physical cause of night waking? If you've ever been anxious, you'll recognize the intense physical discomforts — sweating, fast heartbeat, muscle tension, and more — that come from feeling anxious. Add to that the release of stress hormones that turn on the waking switch and you have a crying, sweating baby standing up rattling his cage when you go in.

Many babies seem to have two developmental stages when they are particularly sensitive to separation anxiety: from six to nine months and from fourteen to eighteen months. Separation anxiety intensifies during a major change in family routine, such as a move, parents' separation, or the temporary absence of one parent. Many parents have told us that their baby seems to be more separation-sensitive at night if they themselves have had a bad day.

We believe there is a natural, inborn developmental reason for the separation anxiety babies feel.

When baby develops the motor abilities to crawl or run away from the security of caregivers, the mind acts as a safety regulator that discourages aloneness. It's as if the body says go, but the mind says no. When baby wakes up alone in a quiet, dark room, aloneness is naturally upsetting to him, and he protests. Those with persistent personalities protest the loudest. Babies with easier temperaments can sometimes self-soothe back to sleep.

At some time or another, most of us have awakened with varying degrees of anxiety. Remember how comforting it is to have someone who loves you sleeping right next to you? Have you ever found it more difficult to go back to sleep if you awaken and your spouse is on a business trip and you are alone in bed? A baby doesn't have all the adult self-help mental mechanisms to soothe himself

back to sleep. When a baby wakes up anxious, his simple mechanism goes like this: "Something is not right here, but my parents can make it right."

POSSIBLE MEDICAL AND PHYSICAL CAUSES OF NIGHT WAKING

If you are having difficulty pinning down why your baby is waking up, go through this checklist:

- ☐ separation anxiety
- ☐ change in family routine
- ☐ hunger
- ☐ gastroesophageal reflux
- ☐ stuffy nose
- ☐ sleep apnea
- ☐ irritating sleepwear
- ☐ teething
- ☐ diaper rash
- ☐ too hot
- ☐ too cold
- ☐ fever
- ☐ a cold
- ☐ food or formula sensitivity
- ☐ nasal irritants:
  - ☐ perfume
  - ☐ powder
  - ☐ hair spray
  - ☐ animal dander
  - ☐ cigarette smoke
  - ☐ dust
  - ☐ mold
- ☐ squeaky crib
- ☐ bedroom or outside noises
- ☐ pinworms

Nighttime Parenting in Special Situations

A S YOU LIVE, SO SHALL YOU sleep. When babies have special needs or when families are going through changes, parents may face more challenging sleep problems. Here is a guide for families with special sleep situations.

NIGHT WAKING AFTER MOTHER RETURNS TO WORK

More and more mothers are continuing to breastfeed after returning to work. This is a big nutritional plus for their babies. And breastfeeding's other benefits multiply the longer mothers nurse, too.

Pumping your breasts while you are away from your baby helps maintain your milk supply. Just as important as having enough milk is nursing your baby frequently during the time you are together. Babies, who are very smart about things as important to them as breastfeeding, make up for their time away from mom by wanting to nurse more often when she is there. Even though they are

drinking mom's own milk from bottles when they are with their substitute caregiver, babies obviously miss the real thing.

Be prepared for your baby to wake up more often at night after you return to work to make up for the nursing and touch time he missed during the day. Night waking and increased night feeding is a reflection of the physiological principle that babies will do what they need to do in order to thrive. Babies need mother's milk and touch to thrive, so they are literally going to "milk" those night nursings for all they can get. Some babies seem to reverse their days and nights after mother returns to work. They nap more and feed less during the day when she is gone and then breastfeed frequently during the evening and through the night. While this sounds exhausting for moms (and sometimes is), most mothers we have interviewed who succeed at combining breastfeeding and working consider this reverse-cycle nursing a plus. Breastfeeding at night helps them unwind, relax, sleep better, and, most important, enjoy their baby more. It also keeps up their milk supply. The challenge is to find enough energy to work during the day and to satisfy baby's need to nurse at night. In our pediatric practice we give mothers who plan to return to work a crash course on working and sleeping. Here's what these mothers have told us helps them the most:

Co-sleep. Sleeping with your baby brings a double perk to working moms: It makes up for both the milk baby has missed during the daytime and the missed "touch time." If you are already co-sleeping, you have no doubt discovered that co-sleeping babies nurse more frequently. Most working and breastfeeding mothers consider co-sleeping a plus. They can nurse the baby several times at night and still get enough sleep themselves. Even mothers who weren't co-sleeping prior to returning to work may end up discovering that co-sleeping is best for themselves and their babies. If you haven't already mastered the art of co-sleeping, it may take you and your baby a while to get used to it. Read chapter 5 on co-sleeping, especially its benefits, page 113. Also read about how to make night nursing easier (in chapter 6), since it will be important for you to find ways to get enough sleep when you are breastfeeding several times a night.

Enjoy an early-morning nursing. Add twenty to thirty minutes of early-morning nursing to your getting-ready-for-work routine. Nurse your baby as soon as you awaken, before you get out of bed and shower and dress. Then nurse baby once more before you leave home or before you leave him at the caregiver's.

One month before going back to work, I started getting up about one and a half hours before he woke up. Sometimes I'd wake up on my own from the engorgement of very full breasts or my husband would wake me up. I would pump off what I had and freeze it. By the time my baby woke up, I'd again have plenty of milk for him. This approach also made the first feeding more pleasant. I didn't have painful breasts to feed him with. By the time I went back to work, I had a big milk bank stored up.

Adjust baby's nap schedule. When you were home on maternity leave, your baby may have had an early-afternoon nap and an early bedtime. Most working mothers find it works better for baby to have a late-afternoon nap and a later bedtime. This allows them to enjoy more quality time with baby during the evening, as well as to get in an extra feeding before bedtime.

Enjoy a happy nursing reunion. Ask your caregiver not to feed your baby during the hour before you arrive. Call ahead if you're going to be early or late. As soon as you arrive home or at the caregiver's, sit down and nurse your baby. Make this relaxing reunion a priority.

My baby loves to be nursed as soon as I get home from work. It also helps me unwind after a tense day of work and fighting the rush-hour traffic. Toward the end of our nursing session, I feel so relaxed.

Plan weekend tank-ups. To build up your milk supply, breastfeed more often on weekends and other nonworking days. Nurse and nap with your baby to catch up on your sleep and to boost your milk production. Working mothers often notice that even if their milk supply dwindles by Friday, a weekend of nursing ensures that they will make extra milk on Monday and Tuesday.

Be flexible. Your baby's sleep patterns will change when you return to work. They may also be affected by changes in the caregiving situation or in your work schedule. Try to understand these changes from your baby's point of view and then be flexible about finding ways to cope. Realistically, you won't be able to do much more than work, breastfeed, and care for your baby and yourself. Avoid other commitments during this time.

Get help! If you are going to continue to produce both milk and income, you are going to need help. When mom works outside the home, dad must share in both the baby care and the running of the household. Delegate as many of the non-baby-related chores as you can, and hire help for the house if possible.

NIGHT WAKING IN A PREMATURE BABY

We're just about ready to take our eight-week-premature baby home from the hospital and wonder what type of sleep patterns we should expect.

A general principle of infant behavior that we have followed during our years in pediatrics is that babies do what they do for basic biological reasons. This principle explains the different sleep patterns of premature babies. In the first few months, preemies may sleep for more total hours (sixteen to eighteen hours a day) than term babies, but they also awaken more frequently. Here's why:

As you learned in chapter 3, there are two main states of sleep: active sleep (also called REM sleep) and quiet or deep sleep (called non-REM sleep). The younger the human being, the greater the percentage of active sleep. The pre-born baby's sleep may be nearly 100 percent active sleep; premature infants (especially micropreemies) may have nearly 90 percent; and term infants 50 to 70 percent. By the time children are two years old, 25 percent of their sleeping time is spent in active sleep. Adolescents and adults spend around 20 percent of their sleep time in active sleep. This shift to a more mature sleep pattern as babies get older is one of the reasons they sleep "better" (that is, wake up less) the older they get.

Why do preemies and younger babies spend so much time in active sleep? Again, they are doing what they do for biological reasons. The last months in the womb and the first months of life are a time of rapid brain development, and sleep researchers believe that REM sleep helps the brain develop. The brain rests during quiet sleep, but it is busily at work during REM sleep. Blood flow to the brain increases during REM sleep, particularly in the area of the brain that automatically controls breathing. During active sleep, the body also increases the manufacture of certain proteins that are the building blocks of the neurons in the brain. So, in a nutshell, all this active sleep is helping preemies' brains grow.

Because of these normal and developmentally beneficial differences in sleep patterns, you should expect your preemie to wake up more frequently than a full-term baby would. It may also take longer for your baby to reach sleep maturity. If your baby was eight weeks early, in theory, you can expect him to continue to wake up frequently for eight weeks longer than you would expect of a term newborn.

Now that you understand your preemie's unique sleep patterns and developmental needs, you can see that you have some nighttime challenges ahead of you. It is especially important for the parents of premature infants to develop a nurturing style of nighttime parenting.

Early Sleep Training — Not for Preemies

While it's wise for all parents to shun the cry-it-out crowd, especially during the early months, this caution is particularly important for preemies. In fact, our general advice of "don't let your baby cry it out" becomes a double-don't for premature infants. Crying wastes energy, oxygen, and food — and preemies need more of all of these things to grow. You may hear someone say, "Crying is good for his lungs." Nonsense. Crying is hard on term babies, and it's doubly difficult for preemies. Excessive crying lowers a baby's level

of blood oxygen, which is already marginal in most premature infants. Babies waste a lot of energy in crying, energy that is needed for catch-up growth. Finally, crying leads to spitting up or reflux. Preemies are prone to reflux and need to keep that food in their tummies.

Consider Co-sleeping

Newborns enter the world with disorganized physiological systems. The brain's control over breathing patterns, heart rates, and waking and sleeping is far from perfect. Preemies are even more disorganized than term newborns. So, co-sleeping, which helps organize baby's physiological systems, has got to be good for growth. What helps preemies grow? More milk, more touch, and less wasted energy. That's exactly what co-sleeping provides. Here are reasons why co-sleeping is particularly beneficial for premature infants:

Preemies grow better. Levels of prolactin, the milk-making hormone, are higher during sleep. There is lots of milk available to co-sleeping babies in the middle of the night. Mothers often produce milk that is higher in fat at night, particularly in brain-building omega-3 fats. Co-sleeping enables you to deliver more "smart milk" and "grow milk" to your preemie.

Preemies sleep safer. Preemies are prone to irregular breathing patterns and stop-breathing episodes, called apnea (see page 226). You probably learned about apnea and apnea monitors while your baby was in the hospital, and you may be using an apnea monitor at home. The co-sleeping mother is like a human apnea monitor. Her presence helps to keep baby breathing. Many parents of preemies in our pediatric practice have reported that their babies seem to breathe more regularly and sound fewer apnea alarms when monitored during co-sleeping.

When my baby was discharged from the hospital, I was told to have her sleep alone in a crib with an apnea monitor. The monitor went off all night long, and it became a nightmare for our whole family. After a while, I left the monitor on her but put her next to me in bed. We both slept wonderfully side by side, and the monitor alarm never sounded. I strongly feel that my presence stimulated her to breathe until she outgrew her stop-breathing tendencies. My touch and closeness were all she needed.

Sleeping close to mommy delivers a therapeutic touch. Increased touch helps babies grow, probably for two physiological reasons: Touch stimulates the release of growth hormone, and it lowers the level of energy-wasting stress hormones.

Co-sleeping babies sleep more peacefully. Videotape studies by sleep researcher Dr. James McKenna revealed that solo sleepers squirm and seem more restless at night than co-sleepers. Instead of wasting energy squirming, your preemie should put that energy into growing.

Mothers sleep better. Research has shown that co-sleeping babies do night-nurse more frequently. Premature babies need to night-nurse

SLEEP TRAINING — NOT FOR PREEMIES

Ban the baby trainers from your home and bookshelf if you have a premature infant. The dictums of baby trainers are: scheduled feedings, not holding baby so much for fear of "spoiling," and letting baby cry it out so that baby learns to sleep through the night. All three of these techniques carry risks for term babies, but they are downright hazardous to the health of preemies. Rigid baby training keeps preemies from thriving and mommies from thriving. Here's why:

Rigid three- or four-hour feeding schedules, as recommended by most baby trainers, will not work for a preemie. Because preemies have tiny tummies and immature digestive systems and tire easily during feedings, they need smaller, more frequent feedings. We've mentioned how the cry-it-out advice keeps babies from thriving. It also keeps mothers from thriving by desensitizing them to the needs of their baby. You need to care for your baby in ways that build up your sensitivity, not tear it down. Baby training makes no physiological sense, especially in the care and feeding of premature infants.

even more frequently. Naturally, co-sleeping is the answer for easier night nursing. Remember the perk of breastfeeding acting like a natural tranquilizer? Nursing your preemie frequently at night naturally stimulates the release of relaxing hormones that help you sleep.

TWINS AND MULTIPLES

We have twins on the way. My friends who also have twins are always complaining that they don't get enough sleep. Are there things I can do to get more sleep but still meet my babies' nighttime needs?

Being blessed with two babies doesn't necessarily mean you will get half as much sleep. If anything, mothers of twins need more sleep than mothers of singletons. Here are some strategies to try so that you can avoid mother-of-twins burnout.

Consider co-bedding. Since they were womb mates for many months, your babies are used to sleeping together. Neonatologists have long observed that twins placed together in the same incubator or bassinet tend to breathe better and grow faster. In a study reported in 2002 in *Clinical Pediatrics,* researchers placed apnea monitors on eleven sets of preterm twins and compared the readings when the twins slept together in the same bassinet and slept separately. The co-bedding twins showed significantly fewer episodes of apnea.

Another perk of co-bedding is that it helps get twin babies on similar sleep schedules, which is particularly helpful if one baby seems to be a "sleeper" and the other one a "waker." You can also try a bedside co-sleeper (see page 126) and have your babies sleep right next to you.

Sometime between four and six months of age, your babies may start moving around and flailing their limbs during sleep, and you may decide it's time for them to try separate sleeping so that they don't wake each other. As they grow, crib mates may become playmates; you may want to separate them at night. You'll also want to keep them apart if one is teething or wakeful for other reasons. Since they're used to sleeping next to a person, this is a good time to consider co-sleeping so they won't be waking up alone.

Consider co-sleeping. Twins benefit from co-sleeping just like single babies do. In fact, they may need the therapeutic touch and other growth-stimulating effects of co-sleeping more, since twins are often born a bit early (see co-sleeping with preemies, above). But is it possible to co-sleep, night-nurse, and still get enough sleep yourself? It has worked for many mothers of twins. Try putting your babies down on their backs in your bed and sleeping between them. A king-size bed is a must with two babies. If bed space is still a problem, consider using a bedside co-sleeper. Co-sleeping is particularly helpful in those early months of marathon night nursing during frequent growth spurts.

In the morning I would move the twins from their co-sleeper into bed with me, one snuggled up on each side. With the warmth and presence of mama, they relaxed and slept more soundly, and so did I. It was really easy to nurse one baby while lying on my side and then roll over and feed the other one.

Double the nighttime parenting. While many mothers of single babies consider nighttime help from their husbands a luxury, for mothers of multiples it's a necessity. Dad can do everything at night that mother can do except breastfeed. And remember, dad can father-nurse a fussy but full baby back to sleep. (See the many nighttime fathering tips in chapter 8.)

Both babies were bottlefed, and we each took an assigned baby for the night. That way we each got up only half as much at night. Then, as one of them started sleeping through, we took turns being the parent on call all night. With this arrangement, we each got to sleep every other night.

Try for the same sleep schedules. "Do everything together" will be your survival motto. Just as you try to get both babies on approximately the same feeding schedules, try to get them on the same sleeping schedule. This may not be possible if they have very different sleep temperaments, but often one twin will take a sleep cue from the other one. If the one who fights sleep sees the easy baby drifting off to sleep, he may imitate his twin. Or he may see this as a chance to get one-on-one time with his parents and try all the harder to stay awake. This is where it really helps to have two sets of arms to get two babies down to sleep at the same time.

Once our twins were four weeks old, I would occasionally pump a little bit before the normal feeding around 6 p.m., and then I'd run to bed. My husband would give them a bottle and play with them in the evening. I would wake up and feed them again at 10 p.m., and then we would all go to sleep.

Do high-needs shift work. Most mothers of twins report that one or the other of their babies will go through a high-need stage and want to be held or nursed more than the other. You may find that sometimes you can put the easier baby to sleep in a crib and then snuggle down with the needy one.

Get double help during the day. If you've got to double the energy you spend holding and nursing your babies, you've got to cut the time you spend doing non-baby-related chores in half. Hire help or delegate the cooking, cleaning, and tidying up to your husband, friends, older children, or willing relatives. Your local Mothers of Twins Club should be able to give you some practical advice. Helpful organizations for parents of twins include the National Organization of Mothers of Twins Clubs (www.nomotc.org) and MOST — Mothers of Supertwins (www.MOSTonline.org). For helpful tips on co-sleeping and night nursing, see La Leche League's book *Mothering Multiples* (www.lalecheleague.org).

I would get set up with pillows while my husband changed one diaper, brought the first baby to me, then changed the second and delivered the second one to me. He'd go back to bed while I nursed them at the same time for twenty to thirty minutes. I cherished the silence, two little nuzzling heads, just the three of us in our little circle. Then my husband and I would put the twins back into their shared crib. We'd just stand over their crib and watch for a few minutes with tears in our eyes. I loved our time together like that!

Consider scheduled feedings, naps, and bedtimes. Most of the parenting advice found in books is focused on parenting one baby at a time. While we usually advise against strict scheduling of feedings and other activities, many of our mothers of multiples have told us scheduling is the only way they survived the first year. As one mom told us, "Feeding on demand is wonderful if you have a singleton, but when you have multiples, feeding on demand means feeding all day."

Once breastfeeding is well established and the babies are thriving through the first few months, it is probably safe to try to schedule feedings in a way that's more predictable for you. This is also true for formula-fed babies if they are not already on a schedule. Your doctor can verify that the babies are gaining adequate weight during this time. One drawback to scheduled breastfeeding is that it means babies will nurse only for nourishment and not for comfort. For many women, offering the breast for comfort is a natural part of the breastfeeding relationship. By nursing for nourishment only, you will help your babies learn other ways to soothe themselves to sleep without relying on the breast. You will also lose the most convenient comforting tool available. You must decide what will work for you. Scheduling the feeds will help you schedule naps and bedtime more predictably and consistently.

Teach self-soothing sleep techniques. Another change that some moms of multiples have found helpful when their babies are around five months old is to teach them to fall asleep without feeding and eventually

with little parental interaction. Review our fading-away self-soothing story on page 101 if you feel that making this transition may work for you. Just as with single babies, we caution parents of multiples to avoid the cry-it-out method of sleep training.

WHEN A CHILD IS SICK

Children often have difficulty sleeping when they are sick. Pain or discomfort gets worse when you're alone in the dark, so children's misery prefers company. When sick, children often cling to their favorite source of comfort and healing, Dr. Mom. Children who usually sleep alone may lobby for sleeping with you in your bed. If illness is zapping their energy, they may take longer naps, fall asleep earlier at bedtime, and then wake up in the wee hours of the morning and be unable to go back to sleep. Just what you need, right?

We have noticed how much more quickly children seem to get better when a parent sleeps close to them. It's that therapeutic power of touch again. Hospitals are recognizing the healing power of parents by routinely providing a cot or a recliner chair so that parents can sleep next to the child's hospital bed.

During the writing of this book, we had to hospitalize three-year-old Madison because of severe asthma. Sandy, an intuitive mother of five, had been down this road many times and knew what worked. She spent many hours a day, and much of the night, snuggling next to Madison in her hospital bed; which helped Madison sleep. The nurses, the

NIGHTTIME PARENTING IN SPECIAL SITUATIONS

mother, and we pediatricians all noticed that the alarm that would sound when Madison's blood oxygen levels fell went off much less when mom slept next to her. That made sense, since sleep relaxes the whole body, including those wheezy breathing passages.

Dr. Bill recalls: The therapeutic effects of relaxing sleep are most evident in the child with croup. One of my most memorable hospital moments was the night I stood by the bedside of nine-month-old Tony, worrying as his croup was getting worse. He was barking like a seal while he struggled to get a breath. I called the ENT specialist and put the operating room on standby, fearing that Tony would need a tracheotomy, an operation in which a tube is inserted into the neck to bypass the swollen vocal cords and allow breathing. I told Tony's mother, "If only he could go to sleep, his croup might get better and he wouldn't need the operation." She said, "Let me try one more thing." She snuggled next to Tony in the tiny bed and nursed him through the opening in the oxygen tent. Tony breastfed himself to sleep, his breathing relaxed, and the surgery was not necessary. Now that he is a teenager, I remind him, especially when he's a little rough on his mom, about how his mother saved him from having a hole in his neck.

WHEN TRAVELING

Children are creatures of habits and routines, and these are disrupted when they travel. Different time zones, different beds, different noises, and different activities can all make it hard to get to sleep. Try these travel tips to help your child sleep better when away from home:

Strive for safety and sameness. New places and new faces are the reason you travel, but try to keep some things the same for baby. New and exciting activities during the day, meeting new family members, and sleeping in a different bed all make it hard for babies and toddlers to wind down at bedtime. Stick to your usual bedtime routine if possible. Take along a bit of "home," such as baby's favorite "lovee" or blanket. If baby is a crib sleeper, be sure that your hotel or vacation place has a suitable and safe crib. (See Safe Crib Sleeping, page 80.) If baby is a confirmed co-sleeper, be sure the adult bed is safe. (See Safe Co-sleeping, page 77.)

Our baby was used to sleeping in his crib at home. On vacation we stayed in a condo that didn't have a crib, so he slept with us. Now that we're home, we can't get him out of our bed. (Smart baby!)

Plan ahead for time-zone changes. While some infants adjust better than adults to time-zone changes, others are upset by them. It often helps to plan ahead and start letting baby go to sleep and wake up at the new times a few days before your trip. Of course, even if you try your hardest to manipulate baby's sleep schedule, she may still outfox you and wake up when the first ray of sunlight comes through the window at 6 a.m. To avoid spending your first day of vacation sleep-deprived, be sure the bedroom is dark.

TRAVEL TIP

To block out the ray of sunlight peering through the slit in the curtains, bring along some metal clips and clip the edges together before you go to bed at night. That may get you an extra hour or two of sleep in the morning. We have found that while most hotels have opaque curtains, they leak rays of sunlight in the morning and need to be clipped together.

WHEN MOVING

Moving to a new home can be stressful for the whole family, infants and toddlers included. This is not usually a good time to make major changes in sleeping routines. With all the excitement and exhaustion involved in moving, your child will need you more during the night, not less. This is not the time to suddenly eject the toddler from your bed and make him sleep in his own. On the other hand, it might be an opportune time to introduce your child to his very own bedroom or a new "big boy" bed. Just don't expect him to sleep there until he feels safe and secure in his new surroundings.

WHEN DAD TRAVELS

My husband travels a lot, and when he's away, our three-year-old is restless and often comes into my room in the middle of the night. How can I get her to sleep better during these times?

A change in family routine, especially one as upsetting as a parent's being gone, often disturbs children's sleep. If you are a closely attached family and your child spends a lot of time with her father, she is going to be upset when he is gone. Also, when dad is away, mom is often tense and tired, and children can sense this.

It's natural for your child to feel anxious when your husband is out of town. In fact, separation anxiety is often considered a psychological strength rather than a weakness. It's often the more securely attached infants and toddlers who are bothered the most by the absence of a parent. Try these extra doses of daytime and nighttime security when one parent is away:

- *Explain the absence.* If one or both parents are away, the child under three may not fully understand that mommy or daddy will be back "in two days." When one or both of us traveled, we softened the separation anxiety by helping our children understand when we would come back. Your child may not comprehend the concept of "two days" or "on Friday." Use concrete terms she can understand: "Today we'll go to the store and then visit Grandma and then go to sleep. Tomorrow we'll play with your friends. One more bedtime after that, and then Daddy will come home." Make a chart or a picture and cross off the events as they happen.

- *Leave a bit of yourself behind.* When you travel, leave a picture of yourself by your child's bedside or a tape recording of your voice reading a favorite story, singing a bedtime song, or just saying "I love you. Good night."

- *Stay connected while apart.* Send your child e-mail about what you are doing on your trip. You can even include pictures of yourself. Your child can dictate replies to send back to you. Phone frequently. Speaking in "word pictures," let your child know what you are doing: "Think about Daddy giving a talk to a whole bunch of people and showing pictures. Imagine me going to bed thinking all about you." Planting these mental images in your child's mind helps her make you a part of her day and night.

Our children used to regard my being on the road as an opportunity to enjoy a family bedroom again. Martha would welcome them in to snuggle with her or put a futon or sleeping bag at the foot of our bed and let them enjoy this "special bed" when daddy was away.

I have a hard time getting our little girl, who is almost three, to go to sleep. Her Navy dad is sailing again after being home for the first three years of her life. What can I do?

Prolonged separation from a military dad on deployment is bound to keep any three-year-old awake, and it is hard on mom, too. This is not the time to be tough on your daughter. She needs the security of knowing you are there for her, night and day. Many military moms find it's best to have their baby or preschool child sleep in their room, or even in their bed, while dad is away. Lie down together on your bed until your child falls asleep and then get up to resume your evening activities. When you retire for the night, you can leave her in your bed, move her onto a mattress at the foot of your bed, or carry her to her own room.

Beware of the sleep trainers who advise you to let her cry it out. Your child has reason for nighttime insecurities right now, and if you respect them, you'll both probably sleep a lot better while dad is away.

SINGLE PARENTS — TWO DIFFERENT BEDS

Depending on the child's age, night waking from night fears may occur more often when children are bounced between two beds in separate homes. The child may get used to a primary sleeping arrangement in the home of the custodial parent and then have to sleep in a different arrangement in the home of the other parent. Or, in cases of dual custody, some children may spend half their time in one bed and half their time in another. Depending on the age and sleep temperament of the child, this may or may not be a problem. If a child is used to sleeping in one arrangement, such as co-sleeping with mom, that child may have difficulty solo sleeping at dad's house. On the other hand, some more adaptable older children have no trouble sleeping in two different beds, and some even enjoy the novelty. It's important that both parents respect their children's individual nighttime needs and not let custody squabbles keep their children awake.

Agree on an approach to nighttime parenting. It helps for both parents to know what bedtime rituals work. If you have found one that works for you, share it with the other parent, and encourage him or her to do likewise. As long as your child is parented to sleep and not just put down to sleep, your child may actually enjoy two different nighttime parenting styles and rituals. For the sake of your child, try to agree on a nighttime parenting philosophy as much as possible.

A common custody squabble that often leads to a legal squabble arises when a toddler is still night-nursing, but dad wants overnights with his child. This is a sensitive situation. Few attorneys and judges understand a toddler's need to night-nurse, and they may misinterpret co-sleeping and night nursing as fostering a dependency, or a ploy to keep dad from enjoying overnights with his child. La Leche League International has a packet of information that professionally discusses this sensitive situation and offers you some helpful guidelines. We have personally been involved as consultants in such custody squabbles.

The bottom line is, What's in the best interest of the child?

NIGHTMARES

Our three-year-old recently began having nightmares. How can I help him through these?

Nightmares occur most commonly in children between two and five years of age. Dreams distort reality. The harmless cartoon character turns into a monster in a child's dream, and this scary image frightens the child awake. Nightmares occur during the light state of sleep, or REM sleep, so children tend to awaken easily from bad dreams. Other sleep disturbances, such as night terrors (also called "sleep terrors"), sleepwalking, and bed-wetting, occur during deep, or non-REM, sleep, and usually these don't wake the child.

Scary dreams can become even more terrifying after a child wakes up, because young children are not yet capable of distinguishing fantasy from reality. It's harder for them to understand that the monster in the dream is not real and is not lurking in a corner of the bedroom. The scary details of the dream linger in the child's mind, and it's hard to go back to sleep.

A principle that's good for parenting — and good for life — is that problems can be viewed as opportunities. Parenting your child through nightmares gives you an opportunity to star as a trusted and helpful resource in your child's emotional life. You'll reap the benefits for many years to come. Here's how:

Comfort your child. When a nightmare strikes, be there to help your child sort out what's real and what's not. Your presence, your touch, and your soothing voice will help your child get through his fear and be ready to go back to sleep. Try to keep your child from being overwhelmed by his fears. Otherwise, the child may become afraid to go to sleep.

Explain nightmares to your child. Help your child understand that dreams are not real. They're just "pictures in your brain." During the daytime, have him practice distinguishing what's real and what's pretend. As your child matures, he will be able to understand that dreams are not real, so he won't be so terrified by them. And he will be old enough to understand that monsters don't really exist.

Minimize scary daytime experiences. Do some detective work to find out what caused the nightmare. Ask your child to explain the content of the dream to see if you can pinpoint the trigger. Take inventory of any new, and possibly scary, events in your child's life, such as a recent move, a new school, or squabbles with friends. In our pediatric practice, we've heard about preschool children who have nightmares after hearing their parents argue in the evening (don't always assume those little ears are totally asleep).

Martha notes: *When Lauren was ten, she told us that when she was little, she would hear us arguing: "You thought I was asleep, but I heard you being mad at each other." Ah, a teachable moment! Lauren surprised us with this news, but Bill was able to turn the problem into an opportunity. He told her, "Even people who love each other feel angry with one another sometimes. When Mommy and Daddy are angry with each other, we have a deal. We always make up and never go to bed angry." We believe children are likely to remember not just the problems but also how their parents solved them.*

Play self-soothing music. If nightmares are a frequent occurrence, try playing a continuous-play tape of your child's favorite lullabies during the night. When he awakens, hearing a familiar lullaby may calm him enough that he can get back to sleep on his own.

Unplug scary TV and other upsetting media images. Obviously, young children should not watch scary, violent movies and television programs. Watch out for other frightening images in the media. The picture of a bleeding soldier on the front page of the paper or a story on the TV news can trigger nightmares. You cannot completely protect your child from learning about the scary things that happen in our world. But children do not need to linger over the details. Children need to be children. They need to know that the adults in their lives love them and will keep them safe.

Provide a secure sleeping environment. Nightmares are especially terrifying to preschoolers who wake up alone. If your preschooler is having nightmares, try letting her sleep in your bed, on a toddler mattress or "special bed" in your room, or with a sibling. Studies have shown that children who sleep with siblings tend to have fewer nightmares than those who sleep solo.

Have a peaceful day. Anything that can cause a change in the circuits of the brain, such as a fever or a disruption in the child's normal sleep patterns, can trigger nightmares or sleep terrors (described below). The best way to lessen nightmares and sleep terrors is to help your child have a peaceful day and fall asleep peacefully at night.

SLEEP TERRORS

Our two-and-a-half-year old daughter wakes up screaming several times a week, but she's not really awake. What's going on, and how can we help her?

These episodes are called sleep terrors or night terrors. While sleep terrors can be frightening for parents to witness, they are less unsettling for the child than nightmares. Children remember nightmares. Even if they don't remember the details, they remember being gripped by fear. Unlike nightmares, which occur during REM, or light, sleep, sleep terrors happen during non-REM, or deep, sleep. Consequently, sleep terrors do not actually awaken the child. Children with sleep terrors don't remember this bizarre phenomenon because they aren't awake during the episodes. Children with sleep terrors don't seem to be sleep-deprived the next day, and they don't develop a fearful attitude about going to sleep. Parents may feel sleep-deprived the next day, but sleep terrors seldom bother children, and they go away with age.

Here's what a typical sleep terror episode looks like: A child suddenly sits up in bed, lets out a piercing scream, looks terrified, and stares straight ahead with eyes wide open. You come running to see what's wrong, and the child continues to cry and breathes heavily. You may feel her heart pounding, her pupils may be dilated, and she may perspire profusely. If you try to wake her, she seems confused and totally disconnected from what's going on. She is oblivious to your attempts to help her. She may even try to push you away when you try to hold her. Don't take it personally. In fact, trying to help may hinder the process of getting through the sleep terror, as some children become more upset if you bother them during an episode. Sleep terrors usually last from five to ten minutes, after which the child — who was never really awake — falls into a deep, calm sleep. The child seems none the worse for wear when she wakes up, but you may be a wreck.

During a sleep terror, a child may bolt out of bed and dart out of the bedroom. Because children can hurt themselves during sleep terrors, it's important to stay with and protect your child until she falls calmly back to sleep. Accident-proof her bedroom, so if she sleepwalks during the terror, she does not trip and hurt herself.

Sleep terrors are considered a quirk in the mysterious neurocircuitry in the brain. Unlike nightmares, which occur toward the end of the night, when the brain is busy dreaming, sleep terrors tend to occur earlier. Sleep terrors usually occur during the first or second deep sleep state of the night, a couple hours after the child goes to sleep. Keep a log of when they occur and you may be able to find a way to prevent them. A time-honored trick for preventing night terrors is to fully awaken your child just before the usual time the night terror occurs, and then cuddle him back to sleep. This helpful parental intervention resets the sleep cycles, which will often prevent an episode of sleep terrors.

Sleep disorder clinics report that the most common trigger of sleep terrors is sleep deprivation. Ensuring that your child gets

SLEEP TERRORS AND NIGHTMARES: HOW TO TELL THE DIFFERENCE

Feature	Sleep Terror	Nightmare
age of child	may occur in toddlerhood, but more common in school-age children	most common between two and five years of age
when they occur	first few hours of night	last few hours of night
sleep cycle	during non-REM, or nondreaming and deep, sleep	during REM, or dreaming and light, sleep
consciousness	does not awaken	fully awakens
activity during	may bolt out of bed and dart out of room	usually stays in bed
memory of event	no memory or even fuzzy recollection	recalls vivid details
comfort needed	none or little	reassured by your comfort
parental help	hands-off	hands-on
danger of injury	high possibility	usually none
tiredness next day	usually none	tired

enough quality sleep is the best home remedy you can offer. Stress can contribute to sleep deprivation. This explains why sleep terrors are more common during illnesses and family upsets that affect your child's sleep pattern. Several children in our practice have experienced sleep terrors during or shortly after a traumatic hospital experience. Also, have your child avoid caffeine-containing drinks, such as sodas, that may disturb her usual sleep patterns. Help your child have peaceful days, and encourage ac-

tive outdoor play that will help her sleep better at night.

It is not always easy to tell the difference between a nightmare and a sleep terror. More important than knowing exactly what's happening is knowing what you can do to help your child. Remain as calm as possible while helping your child resettle. Often, just being there and issuing a reassuring "It's okay . . ." is enough to get your child back to sleep. And once your child senses that you are not afraid, he is less likely to be afraid.

Eleven Tips to Help Parents Sleep Better

MOST OF THE SLEEP TIPS IN this book are designed to help your baby or child sleep better. If your baby sleeps better, you will probably sleep better, too. You can't always control your baby's sleep pattern, but you can control your own sleep choices. The tips in this chapter are designed to help you enjoy a more restful night's sleep, even when your baby does not.

1. MAKE SLEEP A PRIORITY

When you are working around the clock to meet the needs of your baby, it's easy to forget to take care of yourself. Yet parents who do not get enough sleep may not always be effective parents. Your baby needs to sleep well to thrive, but so do you. Remember, your baby needs a reasonably well-rested mother. This means that you must make getting enough sleep a priority — for your own sake and for your baby's.

When a new baby joins the family, parents, especially first-time parents, are often in for a rude awakening — literally. A baby upsets parents' previously predictable lifestyles, especially their sleeping routines. It's important to be realistic about this. During that first year or two of parenting, you're going to need to make some adjustments in your lifestyle to get enough sleep.

Unclutter your daytime life. With a baby to care for, you can't expect to accomplish all the things you used to be able to do in a day and still have time left over to get enough sleep. You will need to set some priorities for your daytime life and let go of what's less important. For some tips on how to accomplish this, see pages 67 to 69.

Basically, I was the sleep problem. When I slept better, our baby slept better and woke up a lot less. I learned to nap during the day. I let the housework go. I needed sleep more than the house needed to be cleaned. If baby went to bed, I did, too!

Go to bed earlier. It's tempting to use those few hours between baby's bedtime and your own bedtime to "finally get something done" or to relax with your spouse. The sense of freedom you feel with baby finally down in bed can entice you into staying up much too late. Try to go to bed at least eight hours before baby's usual morning awake time. If your baby routinely wakes up about 6 a.m., you should be in bed by 10 p.m. The deep and most restful state of sleep occurs in the first third of the night. If you go to bed at midnight and your baby (who went to bed at eight) wakes up at 1 a.m., you are not going to feel very rested in the morning, because your first deep sleep has been interrupted. Going to bed earlier will yield more high-quality sleep time for you at the beginning of the night.

Nurse yourself to sleep after you nurse your baby to sleep. After you have nursed your baby to sleep, you may be tempted to shake off that drowsy, relaxed feeling you get from breastfeeding and get up and do something else. But making your escape from the bedroom prevents you from taking advantage of the breastfeeding hormones that can help you sleep better. While your baby is nursing, your level of prolactin, a sleep-inducing and relaxing hormone, rises, and it peaks forty-five minutes after breastfeeding. This makes it easy to fall asleep. Take advantage of this biological perk to help you fall asleep soon after feeding baby.

The older kids can wait. Permit us to get on our soapbox for a minute. Today's kids are overbooked, overfed, and overcoddled. Just say no! When a new baby comes into the home, older children have to learn the meaning of the word "wait." This is a time when they should learn that moms need to be taken care of, too, and that mom can't always come running whenever anyone needs her. It helps for dad to call a family council together and tell the older children: "This is what mom needs . . ." He can then help the children respect mom's needs by setting an example. Learning that family relationships involve both giving and receiving is an important life lesson. Twenty years or so down the road, your child's future spouse will thank you.

If the older children in the family are still very young, asking them to wait or to solve their own problems may not be appropriate. Toddlers of one, two, or three years of age still need lots of hands-on care and attention, especially when a new baby enters the family. This is a time for dad to pitch in and help with the older child so that mom can rest. Another strategy to give mom a break from the demands of an active young sibling is to hire a teenager to come in a couple afternoons a week to entertain the toddler while mom and baby take a nap.

Martha notes: *Realize that to be a good mom you don't have to operate on all eight cylinders all the time. You can function on six, or even five. I call this the "mom zone"— not bright-eyed and bushy-tailed, but not zombied-out either, though you may be both of those from time to time. In the mom zone, you have plenty of energy to love your child, but not enough to*

SLEEP DEPRIVATION — HAZARDOUS FOR MOMS

The health hazards of sleep deprivation are vastly underrated. New mothers (and fathers) who don't get enough sleep put their health and their ability to care for their families at risk. Here are the most concerning effects of chronic sleep deprivation:

It can make you sick. Sleep deprivation depresses the immune system by reducing white blood cells, which circulate throughout your body on search-and-destroy missions against invading germs. Being sick all the time makes the energy-draining first year of your child's life much harder. Staying healthy helps mothers and fathers maintain a positive attitude toward the stresses of parenting.

It reduces your ability to pay attention. When you don't get enough sleep, it's hard to concentrate, especially during boring and routine tasks such as driving. Falling asleep at the wheel is a common result of sleep deprivation. Also, sleep deprivation slows your reaction time, which also increases your risk of having an accident.

It lessens your enjoyment of your new baby. It is hard to care about things when you are tired all the time. Sleep deprivation dampens your enthusiasm for parenting and keeps you from enjoying special moments with your baby. When you are sleep-deprived, it is more difficult to tune in to your parenting intuition and make those on-the-spot decisions about what your baby needs or why she is crying. It may even affect your judgment and ability to handle emergencies.

It keeps you from enjoying life. Being sleep-deprived will affect your relationship with your spouse, your performance on the job, and your outlook on life in general. Babies need happy, well-rested parents in order to be happy themselves.

Repay Your Sleep Debt

As often as you can, and at least once a week, try to arrange to get an eight- or nine-hour stretch of sleep. Hire help, delegate household responsibilities to your spouse, or do whatever it takes to get out of sleep debt. Even the most bankrupt sleepers find they can get out of sleep debt with one uninterrupted night's sleep.

Dads, help your wife get out of sleep debt. A sleep-deprived mom becomes a burned-out wife, and the whole family suffers. It's amazing how a relaxing day and one un-fragmented night's sleep can restore her well-being. Once a week, arrange for her to have an afternoon relaxing or "just for me" time. Hire help or take over the household chores and as much of the baby care as you can. Setting your wife up for a few hours off call can help restore her well-being, and the whole family benefits. Don't just suggest this to your wife, make it happen: "I've made an appointment for you at the spa. I've already paid for it, and I can't get our money back. I'll drive you there." This setup is especially important to a mother who is of the mind-set "I don't have time to take care of myself because my baby needs me so much."

read Shakespeare or balance your checkbook. You have the energy to read another story, bake a batch of cookies, and maybe cook two vegetables for dinner (but not three), yet not all in the same day. The laundry can wait another day or three. Your mate and your child will get enough of what they need — just maybe not as much as they'd like — that day. The mom zone doesn't go on endlessly. There will be bright and bushy days again. And that thought can keep you cheerful enough to enjoy the feeling at the end of the day that you've been a good-enough mother.

2. EAT TO SLEEP

What and when you eat can affect how you sleep. Some foods work like natural sleeping pills, helping you relax and drift off to sleep. The food-mood connection is vastly underrated. As neurobiologist Michael Gershon, M.D., points out in his book *The Second Brain,* 95 percent of the body's serotonin (the relaxing hormone) is found in the bowels. On page 44 of this book, you'll find which foods are sleepers and which are wakers. Wakers are junk-carb foods that send the brain on a sleepless roller-coaster ride due to rising and falling blood sugar levels, which trigger stress hormones. Carbs that are partnered with protein, fiber, and fat are much better sleep inducers than foods that contain little more than sugar. Ice cream, which has calcium, protein, and fat as well as sugar, is a better bedtime snack than a doughnut.

Don't dine after nine. It's best to eat your evening meal at least three hours before bed-

time. It is harder to fall asleep if your gut is working overtime digesting a heavy meal. The intestines are richly supplied with nerves, and if these nerves in the "gut brain" are revved up, the brain that is trying to fall asleep will be revved up, too. Your body will rest better if your intestines are at rest. Yet don't go to bed hungry. The hormones released when blood sugar is too low can rev up your brain and keep you awake as well.

Research on people who suffer from gastroesophageal reflux (more familiarly, acid reflux or heartburn) shows that early eaters produce less stomach acid than late diners.

Eat easy-to-digest foods. Especially if you suffer from reflux or heartburn, avoid foods that are slow to digest, including foods that are high in fat, spicy foods, and those that you know give you gas. If you are sensitive to certain foods or substances in food, such as the monosodium glutamate (MSG) found in Chinese cooking and other processed foods, be particularly careful to avoid these foods before bedtime.

Take inventory of your nutritional status. In the first six months after giving birth, your body is replenishing nutrients that were depleted during pregnancy. At the same time, breastfeeding makes additional nutritional demands on your body. Be sure to continue to take your prenatal vitamins and minerals as instructed by your doctor. B-vitamins help your brain use the sleep-inducer tryptophan, so that you can sleep better. Iron-deficiency anemia, one of the medical causes of night waking in infants and toddlers, can create a

---

SLEEP-ADE

Dr. Bill's Before-Bed Smoothie

Try our Sears smoothie recipe, which is a blend of the sleep-inducing nutrients tryptophan, calcium, magnesium, and healthy carbs:

- 1 cup milk
- 1 banana
- ½ cup yogurt
- 4 ounces tofu
- 1 tbsp. ground flaxseed meal
- 1 tsp. cinnamon

Blend and enjoy an hour or so before you go to bed.

---

state of hyperanxiety in moms, leading to sleeplessness. Be sure your doctor checks you for anemia during your regular postnatal checkup.

Beware of crash diets. Many women can't wait to return to their prepregnancy weight, but there are many good reasons not to go on a crash diet during the postpartum period. Hunger itself can release hormones that can keep you awake. Be sure to avoid extreme low-carb diets (those that throw the body into a state of metabolic imbalance called chronic ketosis), as they are not healthful for the postpartum mom. Chronic ketosis can cause tiredness and irritability during the day and keep you awake at night. Also, you need

carbs in the bloodstream to partner with the sleep inducer tryptophan and help usher it into brain cells.

Decaf your day. Watch your caffeine intake while your baby is learning how to sleep better and you are adjusting your own sleep habits. Caffeine can stay in your bloodstream for eight hours or longer. Even one cup of coffee in the morning can interfere with your afternoon nap and may even contribute to sleeplessness at night. If you are using large amounts of caffeine during the day (more than the equivalent of five 5-ounce cups of coffee), there may be enough caffeine in your breast milk to interfere with baby's sleep. Caffeine sensitivity is extremely variable. If you are a caffeine-sensitive person, it is best to avoid it entirely at this stage of your parenting.

Avoid alcohol. For most adults, an occasional glass of wine with the evening meal won't adversely affect sleep, but drinking too much too close to bedtime can interfere with your natural sleep cycles. Specifically, alcohol decreases the amount of time you spend in deep sleep, thus decreasing the overall quality of your sleep. In the morning, you may feel like you are in a fog — which is no way to begin the day with a needy baby.

Don't smoke. Nicotine releases stress hormones. It revs up the body by increasing your pulse and blood pressure and revs up the brain because it is a neurostimulant. Besides harming your health and your sleep, nicotine

WHAT ABOUT SLEEPING MEDICATION?

Avoid all over-the-counter and prescription sleeping medications during the time that you are working on getting everyone in the family a good night's sleep. Sleeping medications can be habit-forming, so it may eventually become difficult to fall asleep without medication. Many sleep-inducing drugs (for example, alcohol) interfere with the natural states of sleep. They may help you to fall asleep, but you don't get the same quality of sleep as you would without the drug. Also, some sleep medications may diminish a mother's awareness and sensitivity to her baby's needs at night. There may be medical circumstances that warrant the short-term use of sleep medication for some mothers, but these medications should not be used routinely. **Co-sleeping warning: It's unsafe to sleep with your baby in your bed if you take prescription sleeping medications.**

Some over-the-counter allergy and headache medications contain substances that rev up the system and cause hyper-irritability and sleeplessness. Read labels carefully and avoid medications that contain caffeine. Before taking any over-the-counter or prescription medicine, ask your doctor about its possible effects on sleep.

As an alternative to prescription sleep medications, in consultation with your doctor, try these sleep-inducing natural remedies:

- chamomile tea

- valerian root extract (do not take with sleeping medications or for longer than two weeks at a time)

- tryptophan supplements: 500 to 2,000 milligrams taken with fruit juice an hour before bedtime. In consultation with your doctor, try taking tryptophan for three nights each week. Since tryptophan levels accumulate in the bloodstream, it's safest to give the body a few days off this extra supplement. Tryptophan supplements should be taken only with carbohydrates (such as juice or fruit), since carbs usher the tryptophan into the brain. Don't take them with foods high in protein, since the amino acids in the protein compete with the tryptophan and lessen the amount that gets into the brain. Try the protein-carb-calcium combo foods listed on page 45. As a perk, sleep research has shown that taking extra B-vitamins may increase the sleep effect of tryptophan.

You can get between 500 and 1,000 milligrams of tryptophan naturally in a before-bedtime snack by enjoying our smoothie recipe on the facing page.

is hazardous to your baby's health, increasing the risk of nearly every major disease, especially SIDS (Sudden Infant Death Syndrome).

3. DRESS FOR SLEEP

Cotton clothing is cooler and breathes better than synthetics. Wear a cotton nightgown or pajamas to bed. In warm weather try cotton sheets. In cold weather try flannel ones. Some moms who are co-sleeping and night-nursing prefer nursing nightgowns, with special openings for breastfeeding.

4. EXERCISE FOR SLEEP

Exercising at least an hour a day — in addition to chasing after a busy toddler — can improve the quality of your sleep at night. How does this happen? It's those hormones again! To relax your mind and tone your

muscles, enroll in a yoga or tai chi class. Strenuous exercise improves the quality of deep sleep by stimulating the release of relaxing endorphins and growth hormones, which are natural sleep inducers. Try these tips for getting more exercise every day:

When to exercise? Steal whatever time you can during the day for exercise you enjoy. While exercising anytime during the day can help you sleep better, sleep researchers have found that exercising five to six hours before bedtime has the best effect on sleep. Early-morning exercise will have less impact on how well you sleep at night, since the hormonal effects will wear off during the day. If you exercise vigorously an hour or two before bedtime, you may be too revved up and energized to wind down easily.

How much to move? Try to get between a half hour and one hour of aerobic exercise at least four or five days a week. Work out at a pace that raises your heart and breathing rate enough that you would find it slightly taxing to carry on a long conversation while exercising. Aerobic exercise options include a brisk walk, time on the treadmill or stair stepper, or a fast swim. Some mothers like to put on a CD and dance energetically while baby watches.

5. ENJOY A BEFORE-BED BATH

Sitting in a warm bath or hot tub relaxes not only the body but also the mind for sleep. Twenty minutes in a hot bath will make your

SEARS SLEEP TIP: SLEEPING AND WORKING

If you are a sleep-deprived mom who works outside the home, try having the babysitter arrive a couple hours early one or two mornings a week. The sitter can care for the kids while you grab an extra hour or two of sleep. (This is also a good way for husbands to help out!) During the day, try taking a twenty-minute power nap during your lunch break.

SEARS SLEEP TIP: WALK AND WEAR

Here's a tip we frequently offer new parents. Many babies have their fussiest period between 4 and 6 p.m. Before this "happy hour" strikes, put your baby in a baby sling and take a vigorous walk that lasts at least a half hour. This late-afternoon walk will help you de-stress, and it will calm baby, too. Exercising with mommy and enjoying the great outdoors often reduces late-afternoon fussiness and helps both mothers and babies sleep better at night.

body temperature go up. Then shortly after you go to bed, your body temperature will fall again. This rise and fall in body temperature releases sleep-inducing hormones.

SEARS SLEEP TIP: WAKE AND WRITE

If you just can't fall asleep, or if you wake up and can't get back to sleep, this is a good time to journalize the events of the day, especially pleasant ones. Make a list of scenes that you know relax you and help you sleep, entitled "Scenes to Sleep By." Then, when you can't sleep, using the technique called "restful visualization," fill your mind with instant replays of these scenes to relax your brain off to sleep.

6. TURN OFF THE TUBE

Studies show that children who watch more TV — especially children who have a TV in their bedroom — have more problems with sleep disturbances. Television may have similar effects on many adults. Late-night news shows are enough to keep anyone awake. In addition to the subject matter, the rapid change of images and artificial light patterns on the TV screen rev up the brain and disrupt the process of falling asleep.

7. DON'T WORRY, BE HAPPY!

Remember, sleep is not a state you can force yourself into. But you can create a physical and mental environment that allows sleep to overtake you. In that last hour or so before you go to bed, choose quiet, relaxing activities, such as listening to music, reading a not-too-interesting book, meditating or journalizing, or quietly conversing with your mate. This is a time to think about what went right with your day, not what went wrong. When it's time to turn out the lights, turn your mind to happy thoughts — perhaps recollecting happy moments from your life (or just from your day) or visualizing pleasant scenes, such as a walk along the beach. Try not to muddy your mind with disturbing thoughts.

Late evening is not the time to argue with your spouse, balance the checkbook, or discuss disturbing family matters. Once your mind gets occupied with difficult problems, it's hard to shut off the worrying and fall asleep. Anxiety and anger release stress hormones. The unresolved tension keeps you awake, sometimes for hours, and affects the quality of whatever sleep you do get. Once your mind gets full of disturbing stuff, you then "try" to go to sleep, which only adds to the difficulty of falling asleep. An hour or two later, the tension escalates and you're still awake. Reprogram yourself so that at least an hour or two before you go to bed, you have "happy hour," a time devoted to pleasant conversation and happy thoughts.

Avoiding conflict and tension late at night is more easily said than done, since many new parents find that the only time during the day that they can find to talk to each other is after the baby and the older children are in bed. Perhaps you and your partner can schedule specific times during the week — maybe a weekend breakfast or a Sunday afternoon walk — to discuss family business. When you are both tired and need to talk at night, use your best communication skills to avoid arguments and upset feelings.

Another mental obstacle to getting a good night's rest is what sleep researchers call the "on-call syndrome." We remember experiencing this during our early years of medical training, when we would have trouble sleeping at night if we were on call for emergencies. Even while we slept, some part of our brains was alert, listening for the wake-up call, and this led to a lot of fragmented sleep. Anticipating that baby is going to wake up can have the same effect on parents' sleep. Even on the occasional night when baby sleeps longer stretches, mother may feel like she's on call.

> ## SEARS SLEEP TIP: DON'T WORRY, BE SLEEPY!
>
> When you go to bed, don't think about how soon your baby is going to wake up. Fretting about baby's night waking ("Is this going to be another night of waking up every two hours?") will make it harder to cope. Instead, reflect on the joyful blessings you experienced during the day and the precious little person who also needs you at night.

She wakes up even when baby doesn't and does not sleep as soundly as she could. When you go to bed, try not to think about the night ahead, since those worries are likely to keep you awake. Don't anticipate every peep or cry your baby is going to make during the night. Concentrate on what you need to do, which is relax and benefit from sleep.

Some night training was necessary for me. I had to train myself to go to the bathroom or count to twenty before I went to him, because most times he was able to settle back to sleep without me and I wanted to encourage that behavior.

8. SLEEP MORE THE FIRST MONTH

Many moms enter motherhood already sleep-deprived, thanks to the discomforts and middle-of-the-night trips to the bathroom that are common during the last weeks of pregnancy. Add to this, sleep lost during all-night labors, the birth, and the euphoria that follows, and you have a new mother who badly needs to catch up on her sleep. Unfortunately, during this first month postpartum, newborns often have their days and nights mixed up, and they sleep long stretches during the day (like they did in the womb) and less at night. This is a time for you to sleep "like a baby," even if it means you sleep long stretches during the day yourself. After you've repaid a bit of sleep debt and built up your sleep bank account during the first month, you'll be better able to cope with your baby's daytime and nighttime needs. As your newborn eases into day/night sleep maturity, you will be able to get more of the sleep you need at night, though you may still need an afternoon nap.

9. ENJOY A BEFORE-BED RITUAL

Babies and children aren't the only ones who enjoy bedtime rituals. Adults are creatures of habit, too. Develop your own sleep-inducing routine to help you unwind: a warm bath, massage, music, stories — night-night! Your bedtime ritual may be very similar to your child's wind-down activities. Bedtime sex is also a time-honored and very effective sleep inducer, but many new mothers are too tired to enjoy sex after a long day of infant care. Morning or midafternoon sex is more realistic during that first year with a new baby.

10. NAP WHEN BABY DOES

Easier said than done? Not if you follow tip number 1: Make sleep a priority. Naps are a necessity for new mothers whose sleep is reg-

ularly interrupted by night feedings. Don't be concerned that napping during the day will make it harder for you to sleep at night. Sleep researchers have found that people who nap usually sleep better at night. If you know you can look forward to a nap during the day, you'll worry less about losing sleep at night, and just having that reassurance may help you sleep better.

"But," you say, "I can't fall asleep during the day." Just like at bedtime, you have to create the conditions that allow sleep to overtake you. One way to do this is to work with your body's natural rhythms. Whether you're awake or asleep depends on two systems in the brain: the arousal system (the on switch) and the sleep system (the off switch). Letting sleep overtake you is basically letting the off switch overcome the on switch. Your brain is wired to allow the off switch to predominate over the on switch at different times through a twenty-four-hour day. Sleep researchers have found that during the day, the off switch is most likely to win the competition between one and three o'clock in the afternoon. Take advantage of this natural drive to sleep and have a nap during that time. If you lie down with your baby and breastfeed, the breastfeeding hormones will also help to switch off the part of your brain that wants to stay awake.

11. MAKE NIGHTTIME MOTHERING MORE RESTFUL

Can you actually make waking up at night more restful? Yes, you can. Again, make sleep your priority. Put your energy into getting the sleep you need rather than into fretting about not sleeping. Do everything you can to make your sleeping environment quiet, comfortable, and welcoming. Care for your baby's needs in ways that allow you to get back to sleep quickly. For more ideas to help make nighttime parenting more restful, see these sections:

- Fifteen Ways to Make Night Nursing Easier (page 137)
- Twenty-three Tips for Nighttime Fathering (chapter 8)
- Music to Sleep By (Appendix A)

What helped me get back to sleep was developing a pleasant ritual that I always did after waking up and tending to baby. Rather than toss and turn, I would get up and rub lotion on my feet to help me drift back to sleep.

Surround yourself with darkness. The glow of an alarm clock or the glare from a streetlight outside your window can be very annoying in the wee hours of the morning. Eliminate light sources that bother you. Turn off computers, put a washcloth over an illuminated alarm clock, use blackout shades, and clip the drapes together to block out the early-morning light.

Decorate your bedroom the way you like it. Take the money that you would otherwise have spent on decorating a fancy nursery and

---

SEARS SLEEP TIP: SET YOUR BODY'S CLOCK FOR BEDTIME

Consistent bedtimes are just as important for moms and dads as they are for children. Try to go to bed at about the same time each evening. This will program your body to fall asleep at a predictable time and in a predictable place. Resist the temptation to lie down on the couch in the evening to just take a rest. If you're tired, go to bed. Zoning out on the couch or in your favorite chair won't get you the high-quality rest you need. As soon as you and your baby wake up in the morning, open the blinds or curtains and let natural light come in. Sleep researchers have found that exposure to natural light in the morning sets the body to "awake mode" and helps it transition into "sleep mode" when darkness comes.

---

buying an ornate crib (which your baby won't appreciate anyway) and spend it on your sleep sanctuary. Upgrade your bed to king size, with a good-quality mattress. Buy soft, comfortable bedding in quiet, soothing colors. Make your bedroom a restful environment. Eliminate clutter and stacks of paper that you don't want to look at or think about when you go to bed.

Appendix A: Music to Sleep By

Soothing Moments by Jason and Nolan Livesay. We commissioned our son-in-law, composer Jason Livesay, to compose a medley of music to lull babies (and adults) to sleep. We often go to sleep to the sounds of this soothing CD. Available at *www.AskDrSears.com*.

The following selections can be found on *Night Music*, vol. 1: *Classical Favourites for Relaxing and Dreaming* (box set), Naxos.

Serenade no. 13 for Strings in G Major ("Eine kleine Nachtmusik"), K. 525 Romance, by Wolfgang Amadeus Mozart

Piano Sonata no. 14 in C-sharp Minor ("Moonlight Sontana"), op. 27 Adagio sostenuto, by Ludwig van Beethoven

Symphony no. 40 in G Minor, K. 550 Andante, by Wolfgang Amadeus Mozart

Canon and Gigue for Three Violins; Continuo in D Major Canon, by Johann Pachelbel

Suite Bergamasque for Piano, L. 75 Clair de lune, by Claude Debussy

Concerto for Piano; Orchestra no. 2 in F Minor, op. 21, CT 48 Larghetto, by Frédéric Chopin

The Swan Lake, ballet, op. 20 Andante, by Pyotr Ilich Tchaikovsky

Piano Concerto no. 4 in G Major, op. 58 Andante, by Ludwig van Beethoven

Vocalise, Song for Voice and Piano, op. 34, by Sergey Rachmaninoff

A Midsummer Night's Dream, incidental music, op. 61 Notturno, by Felix Mendelssohn

Pavane for Orchestra and Chorus ad lib in F-sharp Minor, op. 50, by Gabriel Fauré

Symphony no. 1 in C Major, op. 21 Andante cantabile, by Ludwig van Beethoven

L' Arlésienne, Suite I for Orchestra, from the incidental music Adagietto, by Georges Bizet

Piano Concerto no. 21 in C Major ("Elvira Madigan") K. 467 Andante, by Wolfgang Amadeus Mozart

Chant sans paroles ("Song without words," from "Souvenir de Hapsal"), for Piano, op. 2, by Pyotr Ilich Tchaikovsky

Gymnopédies for Piano, by Erik Satie

Preludes and Suite Bergamasque for Piano, by
  Claude Debussy
Prelude to the Afternoon of a Faun, by
  Claude Debussy
Orchestral works of Delius

OTHER SELECTIONS

Serenade for Strings, op. 22, second move-
  ment, by Antonín Dvořák
"Pavane for a Dead Princess," by Maurice
  Ravel
Symphony no. 17 in G Major, K. 129 first
  movement, by Wolfgang Amadeus Mozart
Brandenburg Concerto no. 3, by Johann
  Sebastian Bach

The Well-Tempered Clavier, parts 1 and 2, by
  Johann Sebastian Bach
String quartets by Franz Joseph Haydn
Piano works by Maurice Ravel
String divertimenti and early symphonies by
  Wolfgang Amadeus Mozart
"Dances Sacred and Profane," piano preludes,
  by Claude Debussy

NEW AGE MUSIC IS ALSO VERY GOOD FOR SLEEPING

Yanni (most of his albums are suitable)
John Tesh, *Winter Song*
Drew Tretick, *Serenata, Romantica,* and *A
  Summer Serenade*

Appendix B: Bedtime Books to Sleep By — For Toddlers and Preschoolers

Bedtime for Frances, by Russell Hoban. Harper, 1976.

A Bedtime Story, by Joan Levine. Dutton, 1975.

Blueberries for Sal, by Robert McCloskey. Puffin, 1976.

Can't You Sleep, Little Bear? by Martin Waddell and Barbara Firth. Candlewick Press, 2002.

Goodnight Moon, by Margaret Wise Brown. Harper and Row, 1947.

Guess How Much I Love You, by Sam McBratney. Candlewick Press, 1994.

Harry the Dirty Dog, by Gene Zion. Harper, 1976.

A Hole is to Dig, by Ruth Krauss. Harper, 1952.

The Little Engine That Could, by Watty Piper. Platt, 1961.

Love You Forever, by Robert N. Munsch and Sheila McGraw. Firefly Books, 1986.

Max's First Word, by Rosemary Wells. Dial, 1979.

The Napping House, by Audrey Wood. Harcourt Brace and Company, 1984.

Noah's Ark, by Peter Spier. Doubleday, 1977.

Our Best Friends, by Gyo Fujikawa. Zokeisha, 1977.

Pat the Bunny, by Dorothy Kunhardt. Golden, 1962.

The Poky Little Puppy, by Janette S. Lowrey. Golden, 1942.

Rock-a-Bye Farm, by Diane Hamm. Simon and Schuster, 1992.

Tell Me Something Happy Before I Go to Sleep, by Joyce Dunbar and Debi Gliori. Scholastic, 1998.

Ten in the Bed, by Penny Dale. Discovery Toys, 1988.

There's a Duck in My Closet! by John Trent. Word Publishing, 1993.

The Three Little Pigs, by Paul Galdone. Seabury, 1970.

Tikki Tikki Tembo, by Arlene Mosel. Holt, 1968.

Time for Bed, by Mem Fox. Harcourt Brace and Company, 1993.

Where's Spot? by Eric Hill. Putnam, 1980.

Appendix C: References

1. Ahnert, L., et al. 2004. Transition to child care: Associations with infant-mother attachment, infant negative emotion, and cortisol elevations. *Child Development* 75, no. 3: 649–650.

2. Blair, P. S., P. J. Fleming, D. Bensley, et al. 1999. Where should babies sleep — alone or with parents? Factors influencing the risk of SIDS in the CESDI study. *British Medical Journal* 319: 1457–1462.

3. Brazy, J. E. 1988. Effects of crying on cerebral blood volume and cytochrome aa3. *Journal of pediatrics* 112, no. 3: 457–461.

4. Butler, S. R., et al. 1978. Maternal behavior as a regulator of polyamine biosynthesis in brain and heart of the developing rat pups. *Science* 199: 445–447.

5. Carpenter, R. G., et al. 2004. Sudden unexplained infant death in 20 regions in Europe: Case control study. *Lancet* 363: 185–191.

6. Coe, C. L., et al. 1985. Endocrine and immune responses to separation and maternal loss in non-human primates. In *The psychology of attachment and separation,* ed. M. Reite and T. Fields, 163–199. New York: Academic Press.

7. Crawford, M. 1994. Parenting practices in the Basque Country: Implications of infant and childhood sleeping location for personality development *Ethos,* 22, 1: 42–82.

8. Davies, D. P. 1985. Cot death in Hong Kong: A rare problem? *The Lancet* 2: 1346–1348.

9. Drago, D. A., and A. L. Dannenberg. 1999. Infant mechanical suffocation deaths in the United States, 1980–1997. *Pediatrics* 103, no. 5: e59.

10. Elias, M. F. 1986. Sleep-wake patterns of breastfed infants in the first two years of life. *Pediatrics* 77: 322–329.

11. Field, T., ed. 1995. *Touch in early development.* Mahway, N.J.: Lawrence Earlbaum and Assoc.

12. Forbes, J. F., et al. 1992. The cosleeping habits of military children. *Military Medicine* 157: 196–200.

13. Fukai, S. and F. Hiroshi. 2000. 1999 annual report, Japan SIDS family association. Sixth SIDS International Conference, Auckland, New Zealand.

14. Heron, P. 1994. Non-reactive cosleeping and child behavior: Getting a good night's sleep all night, every night. Master's thesis, Department of Psychology, University of Bristol.

15. Hofer, M. 1983. The mother-infant interaction as a regulator of infant physiology and behavior. In *Symbiosis in parent-offspring interactions,* ed. L. A. Rosenblum and H. Moltz. New York: Plenum.

16. Hofer, M. 1982. Some thoughts on "the transduction of experience" from a developmental perspective. *Psychosomatic Medicine* 44: 19.

17. Hofer, M., and H. Shair. 1982. Control of sleep-wake states in the infant rat, by features of the mother-infant relationship. *Developmental Psychobiology* 15: 229–243.

18. Hollenbeck, A. R., et al. 1980. Children with serious illness: behavioral correlates of separation and solution. *Child Psychiatry and Human Development* 11: 3–11.

19. Karr-Morse, R., and M. Wiley. Interview with Dr. Allan Schore. In *Ghosts from the nursery,* 200. New York: Atlantic Monthly Press.

20. Kaufman, J., and D. Charney. 2001. Effects of early stress on brain structure and function: Implications for understanding the relationship between child maltreatment and depression. *Developmental Psychopathology* 13, no. 3: 451–471.

21. Keller, M. A., and W. A. Goldberg. 2004. Co-sleeping: Help or hindrance for young children's independence? *Infant and Child Development* 13.

22. Kuhn, C. M., et al. 1978. Selective depression of serum growth hormone during maternal deprivation in rat pups. *Science* 201: 1035–1036.

23. Lee, N. P., et al. 1999. Sudden infant death syndrome in Hong Kong: Confirmation of low incidence. *British Medical Journal* 298: 72.

24. Leiberman, A. F., and H. Zeanah. 1995. Disorders of attachment in infancy. *Infant Psychiatry* 4: 571–587.

25. Lewis, R. J., and L. H. Janda. 1988. The relationship between adult sexual adjustment and childhood experience regarding exposure to nudity, sleeping in the parental bed and parental attitudes toward sexuality. *Archives of Sexual Behavior* 17: 349–363.

26. Ludington-Hoe, S. M., et al. 2002. Infant crying: nature, physiologic consequences, and select intentions. *Neonatal Network* 21, no. 2: 29–36.

27. McKenna, J., et al. 1994. Experimental studies of infant-parent co-sleeping: Mutual physiological and behavioral influences and their relevance to SIDS (sudden infant death syndrome). *Early Human Development* 38: 187–201.

28. McKenna, J., and T. McDade. 2005. Why babies should never sleep alone: A review of the co-sleeping controversy in relation to SIDS, bed sharing, and breastfeeding. *Paediatric Respiratory Review* 6: 134–152.

29. Mosenkis, J., 1998. The effects of childhood co-sleeping on later life development. Master's thesis, Department of Cultural Psychology, University of Chicago.

30. Mosko, S., et al. 1994. Infant sleeping position and CO_2 environment during co-sleeping: The parents' contribution. *Pediatric Pulmonology* 18: 394.

31. Nelson, E. A. S., et al. 2001. International child care practices study: Infant sleeping environment. *Early Human Development* 62: 43–55.

32. Perry, B. Incubated in terror: Neurodevelopmental factors in the cycle of violence. In *Children in a violent society.* New York: Guilford Press.

33. Reite, M., and J. P. Capitanio. 1985. On the nature of social separation and social attachment. In *The psychobiology of attachment and separation,* ed. M. Reite and T. Fields, 228–238. New York: Academic Press.

34. Rao, M. R., et al. 2004. Long-term cognitive development in children with prolonged crying. National Institutes of Health. *Archives of Disease in Childhood* 89: 989–992.

35. Richard, C., et al. 1996. Sleeping position, orientation, and proximity in bedsharing infants and mothers, *Sleep* 19: 667–684.

36. Sankaran, A. H., et al. 2000. Sudden infant death syndrome and infant care practices in Saskatchewan, Canada. Program and Abstracts, Sixth SIDS International Conference, Auckland, New Zealand.

37. Schore, A. N. 1996. The experience-dependent maturation of a regulatory system in the orbital prefrontal cortex and the origin of developmental psychopathology. *Development and Psychopathology* 8: 59–87.

38. Sears, W. 1985. The protective effects of sharing sleep. Can it prevent SIDS? Paper presented at the International Congress of Pediatrics, Honolulu.

39. Sears, W. 1995. *SIDS: A parents' guide to understanding and preventing sudden infant death syndrome.* New York: Little, Brown.

40. Sears, W., et al. 1993. The effect of co-sleeping on infant breathing — implications for SIDS. Paper presented at the Eleventh Apnea of Infancy Conference, Rancho Mirage, California.

41. Stifter, C., and T. Spinrad. 2002. The effect of excessive crying on the development of emotion regulation. *Infancy* 3, no. 2: 133–152.

42. Teicher, M. H., et al. 2003. The neurobiological consequences of early stress and childhood maltreatment. *Neuroscience Biobehavior Review* 27, nos. 1 and 2: 33–44.

43. Wolke, D., et al. 2002. Persistent infant crying and hyperactivity problems in middle childhood. *Pediatrics* 109: 1054–1060.

Index

William Sears, M.D., received his pediatric training at Harvard Medical School's Children's Hospital and Toronto's Hospital for Sick Children, where he was Associate Ward Chief of the Newborn Intensive Care Unit. He is currently Associate Clinical Professor of Pediatrics at the University of California, Irvine, and he has practiced as a pediatrician for more than thirty years. Martha Sears is a registered nurse, childbirth educator, and breastfeeding consultant. The Searses are the parents of eight children and coauthors of thirty-two books. Their sons Dr. Robert Sears, father of three, and Dr. James Sears, father of two, are both board-certified pediatricians at the Sears Family Pediatric Practice in San Clemente, California, and coauthors of *The Baby Book* and *The Premature Baby Book*. All four authors live in Southern California.